The Anterior Cruciate Deficient Knee
New Concepts in Ligament Repair

The Anterior Cruciate Deficient Knee

NEW CONCEPTS IN
LIGAMENT REPAIR

DOUGLAS W. JACKSON, M.D.

Medical Director, The Southern California Center for Sports Medicine,
Long Beach, California;
Medical Director, Memorial Bone and Tissue Bank,
Memorial Medical Center, Long Beach, California

DAVID DREZ, Jr., M.D.

Clinical Professor of Orthopaedics, Department of Orthopaedics,
Louisiana State University, School of Medicine, New Orleans, Louisiana;
Director, Louisiana State University,
Knee and Sports Medicine Fellowship Program,
Lake Charles, Louisiana

With 276 illustrations

The C. V. Mosby Company

ST. LOUIS • WASHINGTON, D.C. • TORONTO   1987

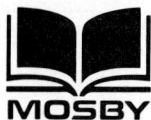

A TRADITION OF PUBLISHING EXCELLENCE

Editor: Eugenia A. Klein
Editorial Assistant: Robin Sutter
Project Editor: Barbara Merritt
Production Editor: Patricia Gayle May
Book Design: Nancy Steinmeyer
Cover Design: Susan E. Lane

Copyright © 1987 by The C.V. Mosby Company

All rights reserved. No part of this publication may be reproduced, stored in a retrieval system, or transmitted, in any form or by any means, electronic, mechanical, photocopying, recording, or otherwise, without prior written permission from the publisher.

Printed in the United States of America

The C.V. Mosby Company
11830 Westline Industrial Drive, St. Louis, Missouri 63146

Library of Congress Cataloging-in-Publication Data

The Anterior cruciate deficient knee.

  Includes bibliographies and index.
  1. Anterior cruciate ligament—Surgery. 2. Ligaments—Transplantation. 3. Ligament prostheses. I. Jackson, Douglas W. II. Drez, David. [DNLM: 1. Knee Injuries—surgery. 2. Knee Joint—surgery. 3. Knee Prosthesis. 4. Ligaments, Articular—surgery. WE 870 A6267]
RD561.A58   1987   617'.582   86-18058
ISBN 0-8016-2411-8

AC/MV/MV 9 8 7 6 5 4 3 2 1 02/D/270

Contributors

JAMES R. ANDREWS, M.D.
Clinical Professor, Section of Sports Medicine,
Department of Orthopaedic Surgery,
Tulane University School of Medicine,
New Orleans, Lousiana;
Director of Orthopaedic Training,
Hughston Orthopaedic Clinic,
Columbus, Georgia

STEVEN PAUL ARNOCZKY, D.V.M., Dipl. ACUS
Associate Professor of Surgery (Comparative Orthopaedics),
Cornell University Medical College;
Director, Laboratory of Comparative Orthopaedics,
Hospital for Special Surgery,
New York, New York

JAMES R. BAIN, M.Sc.
W.L. Gore & Associates, Inc.,
Flagstaff, Arizona

EDMUND N. BIDEN, D. Phil.
Manager/Engineer,
Motion Analysis Laboratory,
Children's Hospital,
San Diego, California

C. WILLIAM BOLTON, D.V.M.
W.L. Gore & Associates, Inc.,
Flagstaff, Arizona

FRANK O. BONNARENS, M.D.
Resident,
Department of Orthopaedics,
Lousiana State University,
New Orleans, Louisiana

WILLIAM C. BRUCHMAN
W.L. Gore & Associates, Inc.,
Flagstaff, Arizona

WILLIAM G. CARSON, Jr., M.D.
Assistant Clinical Professor,
Department of Orthopaedics,
University of Southern Florida,
College of Medicine;
The Sports Medicine Clinic of Tampa,
Tampa, Florida

WILLIAM G. CLANCY, Jr., M.D.
Professor and Head, Section of Sports Medicine,
Division of Orthopaedic Surgery,
University of Wisconsin,
Madison, Wisconsin

DALE M. DANIEL, M.D.
Clinical Associate Professor of Orthopaedic Surgery,
Department of Orthopaedic Surgery,
University of California, San Diego, California;
Staff Orthopedist,
Kaiser Permanente Hospital,
San Diego, California

DAVID DREZ, Jr., M.D.
Clinical Professor of Orthopaedics,
Department of Orthopaedics,
Louisiana State University, School of Medicine,
New Orleans, Louisiana;
Director, Louisiana State University,
Knee and Sports Medicine Fellowship Program,
Lake Charles, Louisiana

DAVID L. FLOOD, M.D.
Director of Sports Medicine,
Department of Orthopaedic Surgery
  and Rehabilitation,
Sharp Rees-Stealy Medical Group,
San Diego, California

BEN GRAF, M.D.
Assistant Professor,
Department of Orthopaedic Surgery,
University of Wisconsin,
University Hospitals,
Madison, Wisconsin

CHRISTOPHER L. IHLE, M.D.
Orthopaedic Surgery and Sports
  Medicine,
Franklin Bone and Joint Clinic,
Franklin, Tennessee;
Williamson Medical Center,
Department of Orthopaedics,
Franklin, Tennessee

DOUGLAS W. JACKSON, M.D.
Medical Director,
The Southern California Center for
  Sports Medicine,
Long Beach, California;
Medical Director,
Memorial Bone and Tissue Bank,
Memorial Medical Center,
Long Beach, California

KEITH L. MARKOLF, Ph.D.
Adjunct Professor,
Department of Orthopaedic Surgery,
University of California, Los Angeles,
Los Angeles, California

GREGG K. McPHERSON, Ph.D.
Laboratory Manager,
Orthopedic Products Division/3M,
St. Paul, Minnesota

**H. VINCENT MENDENHALL,
D.V.M., Ph.D.**
Senior Surgical Research Specialist,
Orthopedic Products Division/3M,
St. Paul, Minnesota

LONNIE E. PAULOS, M.D.
Assistant Clinical Professor,
Division of Orthopaedic Surgery,
University of Utah,
Salt Lake City, Utah

FRANK CORRY PAYNE, III, M.D.
Orthopedic Fellow
Salt Lake City Knee and Sports
  Medicine
Salt Lake City, Utah

J. MICHAEL RAY, M.D.
Team Physician and Orthopedic
  Surgeon
University of Kentucky
Lexington, Kentucky

PAUL R. REIMAN, M.D.
Clinical Instructor in Orthopaedics,
Department of Orthopaedics,
Northeastern Ohio Universities
  College of Medicine,
Akron, Ohio;
Director of Sports Medicine,
Akron General Medical Center,
Akron, Ohio

DANIEL B. ROBERTSON, M.D.
Clinical Instructor,
Department of Orthopaedic Surgery,
University of Texas Southwestern
  Medical School,
Dallas, Texas

THOMAS D. ROSENBERG, M.D.
Assistant Clinical Professor of
  Orthopaedic Surgery
University of Utah School of Medicine,
Salt Lake City, Utah;
Clinical Instructor in Physical Therapy
University of Utah College of Health
Salt Lake City, Utah

TIMOTHY M. SIMON, M.S.
Director of Research,
Research Department,
Southern California Center for Sports
  Medicine,
Long Beach, California

CRAIG L. VAN KAMPEN, Ph.D.
Technical Supervisor,
Orthopedic Products Division/3M,
St. Paul, Minnesota

PHILIP G. WILCOX, M.D.
Knee and Sports Medicine Fellow,
Memorial Medical Center,
Long Beach, California

Preface

Clinicians dealing with the many individual variables presented by a patient with an acute or chronic deficient anterior cruciate ligament have been asking for a clear delineation of guidelines for making the necessary decisions. The challenge in surgically repairing the anterior cruciate ligament disruption is to be more selective in choosing candidates and available procedures, improving surgical results, and decreasing the morbidity and complications of the surgical intervention. The application of basic science to the understanding of anterior cruciate ligament injury has been a significant step forward.

Based on the response to our scientific courses, The Anterior Cruciate—New Concepts, we were requested to put our thoughts and those of the other course faculty members into a text. This is a functional text for the student of the anterior cruciate ligament and for the surgeon who is helping patients make decisions regarding the best treatment for them. These new concepts are coming from many disciplines and are synthesized by experts in the field. References are available for those who wish to pursue specific areas further.

Clinicians involved in the treatment of anterior cruciate ligament injuries should understand basic terms of biomechanics and bioengineering. These terms help explain the principles for success and failure of both the normal and reconstructed anterior cruciate ligament. Restoration of the anatomy, vascularity, and biomechanics of the ligament is correlated with past and present clinical and surgical experience.

New surgical approaches to intra-articular repair and reconstruction have significantly altered patient morbidity. Arthroscopically assisted positioning of osseous tunnels and new graft replacements are the wave of the future and have decreased surgical morbidity. These new concepts are offered for improving surgical technique, evaluating extra-articular procedures, and offering a basis for selecting from the numerous procedures that are now available. The role of intra-articular autografts, allografts, augmentation, and prosthetic replacements are discussed in their current state. The discussions of these potential replacements are meant to show the direction for the future and the questions that must be answered by those proposing the use of the new materials.

No presentation of the anterior cruciate deficient knee is complete without updating the established and changing principles of rehabilitation. Minimizing the deleterious effects of surgery and associated disuse must take place while the desired healing is protected. The patient's rehabilitation and recovery can be enhanced by the use of selective immobilization and bracing. Bracing has become a somewhat controversial area in the management of the anterior cruciate ligament injury. The discussions presented review attempts at prevention of the anterior cruciate injury, postoperative immobilization, and protective bracing.

We have found in the last 3 years that many strides have been made in managing the epidemic problem of the anterior cruciate deficient knee. The next 5 to 10 years will further unravel many of our questions. We have attempted to share with the readers of this text clinically applicable material that represents where we are today and the directions that will continue to develop in the treatment of the anterior cruciate ligament injury.

Douglas W. Jackson
David Drez, Jr.

Contents

1. **The language of knee motion,** 1
   DALE M. DANIEL
   EDMUND N. BIDEN

2. **Anatomy of the anterior cruciate ligament,** 17
   PAUL R. REIMAN
   DOUGLAS W. JACKSON

3. **The vascularity of the anterior cruciate ligament and associated structures,** 27
   STEVEN PAUL ARNOCZKY

4. **Biomechanics of the anterior cruciate ligament,** 55
   BEN GRAF

5. **Clinical examination of the knee for anterior cruciate ligament laxity,** 72
   FRANK O. BONNARENS
   DAVID DREZ, Jr.

6. **Quantitative examination for anterior cruciate laxity,** 90
   KEITH L. MARKOLF

7. **Isometric placement of substitutes for the anterior cruciate ligament,** 102
   BEN GRAF

8. **Fixation of soft tissue,** 114
   DALE M. DANIEL
   DANIEL B. ROBERTSON
   DAVID L. FLOOD
   EDMUND N. BIDEN

9. **Factors affecting choices of anterior cruciate ligament surgery,** 127
   PHILIP G. WILCOX
   DOUGLAS W. JACKSON

10. **Intra-articular surgical considerations,** 142
    CHRISTOPHER L. IHLE
    DOUGLAS W. JACKSON

11. **The role of extra-articular anterior cruciate ligament stabilization,** 168
    JAMES R. ANDREWS
    WILLIAM G. CARSON, Jr.

12 **Anterior cruciate ligament autografts,** 193
WILLIAM G. CLANCY, Jr.
J. MICHAEL RAY

13 **Anterior cruciate ligament allografts,** 211
TIMOTHY M. SIMON
DOUGLAS W. JACKSON

14 **Synthetic augmentation of biological anterior cruciate ligament substitutions,** 226
CRAIG L. VAN KAMPEN
H. VINCENT MENDENHALL
GREGG K. McPHERSON

15 **Biomechanics of artificial ligaments and associated problems,** 239
FRANK O. BONNARENS
DAVID DREZ, Jr.

16 **Design considerations for cruciate ligament prostheses,** 254
WILLIAM C. BRUCHMAN
C. WILLIAM BOLTON
JAMES R. BAIN

17 **Principles of arthroscopic anterior cruciate reconstruction,** 273
DOUGLAS W. JACKSON
PAUL R. REIMAN

18 **Knee braces,** 286
DAVID DREZ, Jr.

19 **Rehabilitation after anterior cruciate ligament surgery,** 291
LONNIE E. PAULOS
FRANK CORRY PAYNE III
THOMAS D. ROSENBERG

20 **The future of anterior cruciate surgery,** 315
DOUGLAS W. JACKSON

1
The language of knee motion

DALE M. DANIEL

EDMUND N. BIDEN

In 1938 Ivar Palmer published his famous thesis *"On The Injuries To The Ligaments Of The Knee Joint."*[9] The paper was based on observations made in "fifty seven selected cases of ligament injuries . . . forty four of those cases underwent surgical treatment." In 1976 Hughston et al.[5] published a classification of knee ligament instability "based on correlation of clinical laxity tests with pathology discovered at the time of surgery." Over that period of 38 years the clinician developed an increasing awareness of the complexity of knee motion and of the ligamentous guidance system.[3,4] During the past two decades we have enticed our engineering colleagues to assist us in the study of knee motion and ligament function. This collaboration brings basic scientists and clinicians together and unquestionably advances our understanding of ligament function and knee motion. Many of the concepts we now hold sacred will be proved false and others will be further developed. Central to the task of placing our understanding, evaluation, and care of knee problems on a stronger scientific foundation is the use of precise terminology. A clear definition of the terms that the clinician has evolved and an understanding and adoption of engineering terms appropriate to the study of knee motion and ligament function will allow us to improve our own thought process and communicate with our engineering colleagues. In this chapter we will discuss terms used in describing knee motion, ligament laxity, and ligament injury.

Knee motion

The motion of the knee or any other system can be described in terms of rotations about or translations along some set of axes. Rotation is simply to turn about an axis, and translation is to slide

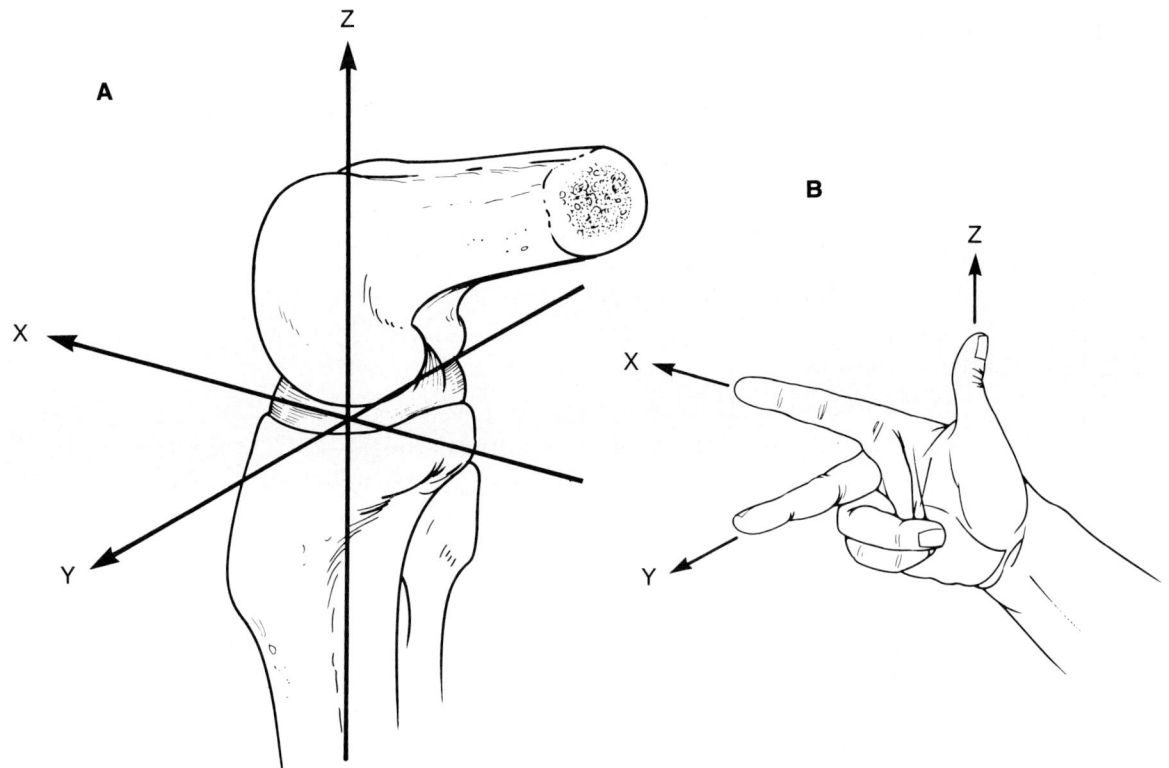

Fig. 1-1 *A, The knee with a conventional three axis system superimposed. B, This sketch of the hand shows a simple way to use the right hand rule. The index finger is pointed along the X axis, the long finger along the Y axis, and the thumb along the Z axis.*

along an axis. Translation is more precisely defined as motion such that all lines in the body remain parallel to their original position. The ability to rotate or translate along or about a particular axis is called a "degree of freedom." Free motion about or along the three mutually perpendicular axes used to define a space represents "six degrees of freedom." In this condition a body is completely free to move. Fig. 1-1 shows a knee with three axes superimposed. Conventionally the axes are arranged to fit the "right hand rule," that is, the X, Y, and Z axes are arranged as the index finger, long finger, and thumb of the right hand as shown in the sketch. Translations in the direction of the fingers or thumb are positive and rotations are positive if they are anticlockwise about an axis viewed from the positive end. In defining motion these translations and rotations are used to describe the movement. For example, knee flexion is a positive rotation about the Y axis.

TABLE 1-1 / Joint axis

AXIS	ROTATION	TRANSLATION	ENGINEERING AXIS
Anteroposterior	Abduction/adduction*	Anteroposterior	X
Mediolateral	Flexion/extension	Mediolateral*	Y
Proximodistal	Internal/external*	Penetration/distraction	Z

*These motions change between left and right knees if the coordinate system of Fig. 1-1 is used.

Axes provide a useful tool to describe motions and positions. Clinically they allow for easy communication and for measurement of joint movement, and they provide a mathematical shorthand to describe the motion. Although it is useful to use conventions, they are merely conventions and, if correctly established, any system that completely describes motion in three dimensions can be transformed into any other similar system.

Motion of the knee usually has been described as motion of the tibia in relation to a fixed femur. The axes are defined in Table 1-1, and their associated motions are commonly used conventions.

Natural knee motions and the motions resulting from clinical laxity tests are not limited to 1 degree of freedom. For example, "knee flexion" during normal gait requires the knee to rotate about the mediolateral axis, translate along and rotate about the anteroposterior axis, and rotate about the proximodistal axis. When an anterior displacement force is applied in performing the 30 degree anterior drawer test, the tibia translates anteriorly and rotates internally. When a posterior displacement force is applied, the tibia rotates externally and translates posteriorly (Fig. 1-2).

A common way of thinking about how the knee flexes is to imagine the *axis of rotation* moving posteriorly. The location of this axis is often called the *instant center* of the knee.[4] Although this is a good description of the view from the sagittal plane, be aware that the instant center is a mathematical concept that is most correctly used to define planar motion. Describing the three dimensional motion of the knee with a mathematical device intended for two dimensions can introduce errors. The errors introduced depend on how sensitive the results of the calculation are to errors introduced by motions or other variables left out in the simplification. Estimating sensitivity is often very difficult, and care must be taken that results from simple tests or simple approximations reflect the subject tested and not the way the test was run.

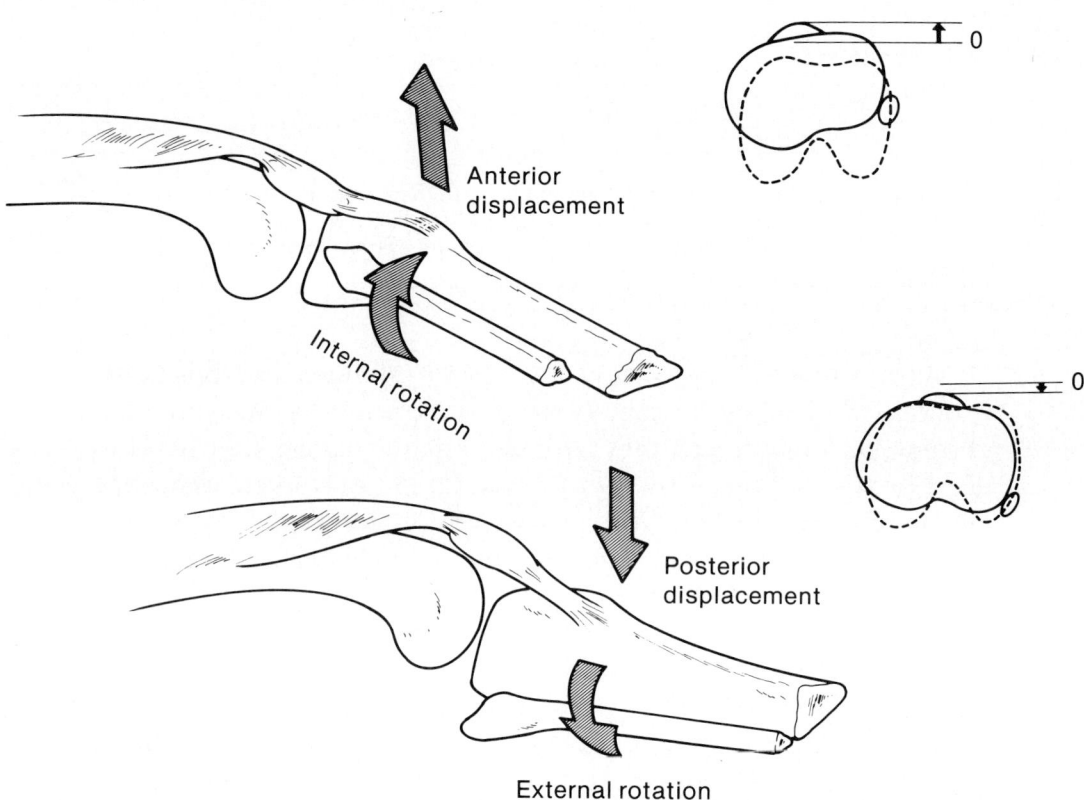

Fig. 1-2 *Coupled motion. Anterior drawer test showing combined anterior translation and internal rotation.*

In general the orthopedists' conventional terminology for knee motion needs little interpretation to make sense to the engineer and vice versa. However, mathematical representations of bodies moving in space often do not have the same neat divisions of motion into rotations and translations as one likes to think of clinically. In cases where complex motions are to be analyzed, it is advisable to carefully define each motion to be measured and to relate it to an established coordinate system.

Constraint and coupled motion

The concepts of constraint and coupled motion are important in understanding the normal movements of the knee. The verb to constrain is often described with words like compel, force, and confine. Couple is described as a link or a joining together. For example, as the knee moves from flexion to extension, the tibia rotates externally on the femur. The extension and external rotation are a

The language of knee motion

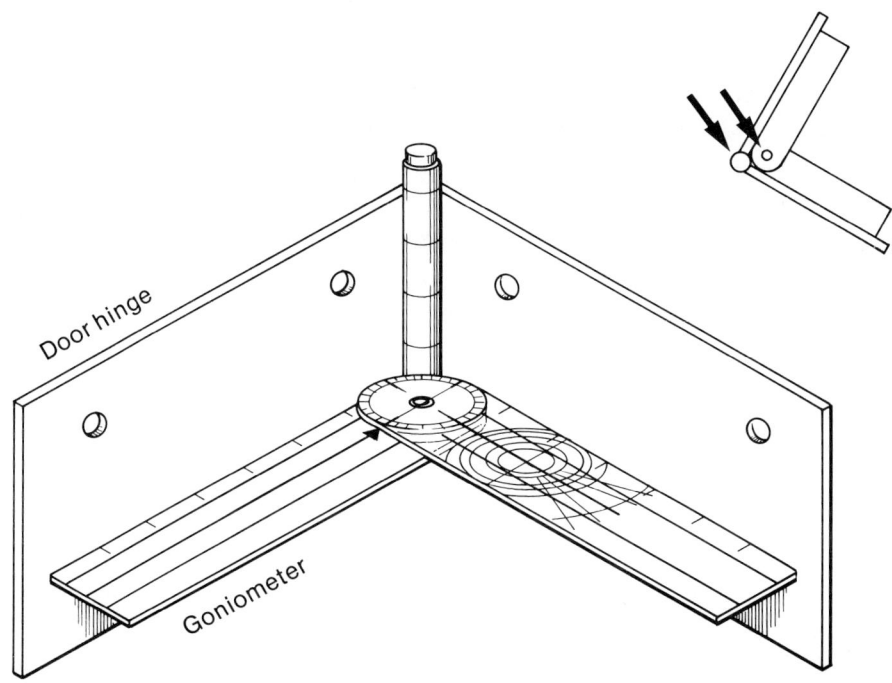

Fig. 1-3 *Testing the range of motion of a door hinge. The offset of the axis of the goniometer and the hinge cause the combination to act like a structure and resist movement.*

coupled motion. The knee is constrained by ligaments, tendons, and the joint capsule to have a range of flexion of from 0 to about 150 degrees. Similarly the soft tissues constrain the rotational motions to a range of 20 to 30 degrees, and movements into abduction or adduction are also limited. The normal knee is constrained in how it can move, and motions are not independent of one another. For example, when the knee moves into extension, the rotation of the tibia on the femur is an obligatory part of the total motion; it is "coupled" to the movement of extension by the way in which the structures of the knee are assembled and by the way in which the ligaments, tendons, and bones share the applied loads.

Let us consider the effects of external constraints on knee motion. Imagine the simple experiment shown in Fig. 1-3. Suppose we decided to measure the range of motion of a door hinge by rigidly attaching a goniometer to it. We would find that the measured range of motion is zero and that although we can arrange the device so that any initial setting of the goniometer can be obtained, the device will not move once the goniometer is attached. This is because the axis of the hinge and the axis of the goniometer are not co-axial; the testing apparatus becomes what engineers would call a "structure" rather than a "mechanism." You may think that this is a silly example, after all, who would do something like that? Yet each time a uniaxial hinged knee brace is prescribed for the "gliding and rolling" knee, some one, whether they appreciate it or not, is attempting to make the knee into a structure because of over constraint.

Whether testing joints in the laboratory or in the clinic one must take care not to provide inappropriate constraint. Joint laxity tests, for example, frequently focus on one motion. The constraint of the testing system on associated motions (coupled motions) may have a major effect on the movement being measured. When performing the 30-degree anterior drawer test, if joint rotation is constrained by the testing system, the tibia's anterior rotation will be significantly diminished.[2,10]

What is the effect of constraining motion? To constrain movement in some fashion requires a force or a moment. (Forces are simply pushes or pulls, and moments are twists.) To restrain motion during the drawer test requires a moment, applied by either the examiners hand or the testing device, to keep the tibia from rotating. Restraining motion in an experimental situation forces the testing device to absorb unexpected and unmeasured forces and moments that may be as important in the control of motion as the "known" loads being applied. In bracing these forces are manifest as "pistoning" of the leg in a brace, torn straps, skin breakdown, and other problems.

Constraint is absolutely essential to the normal function of the knee, to bracing, and to surgical reconstruction. It is important to understand what constraints limit a given motion and where, how, and with what they are applied. Interactions between engineers and orthopedists can provide the orthopedist with useful insights into the engineering what, how, and why of bracing or surgery and can provide the engineer with no end of useful, interesting, and often difficult problems.

Another example of coupled motion is the combined translation and rotation of the femur on the tibia as the knee flexes and extends. Fig. 1-4 shows the femur and tibia in the sagittal plane connected by the cruciate ligaments. If the cruciate ligaments are approximately isometric, that is, if they do not stretch or shorten significantly as

The language of knee motion

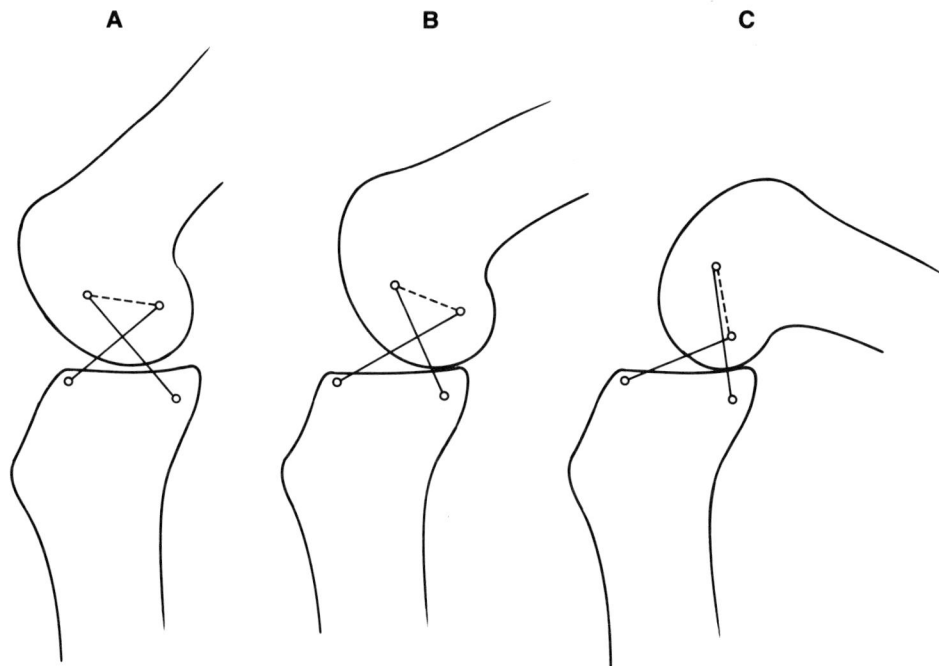

Fig. 1-4 *A through C, Tracing of the femur and tibia showing how the cruciate ligaments change position as the knee flexes.*

the knee bends, then the flexion angle determines the orientation of these ligaments. The cruciate ligaments control the sliding/rolling movement needed to match the long femoral surface to the shorter tibial surface. If a constraint is removed for example, by cutting the anterior cruciate ligament, the coupling between the bones is changed. If a constraint is added, for example, by applying a uniaxial brace, the coupling between the bones changes and new and different loads are applied to the coupling structures.

The interaction of muscle pulls, ligament restraints, and the joint surface contours used to determine joint movement may be compared to a well-pitched tent (Fig. 1-5). The soft tissues resist tensile loads and hard tissues resist compressive loads in the same way that the ropes of a tent resist tension and the poles of a tent resist compression. How the structures are arranged determines how the bones are coupled together, just as the tip of the tent pole is coupled to the motion of the rest of the tent. Thus the structures of the knee are linked by their constraining and coupling functions.

We have used the term *isometric* in describing the cruciate liga-

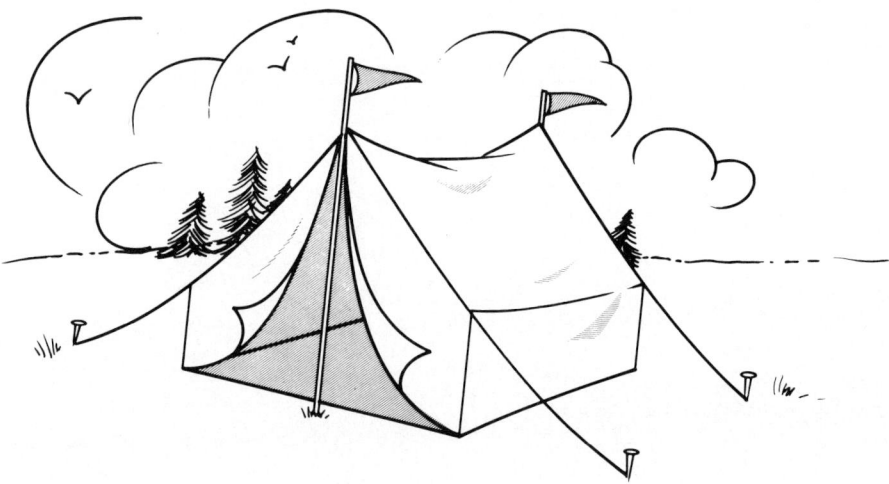

Fig. 1-5 *A well-pitched tent. The poles, like bones, resist compression and the ropes, like ligaments, resist tension.*

ments. In this context isometric is taken to mean of unchanging dimensions; that is, the length of the cruciates is approximately constant throughout the range of flexion. This is a useful concept and can aid in our understanding; however, applying a load to *any* material will cause it to deform. As an extreme example, a fly landing on a metal bar "bends" the bar until the internal stresses in the material equal the load resulting from the fly. That being the case, *no* ligament, tendon, or anything else that bears load can be truly isometric. On the other hand, if the deformations are small, the approximation of isometricity may be the best model.

Ligament laxity

We have discussed some terms used to describe motion of the knee, and in general we have found that the conventional clinical terms have close counterparts in engineering. The description of material properties relies heavily on quite specific engineering terms. In this section we describe some commonly used terms (Table 1-2).

In the study of motion, motions are often described without considering how those motions are changed by deformation of the component parts. In order to describe how tissues react to load, some definitions that describe how materials deform and change

TABLE 1-2 / Units of measurement

TERM	DEFINITION	UNITS
Force	Push or pull	Newtons (pounds)
Moment	Twist	Newton-meters (pound-inches)
Stress	Force/area	Newtons/meter^2 (pounds/inch^2)
Strain	Length change	Meters or meters/meter (inches or inches/inch)

under load must be introduced. This discussion is by no means exhaustive.*

As noted earlier, forces and moments are the essential ingredients of load. Forces are pushes or pulls; moments are twists and are often referred to as torques. Forces and moments can have components in three dimensions and can be manipulated as vectors, that is, they have both magnitude and a direction or line of action. Forces are measured in newtons or in pounds force, and moments are measured in units of force times a distance or newton-meters (pound-inches).

A load applied to a body, such as the piece of tissue shown in Fig. 1-6, is transmitted through the body with the addition of all of the smaller loads born by individual elements of the body. This distribution of load in units of force per area is known as *stress*. Stress is usually expressed in units of newtons per square meter or *pascals* or in the English system as pounds per square inch. The deflection or change in length when the load is applied is referred to as *strain*. Strain is often expressed as the percentage of length change of the body and is given in units of meter of change per meter of original length.

To describe the properties of the material itself, the relationship between stress and strain is usually used. This measure can be applied to a specimen of any size. For physical entities such as a ligament, load/displacement measurements specific to that actual tissue are often used. Examples of load/displacement curves are presented in Fig. 1-7. A specimen is subjected to increasing load while the strain or displacement is measured. Sketches of the typical curves for a linearly elastic material such as steel, for an elastic but

---

*For further study in this area we recommend, Van Cochran: *A Primer of Orthopaedic Biomechanics*,[12] or other books that deal specifically with biomechanics.

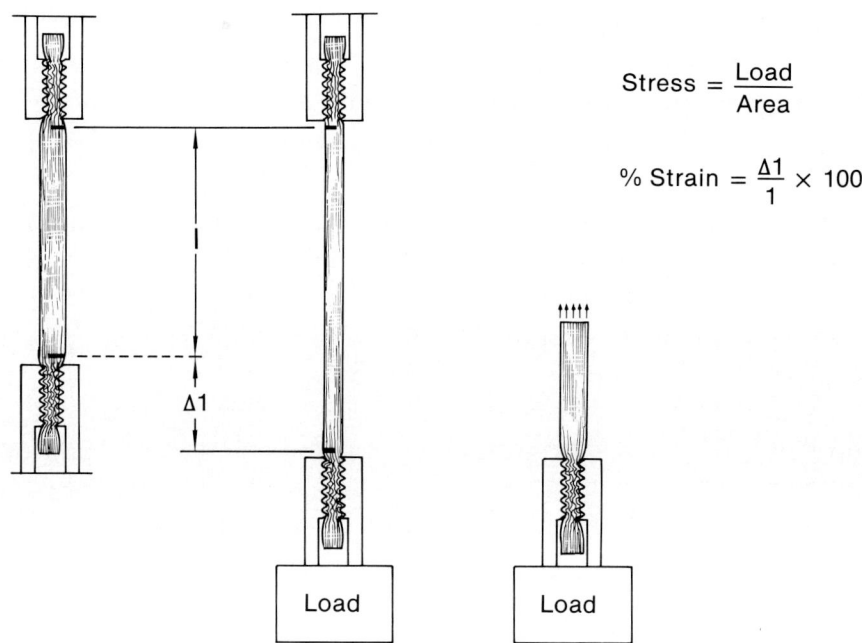

Fig. 1-6 *A tissue specimen loaded in tension. Under load the specimen stretches. The load on the whole specimen is resisted by the sum of the loads in each individual fiber.*

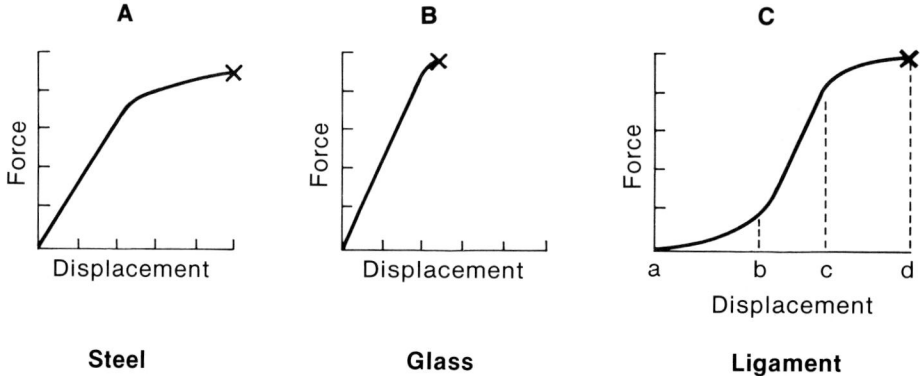

Fig. 1-7 *Load displacement curves for **A**, steel, **B**, glass, and **C**, ligament. The **X** in each marks the failure point. For ligament the area "a-b" is the "toe-in" region and "b-c" is the "linear" region.*

brittle material such as glass, and for a typical ligament are shown. In the first two cases there is an initial period where the increase in strain is directly proportional to the increase in load and where, if the load is removed, the material will assume its original shape. This so-called "elastic region" is the area where most metal components are designed to operate since they can be repeatedly loaded and resume their original geometry. If a brittle material is loaded past its elastic limit, it fails. If a ductile material is loaded past the elastic limit or yield point, the material begins to permanently deform in a process called *plastic deformation*. A plastically deformed body has absorbed some of the deforming energy to change the shape of the body and unlike an elastically deformed body it will not return to its original state if unloaded. The third example, that of the ligament under load, is like neither of the first two examples. If a ligament is stretched, there is an initial "toe-in" region where large deflections occur with very little force followed by a region where the load/displacement curve becomes much steeper and more nearly linear. Without getting into the various mechanisms that produce this effect, suffice to say that the *stiffness* (how hard it is to stretch the ligament a given amount) changes, depending on how much the ligament has already been stretched. From another perspective the *compliance* (how much the ligament stretches under a given increment in load) changes with stretch as well. Ligaments are quite elastic in response to rapidly applied loads but they are not linear in their response.

Even the most elastic material will not return all the energy put into deforming it. This loss is known as *hysteresis.* A typical hysteresis curve is shown in Fig. 1-8. Work is defined as a force times a distance. Thus the area under the load/displacement curve represents work. The work to stretch the specimen is the area under the upper curve and the work recovered in releasing the load is the area below the lower curve. The area between the curves represents work lost to friction. For metals in the elastic range this effect is very small. For materials such as ligaments it can be quite large.

Two other effects we need to mention are creep and relaxation. In Fig. 1-9 loads are placed on a body so that the load is constant and left for a period of time. *Creep* is the effect of the body reorganizing its structure to make it longer, stretching past the initial elastic stretch under the action of a long duration load. This effect is very common in biological materials. The second effect shown is *relaxation.* If a body is stretched or compressed to a fixed length and left

12 *The anterior cruciate deficient knee*

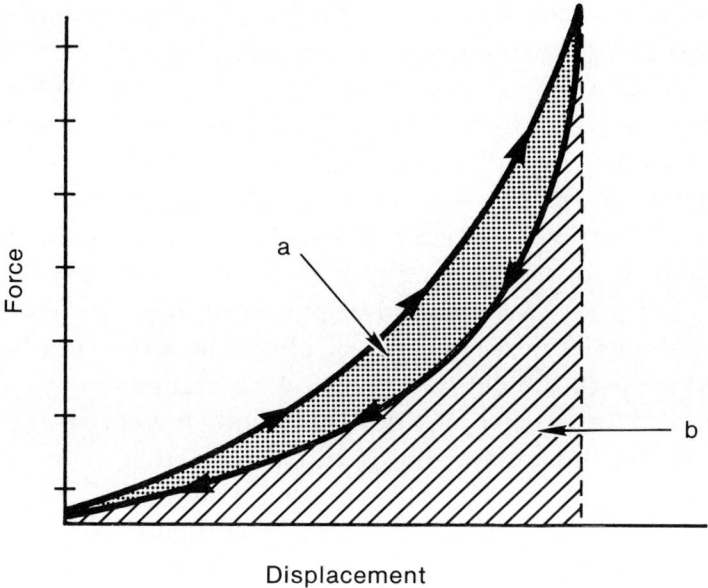

Fig. 1-8 *A load displacement diagram displaying hysteresis. The energy put into stretching the specimen is the sum of the areas marked "a" and "b." Area "b" represents the energy recovered when the load is relaxed. The energy lost during the process is represented by area "a."*

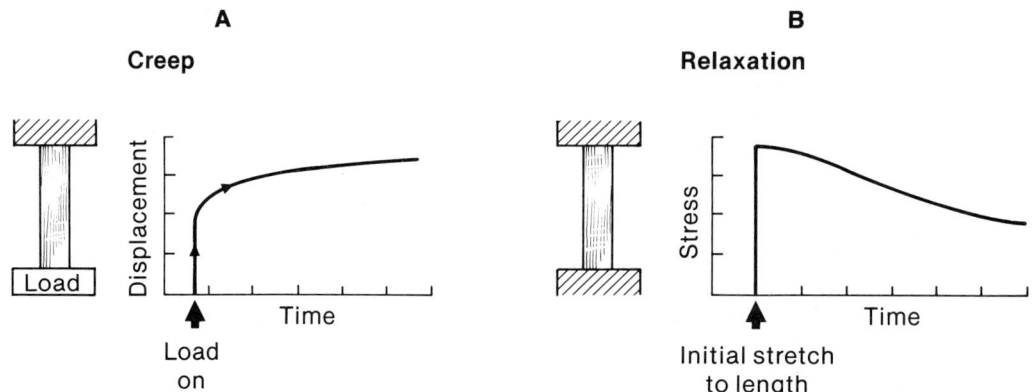

Fig. 1-9 *The effects of creep and relaxation. **A**, A ligament shown under constant load. Creep is the effect of continuous lengthening during application of load. **B**, Relaxation is the decrease in stress with time in a specimen held at constant length.*

and if the stresses in the body decline over time, the body is said to have relaxed. These two effects are combined in a viscoelastic body. In a viscoelastic material creep will be observed under constant force, relaxation will be observed under constant deformation, and the body will act elastically in response to rapid loading. Biological tissues, especially soft tissues, combine these properties in complex ways. They also tend to be materials that are highly anisotropic; that is, they have different properties depending on the orientation of the load, and their response to load is often highly nonlinear and dependent not only on the direction of loading but on the rate as well. A common example of this is a car's shock absorber. Loaded slowly, as when climbing into the car, it provides little resistance to loads, and the car settles until the springs take up the load. Loaded quickly, as by a bump when driving, the shock absorber acts like a rigid bar. Ligaments, consisting as they do of a combination of fibers and fluid, also respond in different ways depending on how they are loaded.

Clinical terminology

Thus far this chapter has dealt principally with engineering definitions and concepts. Clinicians seldom have as much control over their material as does the engineer. The clinician more often has to make his best assessment of the situation based on less well-defined data: the patient's recounting the injury event and discussing his symptoms and disabilities, the evaluation of pain and tenderness, and the "feel of the knee." The clinician has evolved a set of terms and tests based on this data to describe knee ligament injury and the resulting abnormal motion. Some of the terms are listed below. Of particular importance is the recognition that ligament injury grade, clinical laxity grade, joint displacement measurement, and joint instability are not synonymous.* Each term is based on a different set of observations. Ligament injury grade (1 equaling interstitial, 2 equaling partial, and 3 equaling complete) is usually based on indirect evidence of ligament injury, including history and symptoms and signs (swelling, tenderness, laxity) compatible with a ligament injury. If surgery is performed, the grade may be based on direct observation of the ligament. The clinical laxity grade is the clinicians best assessment of abnormal knee joint motion based on the "feel of

*References 1, 2, 5, 6, 8, 10, and 11.

the knee" while applying various deforming forces. Joint displacement measurements are direct measurements of joint translation and/or rotation. The terms stable and instability have been used in two contexts. *Functional stability* and *functional instability* refer to the patient's history of knee function—does the knee "go out," "give way," etc. Stability and instability are also used to describe the results of the clinical laxity examination. *Stability* is defined as a normal laxity examination. *Instability* is equal to a pathological laxity examination. The use of these terms are illustrated by the following example. Patient B.K. had an arthroscopically documented, complete (grade 3) anterior ligament tear. The clinical examination revealed a grade 1 Lachman test and a grade 1 pivot shift test (grade 1 instability). Instrumented measurement revealed anterior tibial displacement of 14 mm in the injured knee and of 8 mm in the normal knee. (Measurement was performed with a 20-pound anterior displacement force applied with the knee in 30 degrees of flexion.) The pathological anterior knee laxity (injured laxity minus normal laxity) is 14 mm − 8 mm = 6 mm. This patient had *no* complaints of functional knee instability.

The following is a list of terms we have found useful in describing ligament injury and the resulting abnormal joint motion.

1. **Injury activity** The activity the patient was involved in at the time of injury; for example, football.
2. **Injury event** The event that resulted in the injury itself; for example, being tackled while playing football.
3. **Injury mechanism** The force/motions thought to cause the injury; for example valgus load on the knee.
4. **Ligament injury grade:**
   First degree Microscopic tearing of the ligament without demonstrable laxity but with signs of ligament injury (pain, swelling, tenderness).
   Second degree Partial ligament disruption with an increase in joint laxity.
   Third degree Complete ligament disruption.
5. **Joint laxity** Joint motion resulting from a displacement force. Laxity measurements have two components: joint displacement and compliance or stiffness.[8]
6. **Clinical laxity grade** (knee stability) The examiner's evaluation of joint motion resulting from a manually applied displacement force. The clinician's evaluation is based on visual discrimination of joint motion and on tactile assessment of joint displacement and "end point stiffness." The injured knee is

compared to the normal knee. The motion is graded as:
Grade zero Normal joint motion = normal stability.
Grade one Mild increase over normal joint motion = 1+ instability.
Grade two Moderate increase over normal joint motion = 2+ instability.
Grade three Marked increase over normal joint motion = 3+ instability.

7. **Joint displacement measurements** Joint displacement measurements obtained from stress x-ray films or instrumented measurement systems.
8. **Displacement force** Force applied to produce a joint displacement. The effect of the force depends on the magnitude, direction, and point of application of the displacing force.
9. **Compliance measurement** The displacement measurement between two displacement loads, for example, 15 and 20 pounds. The inverse of compliance is stiffness, that is, the force divided by the displacement.[2]
10. **Laxity testing conditions** The limb position (hip flexion, knee flexion, internal/external rotation etc.) at the beginning of the test; how the limb is supported and constraint of associated joint motion. These factors as well as the displacement force and the activity of the muscles crossing the joint will affect the resulting joint displacement. Measurements of motions that go in two directions, such as anteroposterior translation, raise the question of how much of the motion is one and how much the other. The answer is dependent on how neutrality is established. If laxity tests to measure ligament integrity are to be compared to the patient's other limb or to some population, it is important that the laxity testing conditions remain constant.
11. **Passive laxity tests** The patient's muscles are relaxed and displacement forces are applied by the examiner or the testing device.
12. **Active laxity tests** Displacement forces result from the patient's muscle activity, for example, the quadriceps active drawer test.
13. **Normal joint laxity** The displacement and compliance measured in an uninjured joint. There is a wide spectrum of normal joint laxity, for example, the 20 pound per 30 degrees (30 pound anterior displaced forced knee in 30 degree flexion) anterior knee laxity varies from 3 to 13 mm. The anterior laxity in 85% of subjects is between 5 and 10 mm. Ninety-two percent of the normal population have a right/left 20 pound per 30 degree anterior displacement difference of no greater than 2 mm.[2,7]

14. **Pathological joint laxity** Joint displacement in a unilaterally injued patient that exceeds the normal right/left difference or an injured knee laxity in a bilaterally injured patient that exceeds the laxity measured in the normal population.[2,7]
15. **Functional instability** A decrease in the control of joint motion. A decrease in the control of joint motion may be secondary to a loss of normal joint surface topography, muscle function, or ligament guidance system.

Summary

Communication is fundamental to any exchange of information. Clear and consistent terminology assists communication by providing a common language. To communicate effectively orthopedists and engineers need to state things clearly and simply.

REFERENCES

1. American Medical Association, Committee on the Medical Aspects of Sports: Standard nomenclature of athletic injuries, 1968, The Association.
2. Daniel, D.M., Malcom, L.L., Losse, G., et al.: Instrumented measurement of anterior laxity of the knee, J. Bone Joint Surg. (Am.) **67:**720-726, 1985.
3. Goodfellow, J., and O'Connor, J.: The mechanics of the knee and prosthesis design, J. Bone Joint Surg. (Br.) **60:**358-369, 1978.
4. Hobson, D., and Torfason, L.: Optimization of four-bar knee mechanism—a computerized approach, J. Biomech. **7:**371-376, 1974.
5. Hughston, J.C., Andrews, J.R., Gross, M.J., et al.: Classification of knee ligament instability, Parts I and II, J. Bone Joint Surg. (Am.) **58:**159-179, 1976.
6. Kennedy, J.C., editor: The injured adolescent knee, Baltimore, 1979, Williams & Wilkins Co.
7. Malcom, L.L., Daniel, D.M., Stone, M.L., et al.: The measurement of anterior knee laxity after ACL reconstruction, Clin. Orthop. **196:**35-41, 1985.
8. Markolf, K.L., Mensch, J.S., and Amstutz, H.C.: Stiffness and laxity of the knee—the contribution of the supporting structures, J. Bone Joint Surg. (Am.) **58:**583-594, 1976.
9. Palmer, I.: On the injuries to the ligaments of the knee joint, Acta. Chir. Scand. (Suppl.) p. 53, 1938.
10. Slocum, D.B., and Larson, R.L.: Rotatory instability of the knee, J. Bone Joint Surg. (Am.) **50:**211-225, 1968.
11. Sullivan, D., Levy, I.M., Sheskier, S., et al.: Medial restraints to anterior-posterior motion of the knee, J. Bone Joint Surg. (Am.) **66:**930-936, 1984.
12. Van Cochran, G.: A primer of orthopaedic biomechanics, New York, 1982, Churchill Livingstone.

2

Anatomy of the anterior cruciate ligament

PAUL R. REIMAN

DOUGLAS W. JACKSON

The success of any surgical procedure begins with a thorough knowledge of the anatomical structures in the region. Reconstructive procedures of the knee have benefited greatly from a number of anatomical and biomechanical studies on the ligaments of the knee.* As detailed knowledge of the structure and function of the anterior cruciate has evolved, the results of surgical reconstruction have improved. The anterior cruciate ligament is one of the most frequently injured structures in the knee. With more surgeons performing arthroscopy, the past decade has seen a greater appreciation of the number of anterior cruciate deficient knees. The surgical techniques for repair and reconstruction of the anterior cruciate have been improving and are based on a more thorough understanding of the anatomical structure and function of the anterior cruciate ligament.

Review of literature

Brantigan and Voshell[4] in 1941 presented detailed anatomical descriptions of the ligamentous structures of the knee. In this same treatise, they proposed the functional significance of each of the ligamentous structures. The association of the collateral ligaments and capsular structures were described by several authors. The pes anserinus tendons, the semimembranosus tendons, and their use in reconstructive procedures as reported by Slocum launched widespread appreciation of rotatory instability of the knee.[17] Hughston provided details regarding the posterior oblique ligament[8] and

*References 1, 3, 4, 6-8, 11, and 13-15.

has added greatly to the knowledge of the posterior lateral corner.[9] Hughston,[9] Jakob,[10] and Seebacher[15] detailed the anterolateral and posterolateral structures and their relation to instability.

Kennedy,[11] Girgis et al.,[7] and Odenstein et al.[14] described the anatomy and функton of the anterior cruciate ligament. Noyes and Grood reported on their studies of the fatigue strength of the anterior cruciate ligament.[13] Arnoczky et al. have provided detailed information on the microvasculature of the cruciate ligaments.[1,3]

Embryology

The knee begins to form from a concentration of mesenchyme in the fourth week of gestation. The formation is rapid, with the appearance of a recognizable knee joint by the sixth week. The anterior cruciate ligament begins to condense during that same period. The anterior cruciate arises from the same blastoma as the semilunar cartilage.[5] The ligament first appears in a ventral position and gradually migrates into the intercondylar notch area. Its structural appearance remains relatively constant as the femoral condyles begin to differentiate. The anterior cruciate ligament remains extrasynovially as it migrates posteriorly during its development.[5,12]

Anatomy

The anterior cruciate ligament courses from its origin on the posterolateral femoral condyle in the intercondylar notch obliquely through the knee joint to its insertion on the anteromedial portion of the tibia. The ligament is a composite of individual fascicles that function collectively so that a portion of the ligament is taut in any position of the knee. This constant tension is possible as a result of the different orientations of the individual fascicles on the femur and tibia.[2]

Femoral origin

The anterior cruciate ligament fibers originate on the posteromedial surface of the lateral femoral condyle near the articular surface. The area of origin has been described as elliptical[7] or oval.[14] The posterior portion of the fibers tend to parallel the articular surface of the lateral femoral condyle. This bony origin is 16 to 24 mm in diameter and is located well posterior in the intercondylar notch (Fig. 2-1). In their study of 33 cadaver knees, Odenstein and Gill-

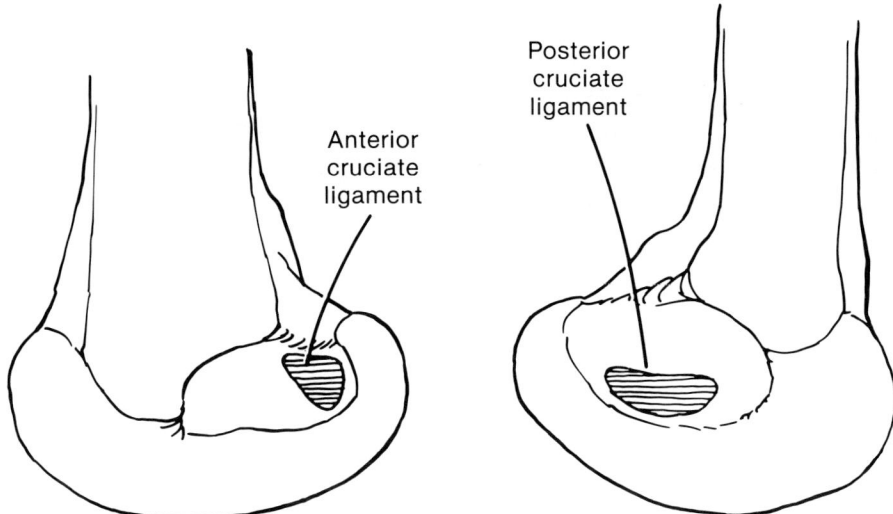

Fig. 2-1 *Schematic drawing of the femur split longitudinally shows the areas of anatomical origin of the anterior and posterior cruciate ligaments. Note the proximity of both origins to the articular surface and the proximity of the origin of the anterior cruciate ligamentous to the posterior aspect of the femur. (Adapted from Girgis, F.G., Marshall, J.L., and Al Monajem, A.R.S.: The cruciate ligaments of the knee joint—anatomical function and experimental analysis, Clin. Orthop. **106**:218, 1975.)*

quist[14] found the center of this bony origin to be 15 mm from the junction between the posterior aspect of the femoral shaft and the most proximal portion of the lateral femoral condyle. Girgis et al.[7] described the area as 24 mm distal to the level of the adductor tubercle or 15 mm anterior to the junction of the roof of the intercondylar notch and the posterior surface of the lateral femoral condyle.

Tibial insertion

The anterior cruciate ligament then courses obliquely in an anteromedial and distal direction to insert into the proximal tibia. The insertion is not onto the anteromedial tibial spine but into a fossa anterior and lateral to the spine (Fig. 2-2). This insertion is broad, with dimensions of 11 mm in width and 17 mm in the anteroposterior direction.[7] The tibial insertion sends variable fibers anteriorly to pass beneath the transverse meniscal ligament. A few fascicles also may insert into the anterior horn of the lateral meniscus. The fibers that insert more posteriorly can also blend with the posterolateral meniscus.[7,14]

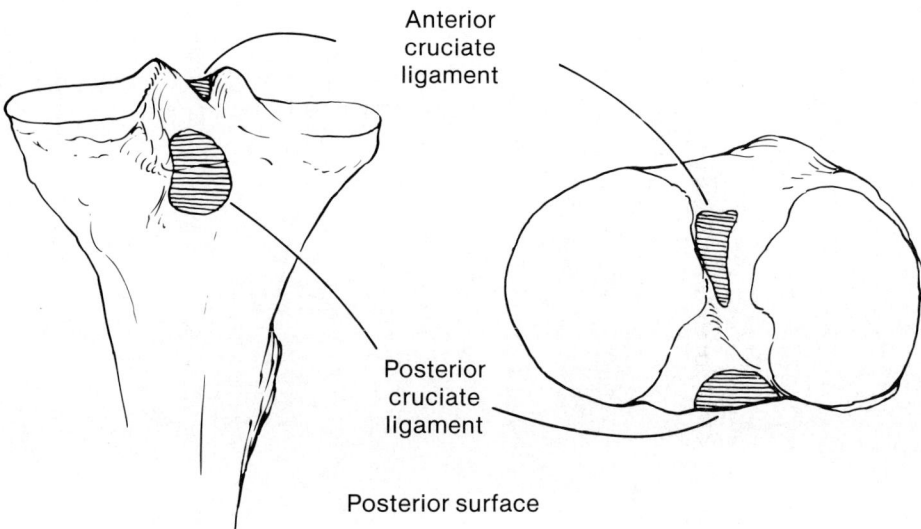

Fig. 2-2 *Schematic drawing of the tibial insertions of the anterior and posterior cruciate ligaments onto the tibia. Note the broad-based insertion of the anterior cruciate into the fossa between the tibial spines. The posterior aspect of the insertion is also located well posterior on the tibia. (Adapted from Girgis, F.G., Marshall, J.L., and Al Monajem, A.R.S.: The cruciate ligaments of the knee joint—anatomical function and experimental analysis, Clin. Orthop. **106**:218, 1975.)*

Interstitial anatomy

The anterior cruciate ligament is enveloped in the synovial membrane, which places the ligament intracapsularly but extrasynovially throughout its course. The location and orientation of the fibers on the tibia and femur determine the lateral spiral twist of the composite ligament in its course through the knee. This orientation results in the fibers arising from the most posteror and proximal portion of the lateral femoral condyle inserting onto the most anterior and medial portion of the tibia. These fibers have been described as the anteromedial bundle. Conversely, those fibers arising from the most anterior and distal portion of the femoral origin insert into the most posterolateral portion of the tibial attachment (Fig. 2-3).[7]

This orientation allows a portion of the anterior cruciate ligaments to be taut during all portions of the range of motion. In extension the posterolateral portion is taut and becomes stressed in hyperextension. In flexion the ligament becomes more horizontal in

Anatomy of the anterior cruciate ligament

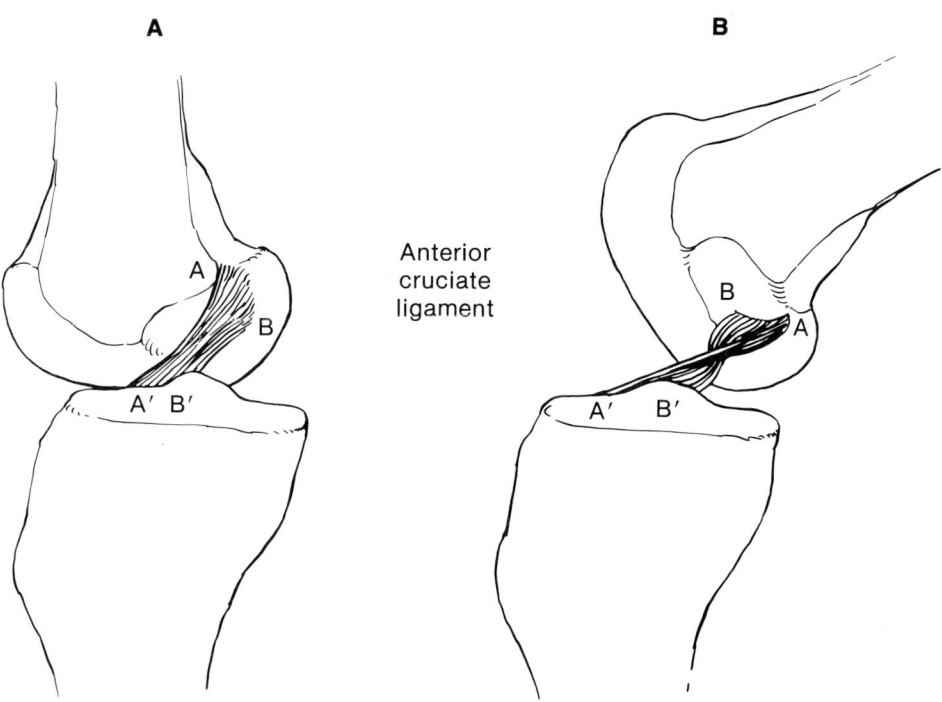

Fig. 2-3 *Diagramatic representation of the anterior cruciate ligament during flexion extension. **A**, Hyperextension. Note the impingement of the roof of the intercondylar notch on the anteromedial bundle (A-A'), as well as the relative tautness of the posterolateral bundle (B-B'). **B**, Ninety-degree flexion. Note the relative tension in the anteromedial bundle (A-A') with relative laxity of the posterolateral bundle (B-B'). There is a continuum of individual fascicles between these two bundles so that a portion of the ligament remains taut during all degrees of flexion. (Adapted from Girgis, F.G., Marshall, J.L., and Al Monajem, A.R.S.: The cruciate ligaments of the knee joint—anatomical function and experimental analysis, Clin. Orthop. **106**:218, 1975.)*

its orientation, placing the anteromedial portion under tension. There is a continuum between the anteromedial and posterolateral portions of the anterior cruciate ligament that results in a portion of the ligament remaining taut at all times. The presence or absence of distinct bundles or subdivisions has been debated extensively. Primarily, subdivisions are proposed to improve the conceptual understanding of the function of the anterior cruciate ligament. The important concepts of the normal anterior cruciate ligament are (1) that each fiber has a unique point of origin and insertion, (2) that the fibers are not parallel and do not have the same length, and (3) that the fibers are not under the same tension at any one point in space.

Odenstein and Gillquist reported that the ligament composite ranged from 25 to 35 mm in length, from 7 to 12 mm in width, and from 4 to 7 mm in depth.[14] Girgis et al. found the ligament to be somewhat larger, with an average length of 38.2 mm and a width of 11.2 mm in the middle third of the ligament.[7] Kennedy et al. found a range between 37 and 41 mm in 10 knees.[11] In full extension, the anterior cruciate ligament takes the form of a broad, flat, homogeneous structure. In flexion, the ligament twists upon itself approximately 90 degrees and thus gives the appearance of multiple bundles. The ligament is narrowest at its most proximal portion near the femoral origin and fans out as it approaches the tibial attachment.

Microstructure

Danylchuk et al. investigated the microstructure of human and bovine cruciate ligaments using scanning electron microscopy.[6] The anterior cruciate ligament is composed of fibrils of collagen of 150 to 250 nanometer (nm) in diameter that interlace to form complex networks. Multiple networks of fibrils from individual fibers of 1 to 20

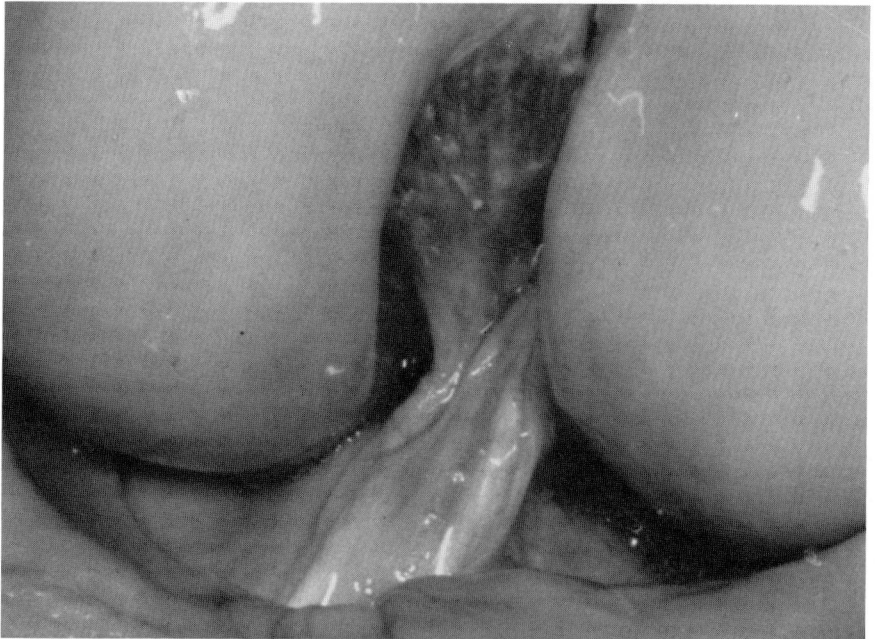

Fig. 2-4 *Anatomical specimen demonstrating the broad-based tibial insertion of the anterior cruciate ligament. Note the twisted appearance of the ligament as a result of the flexed position of the specimen.*

microns (μm) in diameter that tend to parallel the axis of the ligament (Fig. 2-4). Multiples of the collagen fibers coalesce to form subfascicular units 100 to 250 μm in diameter. Surrounding each subfascicular unit is a thin band of loose connective tissue, the endotendineum. Danylchuk et al. exhibited three to twenty subfascicular units coalescing to form visible fasciculi of varying sizes. Each fasciculus is surrounded by epitendineum, which is thicker than the endotendineum. The epitendineum is more loosely and randomly oriented than the fascicles. The entire ligament is then surrounded by both a paratenon and a synovial sheath (Fig. 2-5).[6]

Kennedy et al. investigated the neural structures of the knee and found neural elements within the anterior cruciate ligament.[11] These

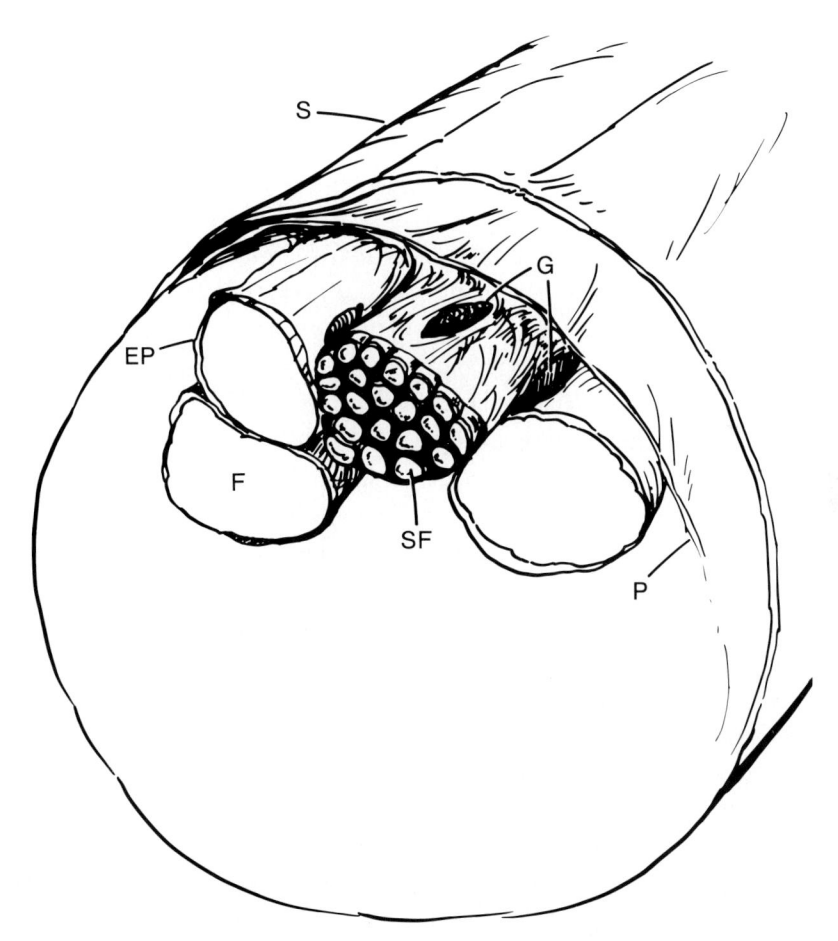

Fig. 2-5 *Schematic representation of the microstructure of the anterior cruciate ligament at the fascicular level. (S, synovial sheaths; P, paratenon; G, Golgi tendon organs; F, Fasciculus; SF, Subfasciculi; EP, epitendineum.)*

elements were primarily found within invaginations in the ligament near the tibial insertion of the anterior cruciate. Neural structures were also present in the synovial tissue surrounding the anterior cruciate ligament. Of significance was the identification of Golgi-like tension receptors in the posterior cruciate ligament. These were found near the origin of the posterior cruciate along with neural elements similar to those found in the anterior cruciate ligament.

Schultz et al. reviewed ten fresh specimens of anterior cruciate ligaments from knees that were free of disease. The ages of the specimens ranged from 1 week to 18 years. Each of the anterior cruciate ligaments contained fusiform neural structures consisting of a single axon wrapped in a fibrous capsule—similar to a Golgi tendon organ. The long axis of the structure was parallel to the ligament, and the structure was found in the fibrous-fatty paratenon.[16] Further studies on the functional significance of these receptors would add greatly to the understanding of pre- and post-injury knee kinematics.

Surgical relevance

Reconstruction of the anterior cruciate ligament has for many years emphasized reconstruction and reproduction of the normal anatomical locations of the anterior cruciate ligament. However, one must not only understand the static anatomy of the joint but must have an appreciation of knee joint kinematics. The anterior cruciate ligament, like all ligaments, guides joint motion by constraining abnormal motion. This guidance of the kinematics is evidenced by the relative tension seen in the various fascicles of the composite anterior cruciate ligament. While under tension, the individual fascicles exert a restraining effect against abnormal motion. Only by reconstructing each of the individual fascicles could the original anatomy be reproduced exactly.

Therefore the goals of reconstruction must be somewhat modified. Of greatest importance is reproduction of the functions of the normal anterior cruciate ligament. The function of the anterior cruciate ligament most often recognized is the resistance of anterior tibial translation on the femur. However, the anterior cruciate ligament also resists hyperextension of the knee and excessive internal tibial rotation. Secondary functions of the anterior cruciate are restraining of both varus and valgus stresses and guidance of the tibia in the screw-home mechanism of the joint during terminal extension maneuvers. This deficiency is seen most commonly in the athlete who is changing directions or decelerating. Thus the reconstruction of an anterior cruciate deficient knee must attempt to reproduce not only normal anatomy by using the isometric points within the femoral origin and tibial insertion of the original ligament, but also to reproduce the function by using a substitute of appropriate material properties. Extra-articular reconstructive procedures can be used to modify and/or enhance the secondary restraints of the anterior cruciate ligament deficient knee. The challenge of the future is to duplicate the constraints of the anterior cruciate ligament on the translation and rotation movements during knee motion.

Summary

The anterior cruciate ligament is a complex ligamentous structure that begins its formation early in gestation. The ligament is composed of multiple fascicles that function collectively to restrain both anterior displacement and rotational forces on the knee. Reproduction of the exact anatomy of the anterior cruciate by surgical reconstruction is difficult because of the multifascicular structure of the ligament. Further studies into the anatomy of the individual fascicles and their vascularity and neurological innervations will contribute to our understanding of the function of the anterior cruciate ligament.

REFERENCES

1. Arnoczky, S.P., Rubin, R.M., and Marshall, J.L.: Microvasculature of the cruciate ligaments and its response to injury, J. Bone Joint Surg. (Am.) **61:**1221-1229, 1979.
2. Arnoczky, S.P.: Anatomy of the anterior cruciate ligament, Clin. Orthop. **172:**19-25, 1983.
3. Arnoczky, S.P.: Blood supply to the anterior cruciate ligament and supporting structures, Orthop. Clin. North Am. **16:**15-28, 1985.
4. Brantigan, O.L., and Voshell, A.F.: The mechanics of the ligaments and menisci of the knee joint, J. Bone Joint Surg. **23:**44-46, 1941.
5. Crelin, E.S.: Development of the musculoskeletal system, Ciba Found. Symp. vol. **33**(1), 1981.
6. Danylchuk, K.D., Finlay, J.B., and Krcek, J.P.: Microstructural organization of human and bovine cruciate ligaments, Clin. Orthop. **131:**294-298, 1978.
7. Girgis, F.G., Marshall, J.L., and Al Monajem, A.R.S.: The cruciate ligaments of the knee joint—anatomical, functional, and experimental analysis, Clin. Orthop. **106:**216-231, 1975.
8. Hughston, J.L. and Eilers, A.F.: The role of the posterior oblique ligament in repair of acute medial tears of the knee, J. Bone Joint Surg. (Am.) **55:**923-940, 1973.
9. Hughston, J.L., and Norwood, L.A.: The posterolateral drawer test and external rotational recurvatum test for posterolateral rotatory instability of the knee, Clin. Orthop. **147:**82-87, 1980.
10. Jakob, R.P.: Observations on rotatory instability of the lateral compartment of the knee, Acta. Orthop. Scand. **191:**1-32, 1981.
11. Kennedy, J.C., Weinberg, H.W., and Wilson, A.S.: The anatomy and function of the anterior cruciate ligament, J. Bone Joint Surg. (Am.) **56:**223-235, 1974.
12. Muller, W.: The knee, form, function, and ligament reconstruction, Berlin, 1983, Springer, Verlag.
13. Noyes, F.R., and Grood, E.S.: The strength of the anterior cruciate ligament in humans and rhesus monkeys, J. Bone Joint Surg. (Am.) **58:**1074-1082, 1976.
14. Odenstein, M., and Gillquist, J.: Functional anatomy of the anterior cruciate ligament and a rationale for reconstruction, J. Bone Joint Surg. (Am.) **67:**257-262, 1985.
15. Seebacher, J.R., Inglis, A.E., Marshall, J.L., et al.: The structure of the posterolateral aspect of the knee, J. Bone Joint Surg. (Am.) **64:**536-541, 1982.
16. Schultz, R.A., Miller, D.C., Kerr, C.S., et al.: Mechanoreceptors in human cruciate ligaments, J. Bone Joint Surg. (Am.) **66:**1072-1976, 1985.
17. Slocum, D.B., and Larsen, R.L.: Rotatory instability of the knee—its pathogenosis and a clinical test to determine its presence, J. Bone Joint Surg. (Am.) **50:**211-225, 1965.

3
The vascularity of the anterior cruciate ligament and associated structures
Its role in repair and reconstruction

STEVEN PAUL ARNOCZKY

The structure, function, and injury of the anterior cruciate ligament have long been topics of interest and debate among orthopedic surgeons. Recently, these discussions have also focused on the blood supply of this structure in both the normal and injured state.

Isolated within the intra-articular environment of the knee, the cruciate ligaments possess a somewhat "fragile" blood supply as compared with extra-articular tissues. Following injury to the anterior cruciate ligament this intra-articular blood supply may be compromised and thus reparative or reconstructive procedures may be at risk. Treatment of anterior cruciate ligament injuries, therefore, must not only be concerned with the recreation of a functional structure but also with the reestablishment of the normal physiology of the tissues. Thus knowledge of the intra-articular vascular anatomy of the knee is of paramount importance in the surgical repair and reconstruction of cruciate ligament injuries.

This chapter examines the vascular anatomy of the anterior cruciate ligament and its associated structures and focuses on the role of this vascularity in anterior cruciate ligament repair and reconstruction.

Cruciate ligaments

The major blood supply to the anterior and posterior cruciate ligaments arises from the ligamentous branches of the middle genic-

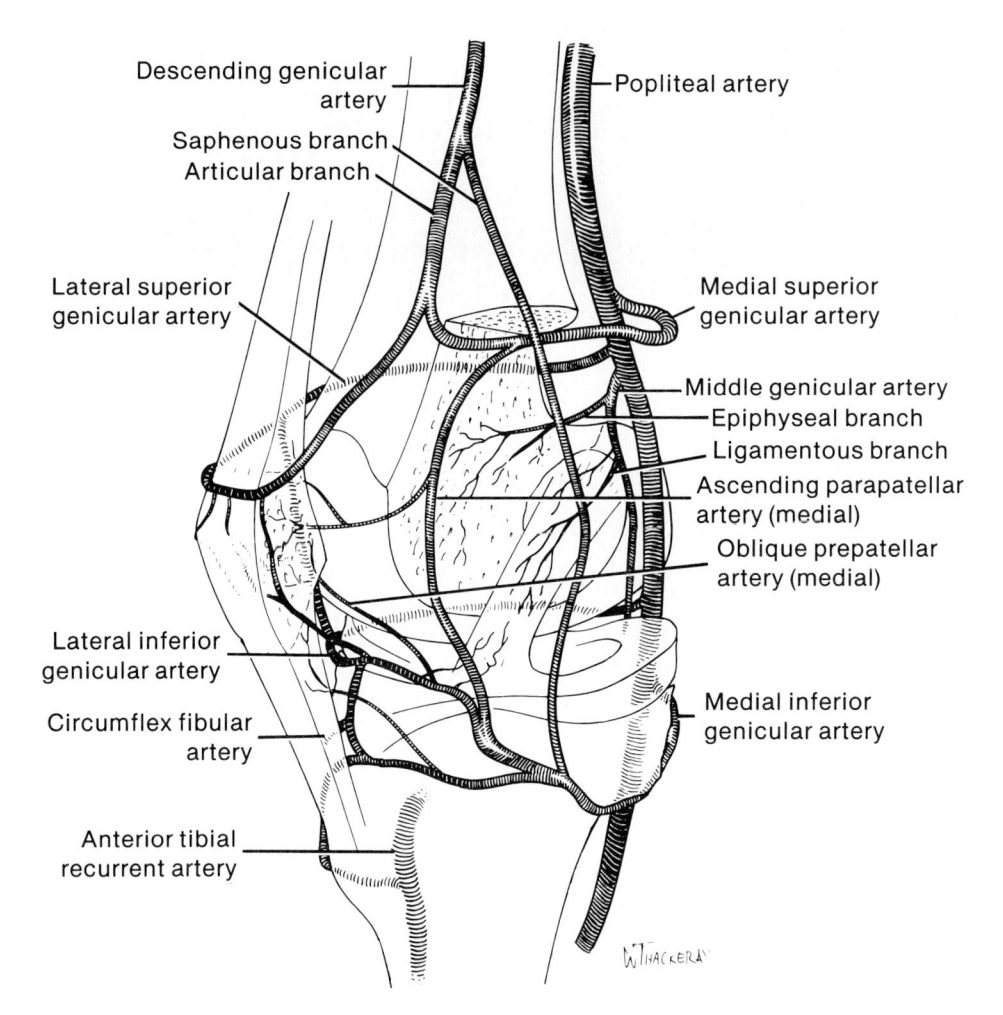

Fig. 3-1 *Schematic drawing of the knee illustrating the location and course of the major arteries that supply the joint. (From Arnoczky, S.P.: Blood supply to the anterior cruciate ligament and supporting structures, Orthop. Clin. North Am.* **16:**15-28, 1985.)

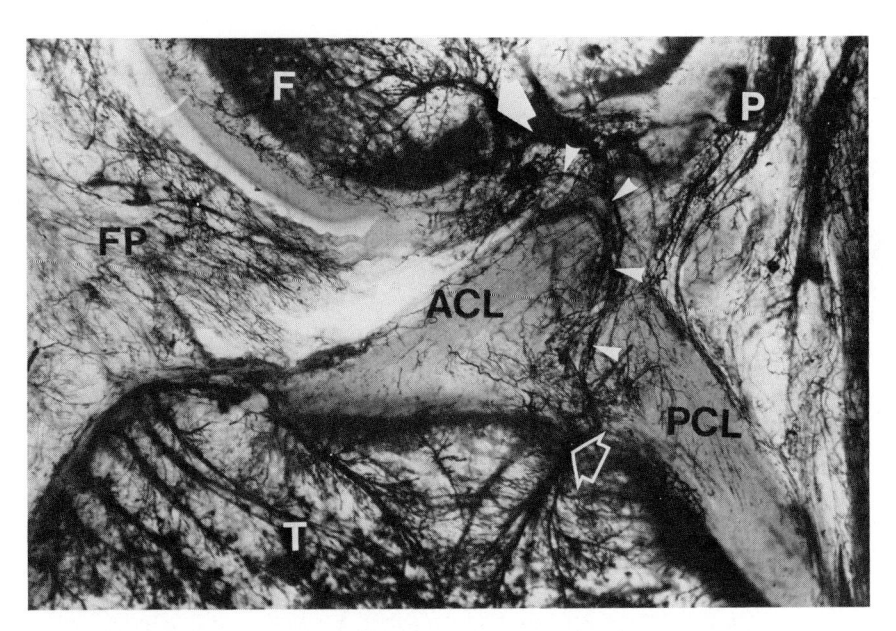

Fig. 3-2 *A 5-mm thick sagittal section of a human knee (Spalteholz technique) showing the branches of the middle genicular artery that supply the distal femoral epiphysis* (large white arrow), *the proximal tibial epiphysis* (large open arrow), *and the cruciate ligaments* (small white arrowheads). (F, *femur;* T, *tibia;* FP, *fat pad;* P, *popliteal artery;* ACL, *anterior cruciate ligament;* PCL, *posterior cruciate ligament.*) *(From Arnoczky, S.P.: Blood supply to the anterior cruciate ligament and supporting structures, Orthop. Clin. North Am.* **16**:*15-28, 1985.)*

ular artery as well as from some terminal branches of the medial and lateral inferior genicular arteries (Figs. 3-1 and 3-2).*

The cruciate ligaments are covered by a synovial fold that originates at the posterior inlet of the intercondylar notch and extends to the anterior tibial insertion of the ligament where it joins with the synovial tissue of the joint capsule distal to the infrapatellar fat pad. This synovial membrane, which forms an envelope about the ligaments, is richly endowed with vessels that originate predominantly from the ligamentous branches of the middle genicular artery (Fig. 3-3). A few smaller terminal branches of the lateral and medial inferior genicular arteries also contribute some vessels to this synovial plexus through its connection with the infrapatellar fat pad. The synovial vessels arborize to form a weblike network of periliga-

*References 7, 8, 11, 14, 16, 18, 22, 25, 30, and 32.

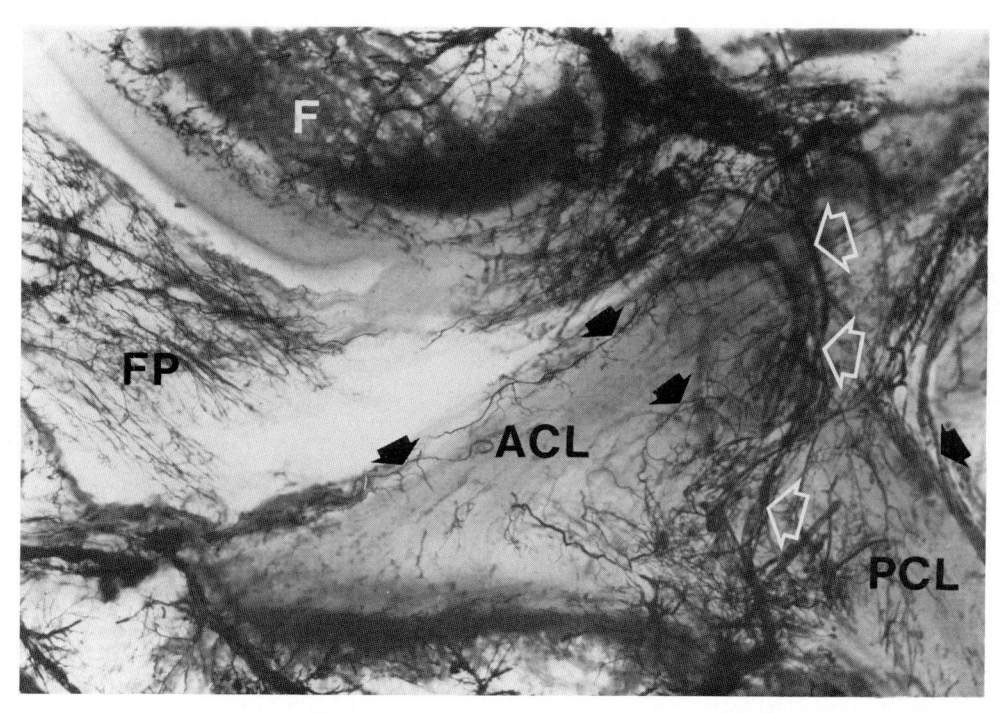

Fig. 3-3 *A 5-mm thick sagittal section of a human knee joint (Spalteholz technique) showing the vascularity of the anterior cruciate ligament. The ligamentous branch of the middle genicular artery and its divisions* (open arrows) *can be seen supplying the periligamentous branches* (black arrows) *of the synovial covering of the anterior cruciate ligament* (ACL). (F, *femur;* FP, *fat pad;* PCL, *posterior cruciate ligament.*) *(From Arnoczky, S.P.: Anatomy of the anterior cruciate ligament, Clin. Orthop.* **172:**19-25, 1983.)

mentous vessels that ensheath the entire ligament (Fig. 3-4). These periligamentous vessels then give rise to smaller connecting branches that penetrate the ligament transversely and anastomose with a network of endoligamentous vessels (Fig. 3-5). These vessels, along with their supporting connective tissues, are oriented in a longitudinal direction and lie parallel to the collagen bundles within the ligament.[7,8,16,25]

The blood supply of the anterior and posterior cruciate ligaments is predominantly of soft tissue origin. While the middle genicular artery gives off additional branches to the distal femoral epiphysis and proximal tibial epiphysis, the ligamentous-osseous junctions of the cruciate ligaments do not contribute significantly to the vascular scheme of the ligaments themselves (Fig. 3-6).[7,8,25]

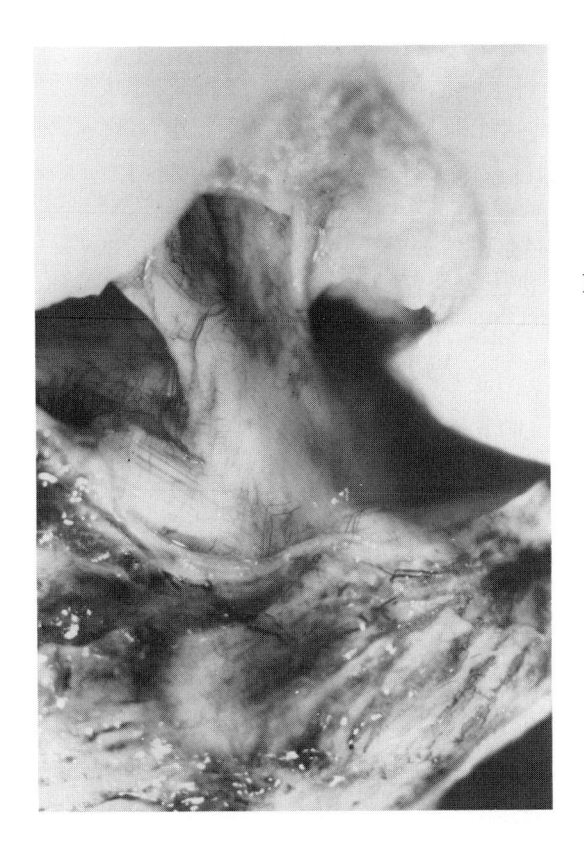

Fig. 3-4 *Photograph of a human knee specimen injected with India ink demonstrating the synovial (periligamentous) vasculature on the surface of the anterior cruciate ligament. (Note that the infrapatellar fat pad has been removed for better visualization.) (From Arnoczky, S.P.: Blood supply to the anterior cruciate ligament and supporting structures, Orthop. Clin. North Am. **16**:15-28, 1985.)*

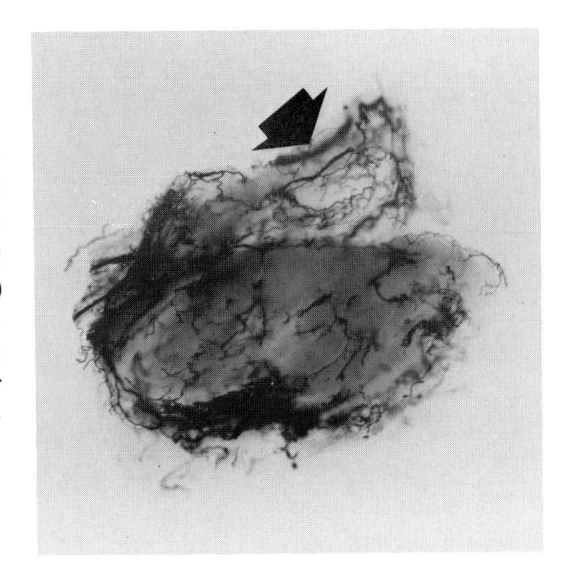

Fig. 3-5 *Cross section of a human anterior cruciate ligament (Spalteholz technique) demonstrating the periligamentous as well as endoligamentous vasculature. The fold of the synovial membrane (arrow) can be seen supplying vessels to the synovial covering of the ligament. (From Arnoczky, S.P.: Anatomy of the anterior cruciate ligament, Orthop. Clin. **172**:19-25, 1983.)*

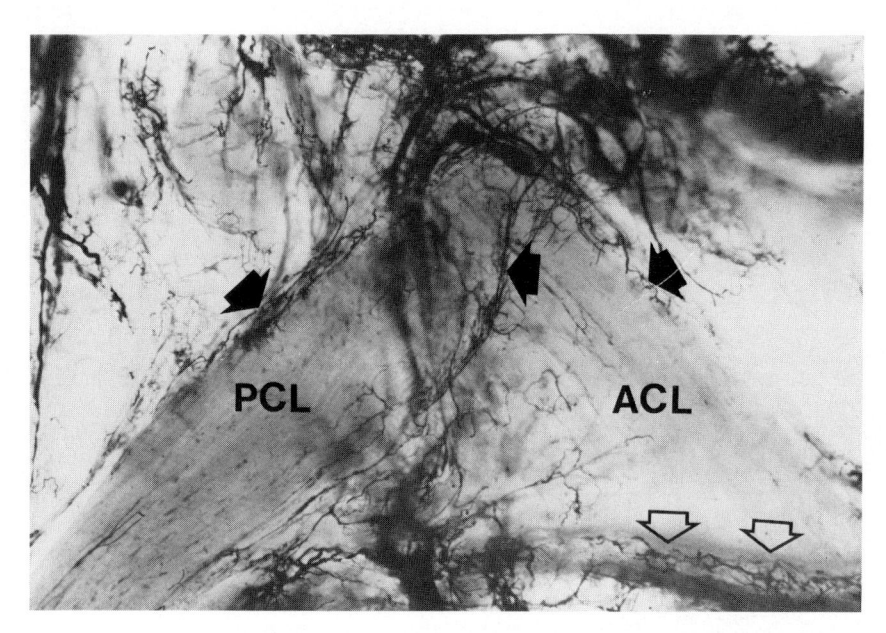

Fig. 3-6   *A 5-mm thick sagittal section of a human knee joint (Spalteholz technique) showing the periligamentous vasculature of the anterior (ACL) and posterior (PCL) cruciate ligaments* (closed arrows). *Note the absence of vessels crossing the ligamentous osseous attachment of the anterior cruciate ligament* (open arrows). *(From Arnoczky, S.P.: Blood supply to the anterior cruciate ligament and supporting structures, Orthop. Clin. North Am.* **16**:*15-28, 1985.)*

Although the location of the posterior cruciate ligament places it in intimate contact with the ligamentous branches of the middle genicular artery and the vascular synovial tissue of the posterior joint capsule, there is no evidence to suggest that the posterior cruciate ligament has a better vascular supply than the anterior cruciate ligament.[7,8]

Infrapatellar fat pad

As noted earlier, the infrapatellar fat pad plays an important role in the vascular scheme of the cruciate ligaments. The infrapatellar fat pad is supplied by the transverse infrapatellar anastomosis of the medial and lateral inferior genicular arteries. These arteries arborize into a weblike network of vessels that permeates the entire infrapatellar fat pad. The extent of this vascularization is variable and is dependent on the size of the infrapatellar fat pad (Fig. 3-7).[7,8,16,30]

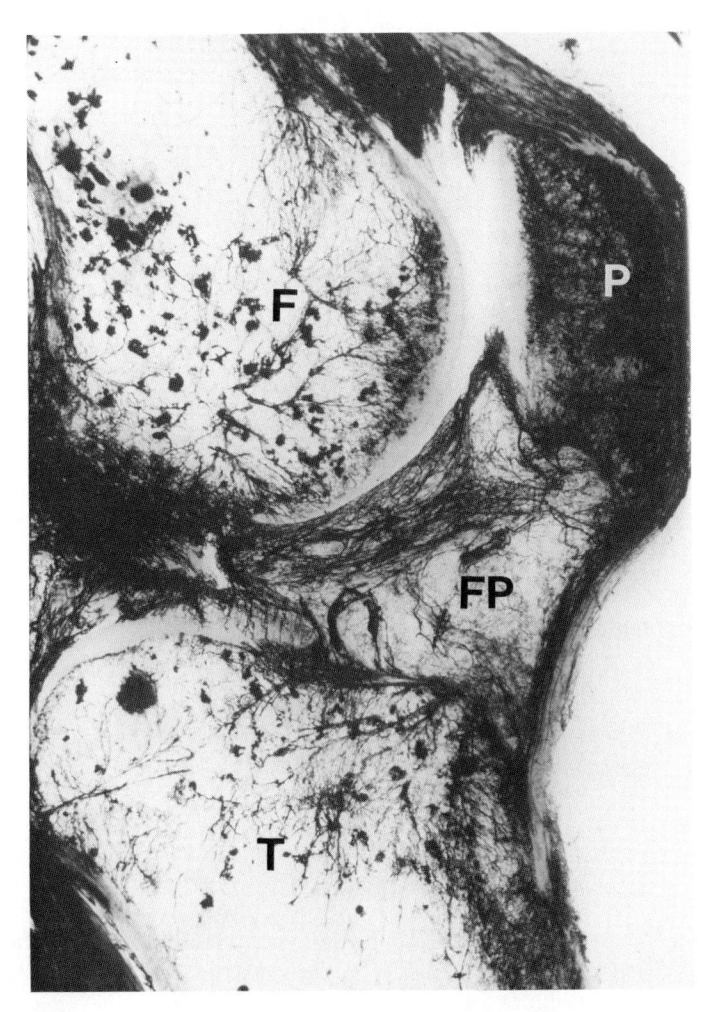

Fig. 3-7 *A 5-mm thick sagittal section of a human knee joint (Spalteholz technique) showing the extent and distribution of the vasculature of the infrapatellar fat pad (FP). (F, femur; T, tibia; P, patella.) (From Arnoczky, S.P.: Blood supply to the anterior cruciate ligament and supporting structures, Orthop. Clin. North Am. **16**:15-28, 1985.)*

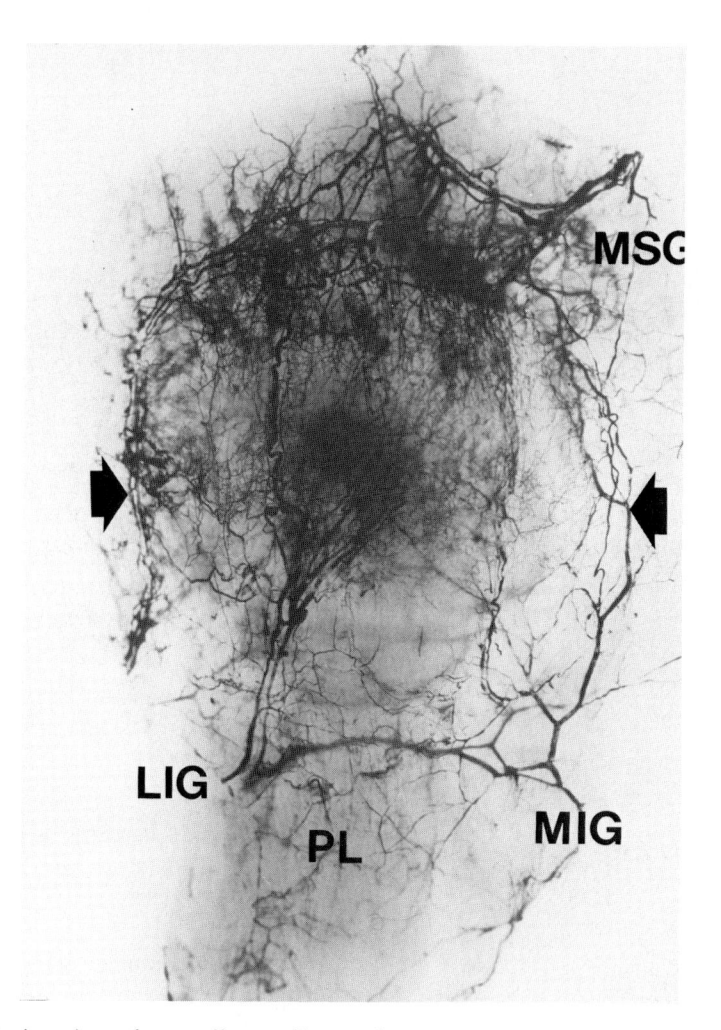

Fig. 3-8 *Anterior view of a patella-patellar tendon specimen (Spalteholz technique) illustrating the location and course of the vascular plexus that encircles the patella. Branches of the lateral inferior genicular artery (LIG) and the medial inferior genicular artery (MIG) can be seen anastomosing deep to the patellar ligament (PL). The medial and lateral ascending parapatellar arteries (arrows) complete the circle and join the superior and inferior genicular arteries. The medial inferior genicular artery (MIG) can be seen providing a "vascular leash" to the medial aspect of the patella-patellar ligament complex. (From Arnoczky, S.P.: Blood supply to the anterior cruciate ligament and supporting structures, Orthop. Clin. North Am. **16**:15-28, 1985.)*

Patellar ligament

The patellar ligament receives its blood supply from two major sources—the infrapatellar fat pad and the retinacular tissues. The retinaculum is supplied by the medial inferior genicular artery and the recurrent tibial arteries. As noted previously, the infrapatellar fat pad is supplied by the inferior medial and lateral genicular arteries, which anastomose with each other within the infrapatellar fat pad on the posterior surface of the patellar ligament.[8,14,30]

The anterior portion of the patellar ligament is supplied throughout its length by vessels from the retinaculum, and the posterior portion of the ligament receives vessels from the infrapatellar fat pad (Fig. 3-8). These vessels originate at the proximal and midportion of the patellar ligament and course inferiorly on the posterior surface of the ligament.[8,30]

A "vascular leash" that supports the medial portion of the patella-patellar ligament complex has been described.[21,29] This vascular bundle is made up of vessels from the medial inferior genicular artery and provides vessels to both the anterior and posterior surfaces of the medial third of the patellar ligament (Fig. 3-9).

Vascular response of the anterior cruciate ligament to injury and repair

Primary repair of cruciate ligament injuries in the knee is often difficult and yields inconsistent results. The specific biological factors that may contribute to the problem are not clearly understood. Considerable experimental work has been done on cruciate ligament healing, but the role of the ligamentous vasculature has only been implied.[28] Experimental studies have shown that, in the dog, a surgically created lesion of the anterior cruciate ligament results in a significant vascular response throughout the ligament (Fig. 3-10).[5] This vascular response arises from the soft tissues (infrapatellar fat pad and synovium) that surround the ligament.[5] When these vascular soft tissues are removed at the time of injury the intraligamentous vascular response is minimal and delayed (Fig. 3-11).[5] These findings would suggest the preservation and use of the soft tissue of the joint in the repair of anterior cruciate lesions in an attempt to optimize the vascular response of the ligament.

Studies have also shown that although the anterior cruciate ligament is capable of a vascular response following injury, spontane-

Text continued on p. 40.

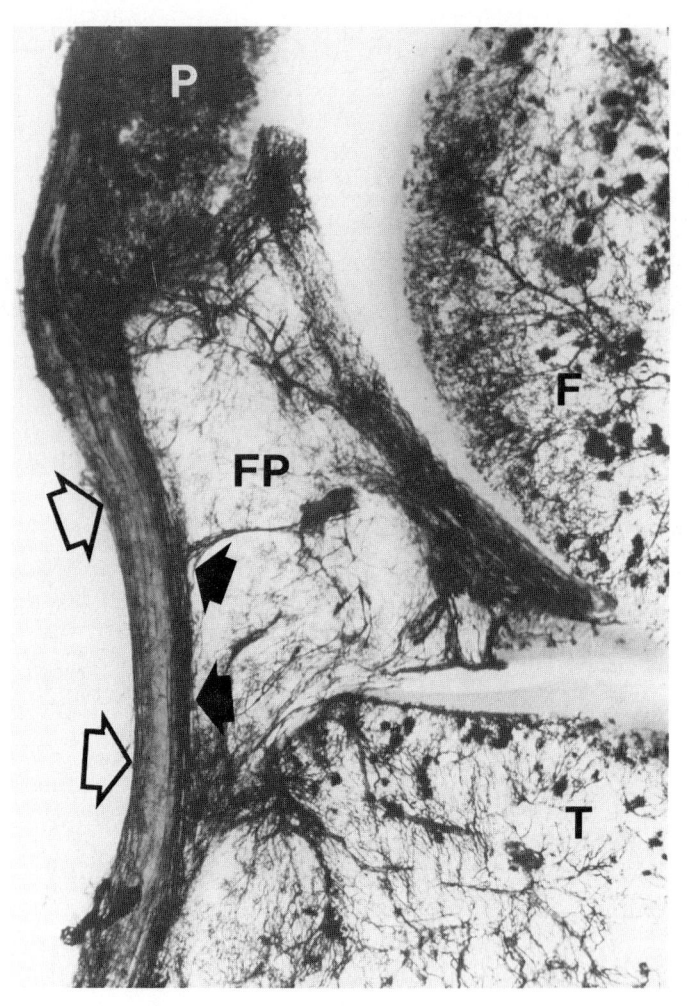

Fig. 3-9 *A 5-mm thick sagittal section of a human knee joint (Spalteholz technique) showing the vascular supply to the patellar ligament and infrapatellar fat pad (FP). The retinacular vessels (open arrows) overlie the patellar ligament and supply its anterior aspect; vessels from the infrapatellar fat pad supply the posterior portion of the patellar ligament (closed arrows). Vessels from the fat pad originate at the proximal and midportion of the patellar ligament and course inferiorly on the posterior surface of the ligament. (P, patella; F, femur; T, tibia.) (From Arnoczky, S.P.: Blood supply to the anterior cruciate ligaments and supporting structures, Orthop. Clin. North Am. **16**:15-28, 1985.)*

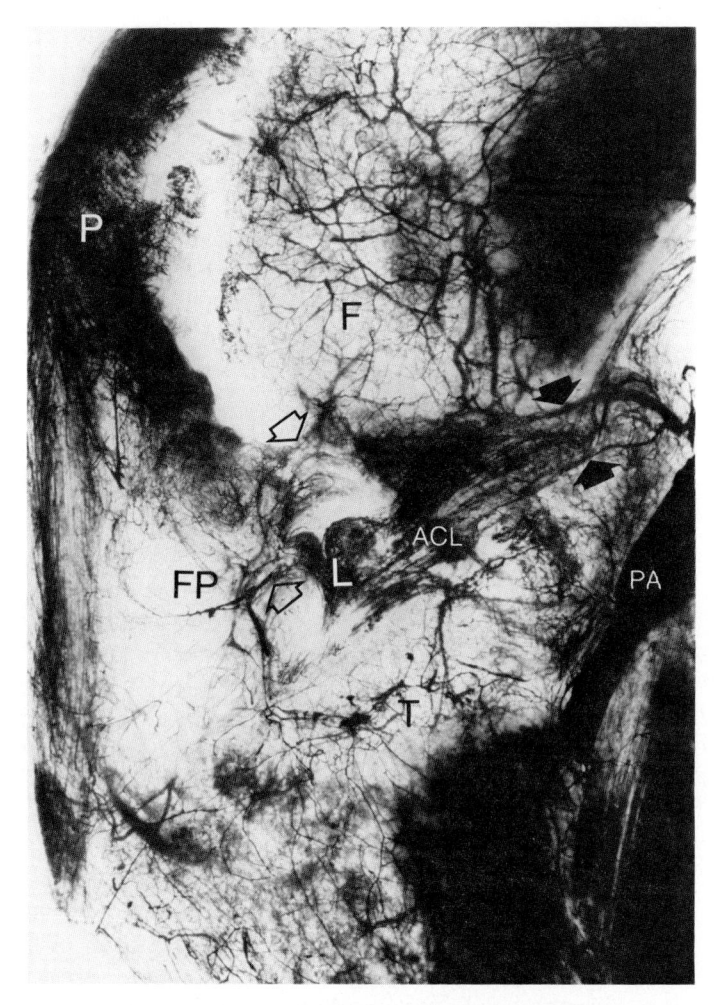

Fig. 3-10 *A 5-mm thick section of a dog's knee, 2 1/2 weeks after partial surgical transection of the anterior cruciate ligament (ACL) (Spalteholz technique). Note the rich vascular reaction at the site of the lesion (L) and throughout the entire anterior cruciate ligament. Vessels from the infrapatellar fat pad (open arrows) and branches of the middle genicular artery posteriorly (closed arrows) appear to contribute to the vascular response. (PA, popliteal artery; F, femur; T, tibia; P, patella; FP, fat pad.) (From Arnoczky, S.P., Rubin, R.M., and Marshall, J.L.: Microvasculature of the cruciate ligaments and its response to injury: an experimental study in dogs, J. Bone Joint Surg. [Am.] 61:1221-1229, 1979.)*

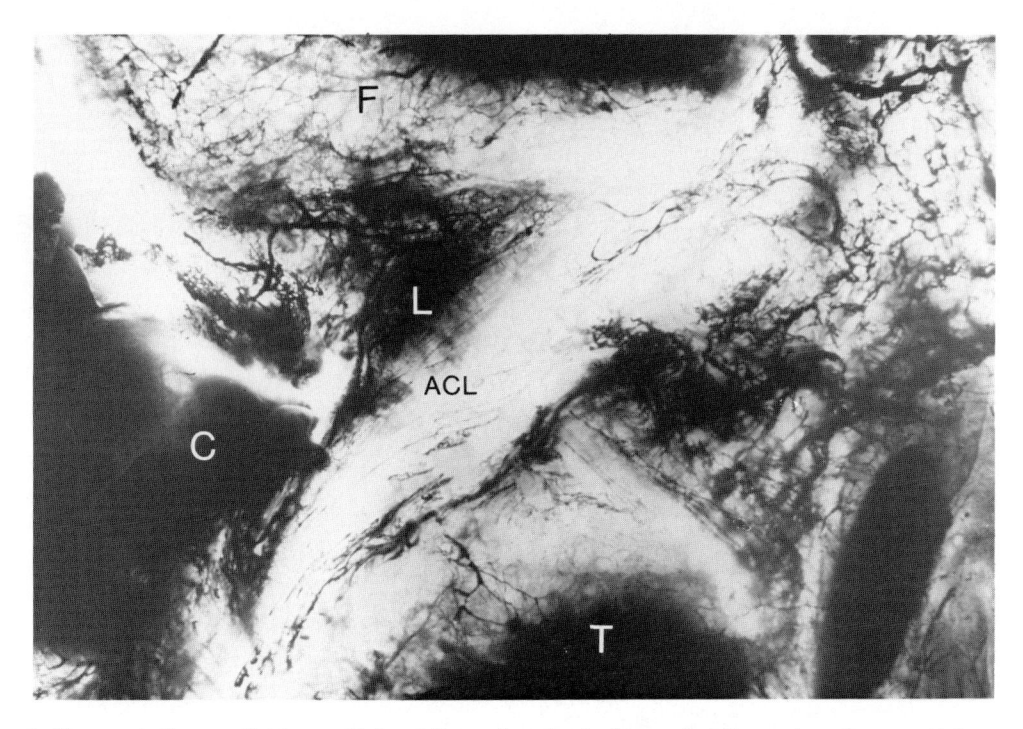

Fig. 3-11 *A 5-mm thick sagittal section of a dog's knee, 2 1/2 weeks after partial surgical transection of the anterior cruciate ligament (ACL) and resection of the infrapatellar fat pad and synovium (Spalteholz technique). Note the abundance of vessels at the site of the lesion (L). The intraligamentous vascular response of the anterior cruciate ligament appears less robust than the response seen in the specimen without synovectomy and resection of the fat pad. The clot (C) in the area of the resected fat pad, when dissected out, appeared to be densely adherent to the anterior cruciate ligament. (F, femur; T, tibia.) (From Arnoczky, S.P., Rubin, R.M., and Marshall, J.L.: Microvasculature of the cruciate ligaments and its response to injury: an experimental study in dogs, J. Bone Joint Surg. [Am.] 61:1221-1229, 1979.)*

The vascularity of the anterior cruciate ligament and associated structures 39

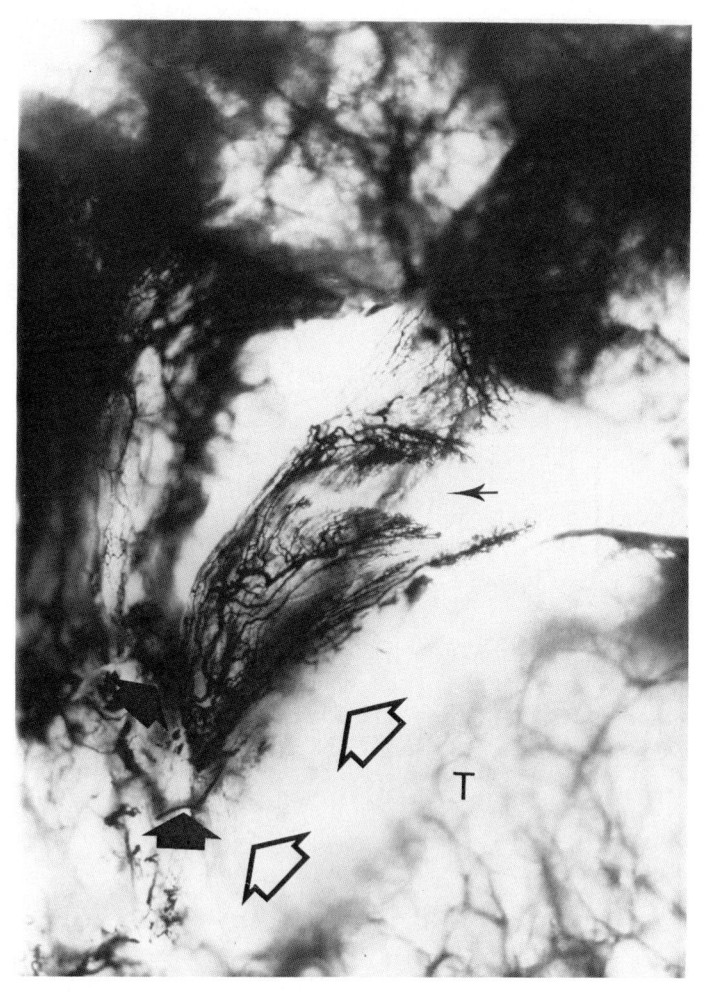

Fig. 3-12 *A 5-mm thick sagittal section of a dog's knee 8 weeks after partial surgical transection of the anterior cruciate ligament, leaving the infrapatellar fat pad and synovial membrane intact (Spalteholz technique × 5). A portion of the infrapatellar fat pad has been dissected to permit better visualization of the anterior cruciate ligament. The incision in the anterior cruciate ligament can be seen as a defect* (small arrow) *that, even at 8 weeks, has not filled in. The vigorous and extensive intraligamentous vasculature of the anterior cruciate ligament outlines the borders of the lesion. These intraligamentous vessels appear to be derived from the soft tissues (intrapatellar fat pad and synovial tissue). Several so-called "feeder vessels"* (larger closed arrows) *are visible at the base of the ligament. No reactive vessels cross the ligamentous-osseous attachment site* (open arrows) *on the tibia (T) at the anterior cruciate ligament. (From Arnoczky, S.P., Rubin, R.M., and Marshall, J.L.: Microvasculature of the cruciate ligaments and its response to injury: an experimental study in dogs, J. Bone Joint Surg. [Am.]* **61:***1221-1229, 1979.)*

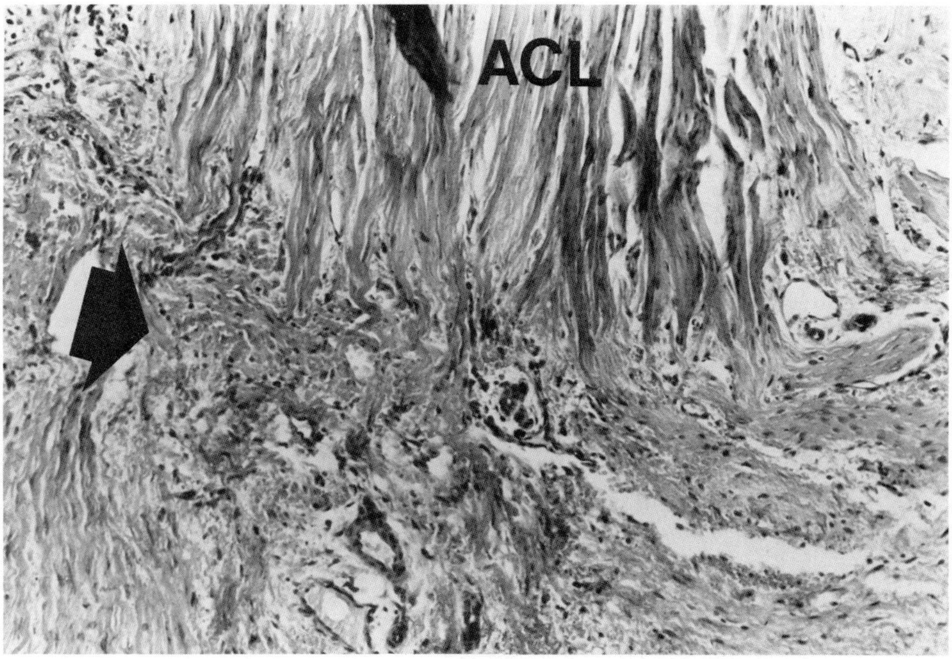

Fig. 3-13 *Photomicrograph showing the repair site of an anterior cruciate ligament of a dog 6 weeks following transection and primary repair. Note the fibrovascular scar tissue present at the repair site (arrow) and the adjacent normal ligamentous tissue of the anterior cruciate ligament (ACL). (Hematoxylin and eosin × 100.)*

ous repair (or healing by second intention) does not occur (Fig. 3-12).[5,28] This may result from the fact that synovial fluid dilution of the hematoma following injury prevents the formation of a fibrin clot and thus the initiation of the healing mechanism.[28] Another theory suggests that the dynamic nature of the fascicles of the anterior cruciate ligament through the range of motion prohibits the spontaneous union of these fibers.[5]

The observations stated above have given support to the primary repair of certain anterior cruciate ligament lesions. Although the long-term efficacy of such procedures is still a matter of debate, clinical and experimental evidence demonstrates that following primary repair the anterior cruciate ligament heals by the formation and organization of a fibrovascular scar (Fig. 3-13). Like the vascular response that initiates healing, this repair tissue originates extrinsically from the adjacent soft tissues of the knees, primarily the infrapatellar fat pad. Although this healing response can be quite extensive, the maturation of this fibrovascular scar tissue into a functional ligament may take many months.

Revascularization of anterior cruciate ligament replacements

Autografts

Intra-articular transplantation of autogenous tissues has long been advocated as a method for replacement of the anterior cruciate ligament.* The success of these transplants is dependent, in large part, on the ability of these tissues to survive and function in the intra-articular environment of the knee. Several studies have demonstrated that patellar tendon grafts used to replace the anterior cruciate ligament are essentially avascular at the time of transplantation (Fig. 3-14).[3,6,12] Thus these tissues must be revascularized if they are to remain viable within the joint. Experimental studies have shown that following transplantation, patellar tendon grafts are initially enveloped with a vascular synovial tissue that originated from the soft tissues of the knee (infrapatellar fat pad and synovium) (Fig. 3-15).[3,6,12] This "synovialization" process occurs during the first 4 to 6 weeks following transplantation. During that time, the central avascular core of the graft is undergoing a process of ischemic necrosis. Thus the graft plays an innocent role in a race between avascular necrosis and revascularization. Fortunately the soft tissues that initiated the "synovialization" of the graft also provide the source for an intrinsic revascularization response in which vessels from the infrapatellar fat pad and synovium penetrate the connective tissue "scaffold" of the graft and revascularize the transplanted tissue (Fig. 3-16). This revascularization response is accompanied by a cellular proliferation that eventually repopulates the graft with new cells (Fig. 3-17). Although the complete revascularization of the patellar tendon grafts can take as long as 20 weeks (Fig. 3-18) even more time is required for the graft to remodel and take on the structural and mechanical characteristics of a ligament.

*References 2-4, 13, 23, and 27.   *Text continued on p. 47.*

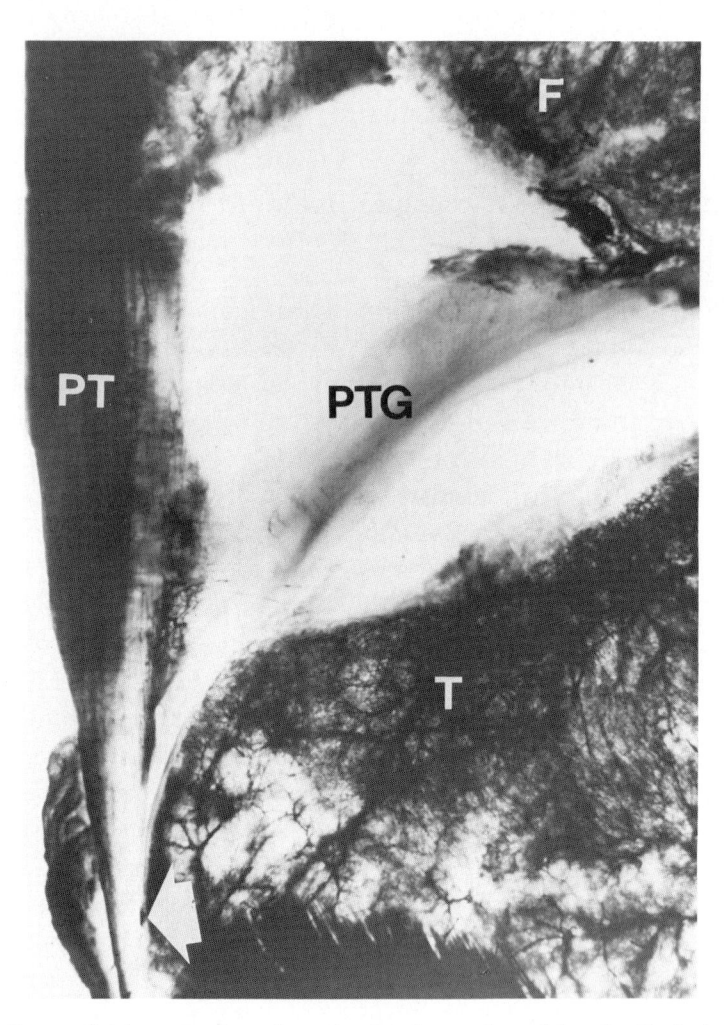

Fig. 3-14 *A 5-mm thick sagittal section of a dog knee cleared by the Spalteholz technique, 2 weeks after replacement with a patellar tendon graft (× 2). The patellar tendon graft (PTG) shows no evidence of perfused vessels. Note the absence of vessels crossing the tibial attachment of the graft (arrow). (The infrapatellar fat pad and the posterior cruciate ligament were removed after clearing to permit better visualization.) (F, femur; T, tibia; and PT, patellar tendon.) (From Arnoczky, S.P., Tarvin, G.B., and Marshall, J.L.: Anterior cruciate ligament replacement using patellar tendon: evaluation of graft revascularization in the dog, J. Bone Joint Surg. [Am.] **64:**217-224, 1982.)*

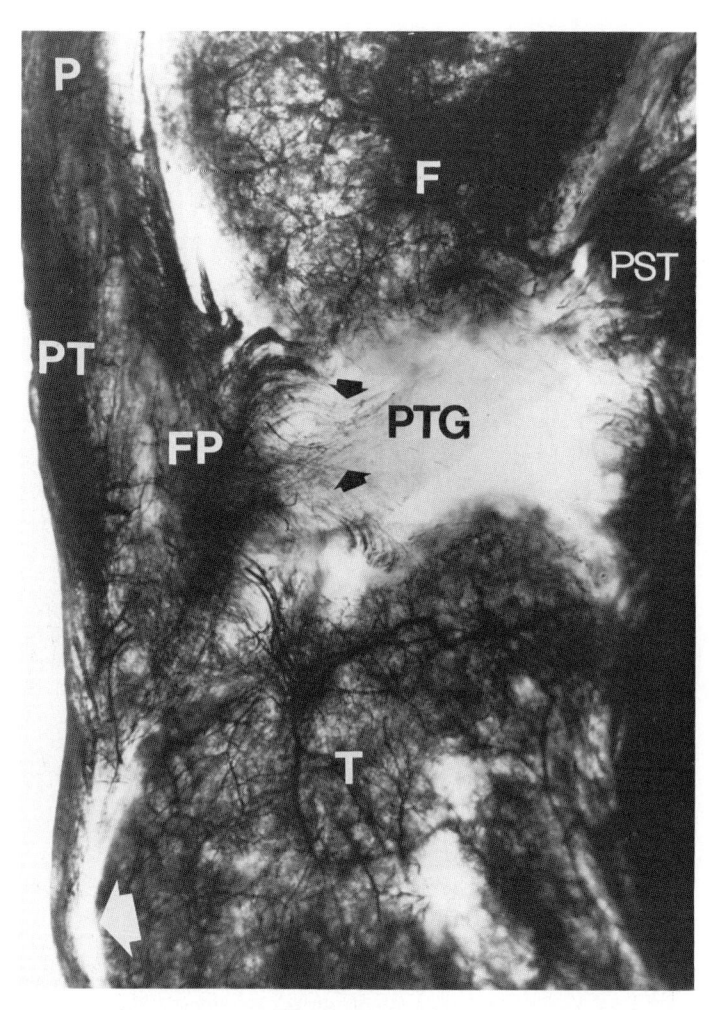

Fig. 3-15 *A 5-mm thick sagittal section of a dog's knee 6 weeks after replacement of the anterior cruciate ligament with a patellar tendon graft (PTG). Note the vascular response of the infrapatellar fat pad (FP) and posterior soft tissues (PST). Vessels from the fat pad can be seen extending over the surface of the patellar tendon graft (black arrows) and are part of the vascular synovial envelope. Note that the tibial attachment of the graft (white arrow) does not contribute any vessels to the graft. (F, femur; T, tibia; PT, patellar tendon; and P, patella.) (From Arnoczky, S.P., Tarvin, G.B., and Marshall, J.L.: Anterior cruciate ligament replacement using patellar tendon: an evaluation of graft revascularization in the dog, J. Bone Joint Surg. [Am.] 64:217-224, 1982.)*

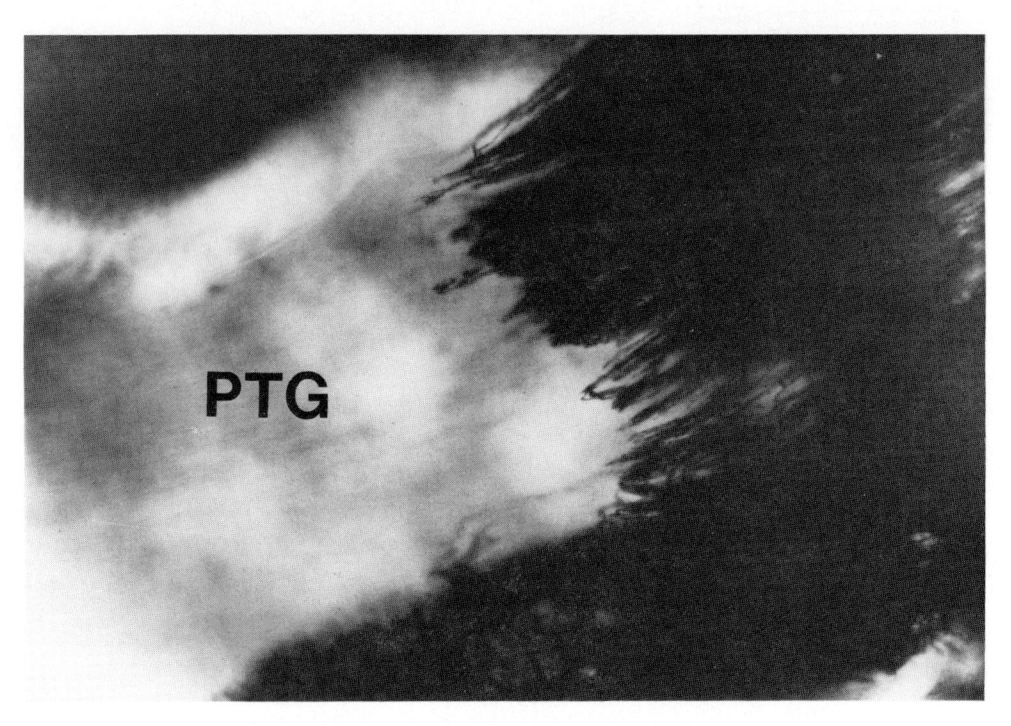

Fig. 3-16 *A 5-mm thick sagittal section of a dog's knee 10 weeks after replacement of the anterior cruciate ligament with a patellar tendon graft (PTG) (Spalteholz technique × 20). Note the advancing brushlike border of the intrinsic vascular response. These terminally looped capillaries are migrating within the substance of the avascular patellar tendon. (From Arnoczky, S.P., Tarvin, G.B., and Marshall, J.L.: Anterior cruciate ligament replacement using patellar tendon: an evaluation of graft revascularization in the dog, J. Bone Joint Surg. [Am.] 64:217-224, 1982.)*

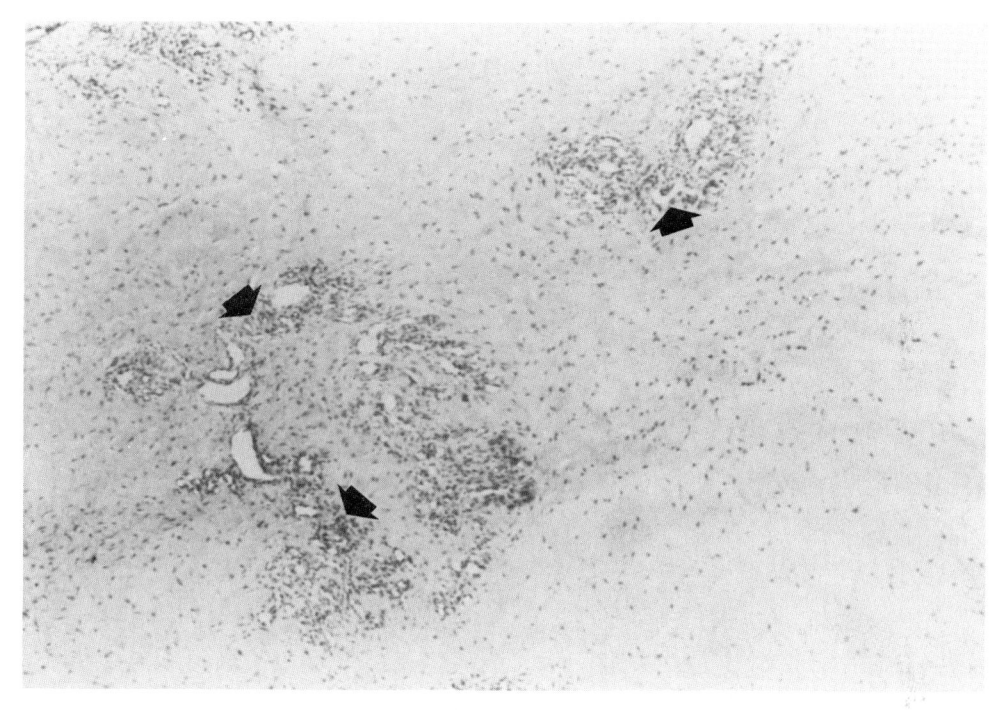

Fig. 3-17 *Photomicrograph of a longitudinal section of a patellar tendon graft 10 weeks after replacement of the anterior cruciate ligament. There is an invasion of capillary buds* (arrows) *into the avascular graft. Note the cellular proliferation that accompanies the vascular ingrowth (Hematoxylin and eosin × 100). (From Arnoczky, S.P., Tarvin, G.B., and Marshall, J.L.: Anterior cruciate ligament replacement using patellar tendon: an evaluation of graft revascularization in the dog, J. Bone Joint Surg. [Am.]* **64:***217-224, 1982.)*

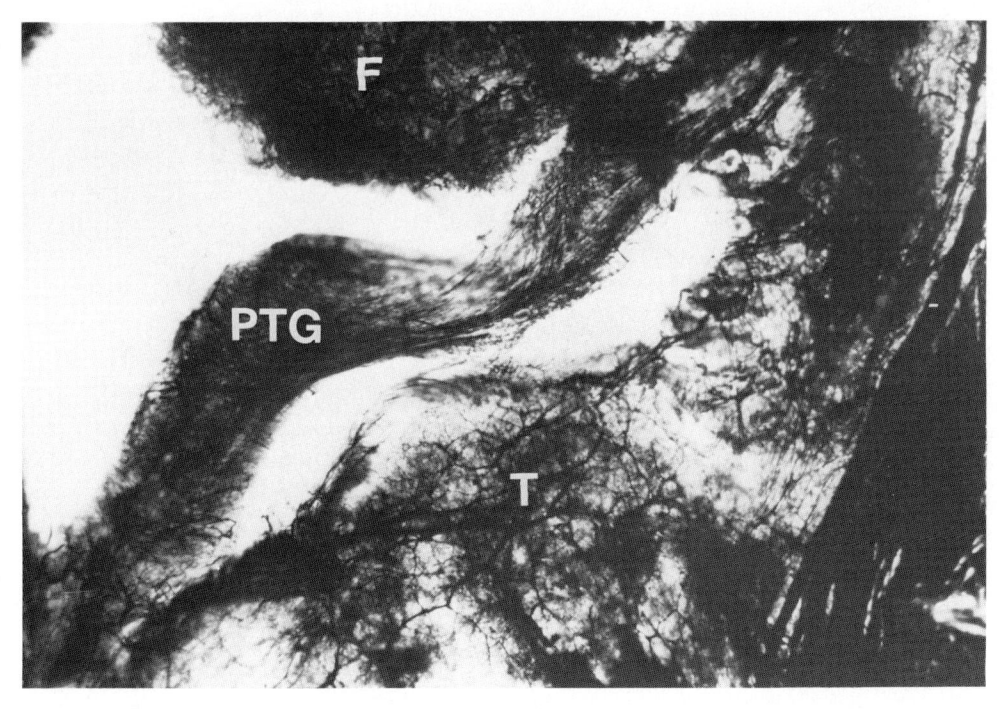

Fig. 3-18 *A 5-mm thick sagittal section of a dog's knee 20 weeks after replacement of the anterior cruciate ligament with a patellar tendon graft (PTG) (Spalteholz technique × 5). Note the complete and profuse vascularization of the entire graft. The infrapatellar fat pad and posterior cruciate ligament were removed after clearing to permit better visualization. (F, femur; T, tibia.) (From Arnoczky, S.P., Tarvin, G.B., and Marshall, J.L.: Anterior cruciate ligament replacement using patellar tendon: an evaluation of graft revascularization in the dog, J. Bone Joint Surg. [Am.] **64**:217-224, 1982.)*

Vascularized patellar tendon grafts

In an effort to eliminate the period of ischemic necrosis and revascularization following patellar tendon transplantation, operative procedures have been described that preserve a portion of the graft's blood supply.[13,29] In one technique, the central third of the patellar ligament along with its infrapatellar blood supply is used as a vascularized graft (Fig. 3-19).[13] Another technique uses the medial third of the patellar ligament, preserving its "vascular leash" within the medial retinacular tissues (Fig. 3-20).[29] By preserving the blood supply of the graft, tissue viability is maintained throughout the postoperative period and the process of ischemic necrosis and graft revascularization usually associated with patellar tendon grafts is minimized or avoided. Although the use of vascularized patellar tendon (VPT) grafts was also thought to enhance the material properties of the graft (over avascular grafts), experimental evidence has shown no difference in the material properties of avascular patellar tendon grafts and vascularized patellar tendon grafts following transplantation.[19]

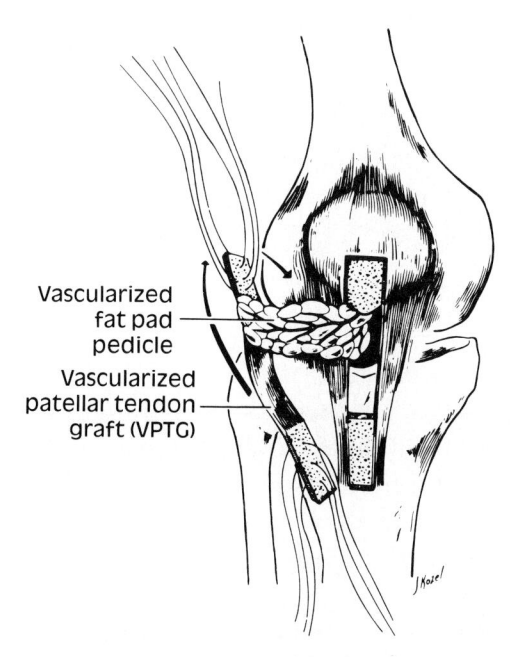

Fig. 3-19 *Drawing of the knee showing the central third of the patella with its vascular supply intact harvested as an anterior cruciate ligament replacement. (From Clancy, W.G., Jr.: Anterior cruciate ligament functional instability: a static intra-articular and dynamic extra-articular procedure, Clin. Orthop. **172**:102-106, 1983.)*

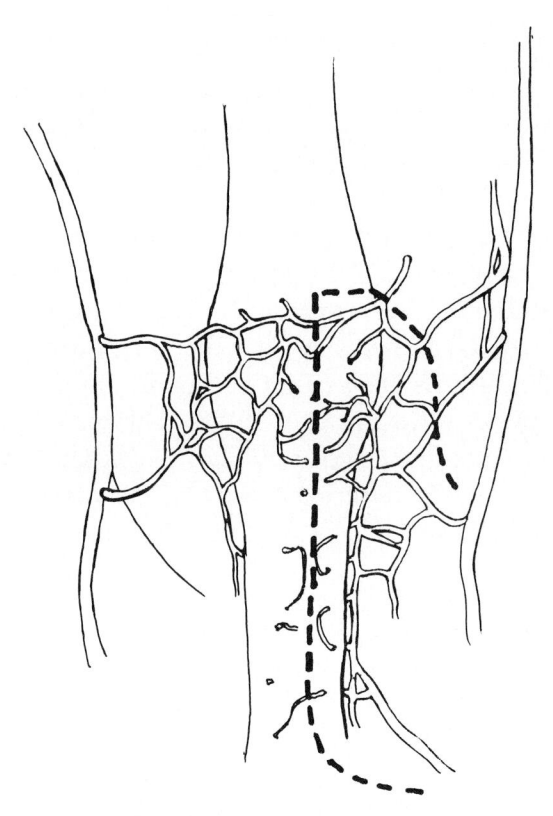

Fig. 3-20 *Drawing of the vascularized patellar tendon graft based on the inferior medial geniculate artery. (From Paulos, L.E., Butler, D.L., Noyes, F.R., and Grood, E.S.: Intra-articular cruciate reconstruction. Part II. Replacement with vascularized patellar tendon, Clin. Orthop. 172:78-84, 1983.)*

Allografts

The success of autogenous tissues as anterior cruciate ligament substitutes and the fact that these grafts are avascular "free" grafts at the time of transplantation has led to the concept of using allograft tissues for anterior cruciate ligament replacement. As with autogenous tissues, these allografts must be revascularized and revitalized if they are to remain functional within the joint. Because preservation techniques such as freeze-drying or deep-freezing are required to destroy the cellular components of the graft and thus make them less immunogenic, the allografts are essentially inert collagen scaffolds that must be revascularized and remodeled with host tissue. Recently, several experimental studies have examined the biology of allograft tissues used to replace the anterior cruciate ligament.[9,15,31] It has been shown that following transplantation, deep-frozen patellar tendon allografts undergo a revascularization process similar to that observed in patellar tendon allografts.[9,31] The vascular tissues of the infrapatellar fat pad and synovium provide a vascular synovial envelope around the graft and supplied the origin for the intrinsic revascularization and cellular proliferation within the allograft. As in the autogenous patellar tendon grafts this revascularization process was complete at 5 months, and by 6 months the allograft resembled a normal ligament.[9]

Synthetic prostheses

Although biological tissues are the most commonly used grafts to replace the anterior cruciate ligament, synthetic materials such as dacron,[10,25,33] polypropylene,[23] and carbon fibers[1,17,20] are being investigated as potential graft materials. In many instances these synthetic materials are intended to act as a "scaffold" on which connective tissue can proliferate and form a "neoligament."[10,17] In these cases the ability of the material to support and induce vascular and cellular ingrowth is critical to the success of the prosthesis. Thus, as in the case of the biological grafts, these synthetic "scaffolds" must be "revascularized" for a neoligament to develop. Experimental studies have shown that following transplantation most synthetic grafts are surrounded by vascular synovial tissue that arises from the infrapatellar fat pad and synovium of the knee joint (Fig. 3-21).[10] This vascular synovial tissue completely envelopes the prosthesis and, depending on the synthetic material and its fabrication, the vessels may penetrate the entire graft (Fig. 3-22).[10] These vessels, of course, also bring in cells that eventually will contribute to the formation of the neoligament (Fig. 3-23).[10]

The role of the vascular soft tissues of the knee (infrapatellar fat pad and synovium) in contributing to the formation of a neoligament on a synthetic or biological scaffold is an important one. It must be remembered, however, that many factors, such as the material properties of the scaffold and the mechanical forces placed across it, ultimately determine the character and quality of the neoligament. The vascular soft tissues of the knee merely provide the biological support for this process. Thus, although these soft tissues should be preserved and utilized in the reconstruction of the anterior cruciate ligament, they are but one of several important factors in the ultimate success of the procedure.

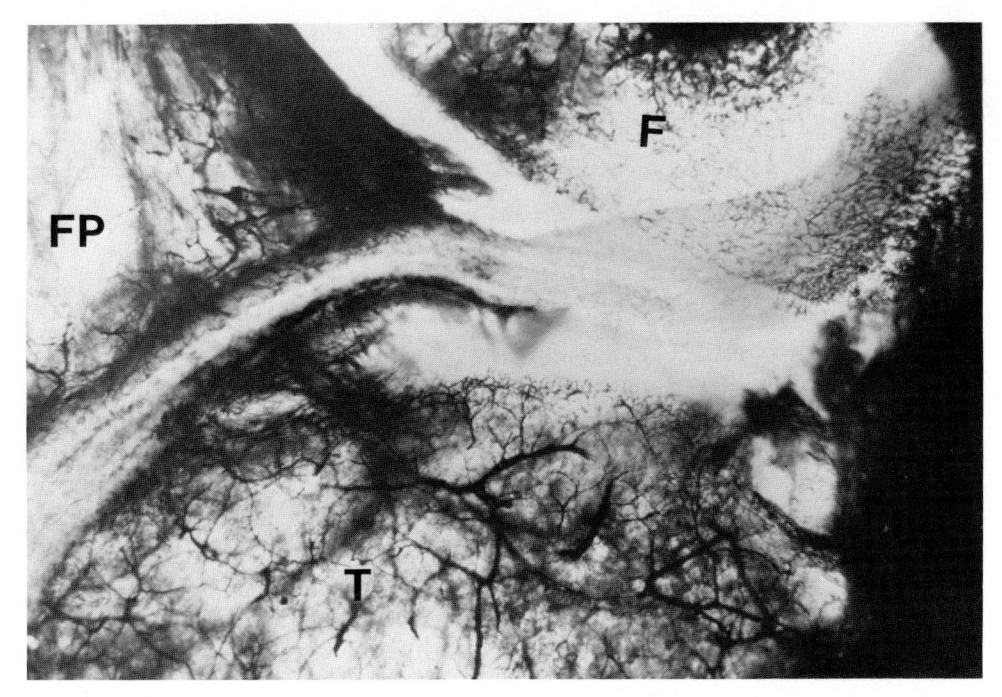

Fig. 3-21 *A 5-mm thick sagittal section of a dog's knee 6 months following replacement of the anterior cruciate ligament with a dacron prosthesis (Spalteholz technique × 2). Note the marked vascular encapsulation and ingrowth in the areas of the infrapatellar fat pad (FP). (F, femur; T, tibia.) (From Arnoczky, S.P., Warren, R.F., and Minei, J.P.: Replacement of the anterior cruciate ligament using a synthetic prosthesis: an evaluation of graft biology in the dog, Am. J. Sports Med.* **14:***1-6, 1986.)*

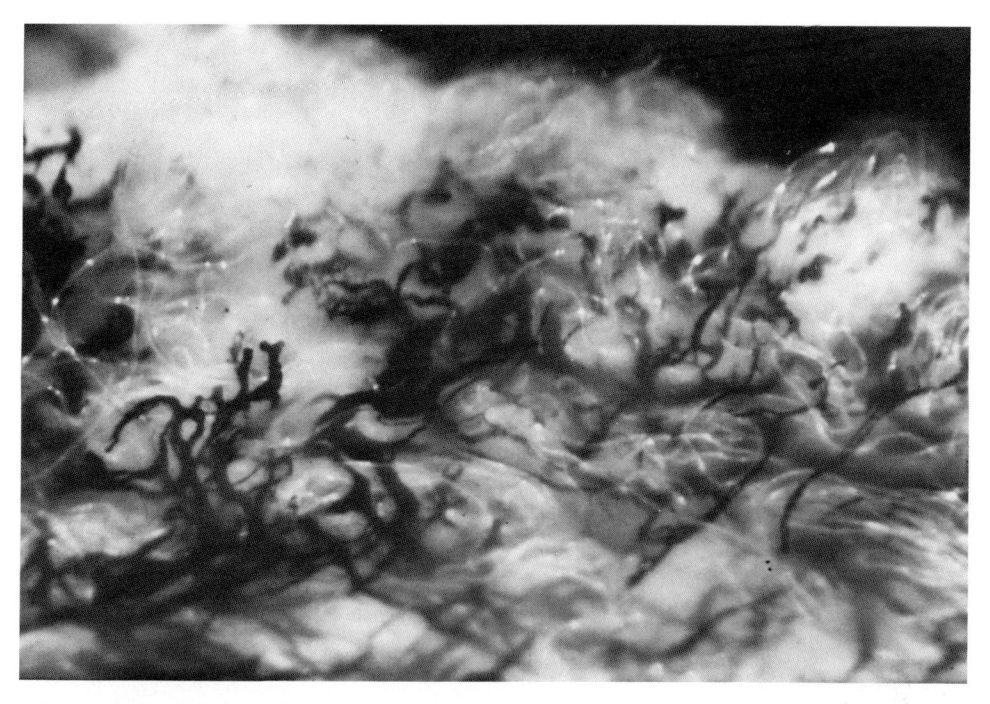

Fig. 3-22 *India-ink injection specimen showing the vascular ingrowth into the interstices of a dacron prosthesis used to replace the anterior cruciate ligament of a dog (3 months postoperatively). (From Arnoczky, S.P., Warren, R.F., and Minei, J.P.: Replacement of the anterior cruciate ligament using a synthetic prosthesis: an evaluation of graft biology in the dog, Am. J. Sports Med.* **14:***1-6, 1986.)*

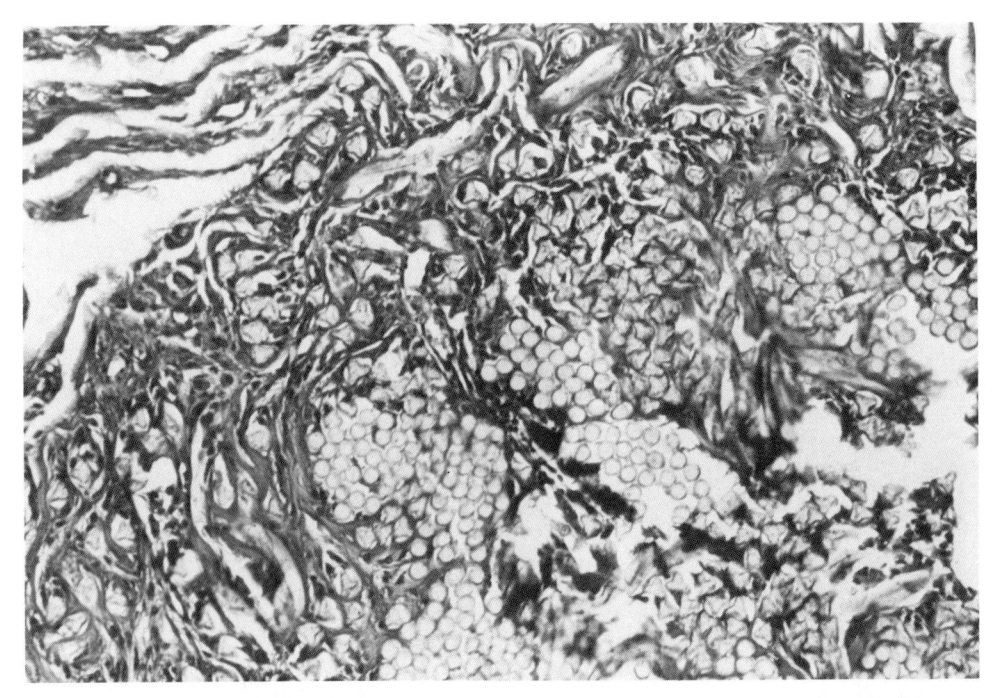

Fig. 3-23 *Photomicrograph of a transverse section of a dacron graft 3 months following implantation to replace the anterior cruciate ligament in a dog. Connective tissue cells can be seen surrounding the deeper fibers of the graft. (Hematoxylin and erosin × 100.) (From Arnoczky, S.P., Warren, R.F., and Minei, J.P.: Replacement of the anterior cruciate ligament using a synthetic prosthesis: an evaluation of graft biology in the dog, Am. J. Sports Med. **14:**1-6, 1986.)*

Summary

Although the importance of cruciate anatomy and function is obvious when evaluating ligamentous injury, the biological aspects of ligamentous blood supply and viability are equally important when contemplating primary repair and reconstruction.

The vascular origins of the cruciate ligaments are in the soft tissues. Therefore the use and preservation of these soft tissues during surgical repair or reconstruction is paramount if ligament (or graft) viability is to be optimized.

Perhaps it is appropriate to recall Girdlestone's observation in 1932 on the role of soft tissues in the healing of bone:

"... union cannot be imposed but may have to be encouraged. For a bone is a plant with its roots in the soft tissue and when its vascular connections are damaged it often requires not the mechanical technique of a cabinetmaker but the patient care and understanding of a gardener."[24]

The cruciate ligaments are also plants whose vascular roots lie in the soft tissues of the knee. In repairing or reconstructing these ligaments, therefore, the surgeon must not only restore the structural integrity of the ligaments but also use the soft tissues to reestablish their vascular roots.

REFERENCES

1. Alexander, H., Parsons, J.R., Smith, G., et al.: Anterior cruciate ligament replacement with filamentous carbon, Trans. Ortho. Res. Soc. **7**:45, 1982.
2. Alm, A.: Survival of part of patellar tendon transposed for reconstruction of anterior cruciate ligament. Acta Chir. Scand. **139**: 443-447, 1973.
3. Alm, A., Liljedahl, S.O., and Stromberg, B.: Clinical and experimental experience in reconstruction of the anterior cruciate ligament, Orthop. Clin. North Am. **7**:181-189, 1976.
4. Alm, A., and Stromberg, B.: Transposed medial third of patellar ligament in reconstruction of the anterior cruciate ligament: a surgical and morphologic study in dogs, Acta Chir. Scand. (Suppl.) **445**:37-49, 1974.
5. Arnoczky, S.P., Rubin, R.M., and Marshall, J.L.: Microvasculature of the cruciate ligaments and its response to injury, J. Bone Joint Surg. (Am.) **61**:1221-1229, 1979.
6. Arnoczky, S.P., Tarvin, G.B., and Marshall, J.L.: Anterior cruciate ligament replacement using patellar tendon: an evaluation of graft revascularization in the dog, J. Bone Joint Surg. (Am.) **64**:217-224, 1982.
7. Arnoczky, S.P.: Anatomy of the anterior cruciate ligament, Clin. Orthop. **172**:19-25, 1983.
8. Arnoczky, S.P.: Blood supply to the anterior cruciate ligament and supporting structures, Orthop. Clin. North Am. **16**:15-28, 1985.
9. Arnoczky, S.P., Warren, R.F., and Ashlock, M.A.: Anterior cruciate ligament replacement using a patellar tendon allograft: an experimental study in the dog, J. Bone Joint Surg. (Am.) **68**:376-385, 1986.
10. Arnoczky, S.P., Warren, R.F., and Minei, J.P.: Replacement of the anterior cruciate ligament using a synthetic prosthesis: an evaluation of graft biology in the dog, Am. J. Sports Med. **14**:1-6, 1986.
11. Bousquet, M.G.: The traumatic rupture of the cruciate ligaments of the knee, Thesis, Lyon, France, 1969.
12. Clancy, W.G., Jr., Narechania, R.G., Rosenberg, T.D., et al.: Anterior and posterior cruciate ligament reconstruction in rhesus monkeys: a histologic, microangiographic, and biomechanical analysis, J. Bone Joint Surg. (Am.) **63**:1270, 1981.
13. Clancy, W.G., Jr.: Anterior cruciate ligament functional instability: a static intraarticular and dynamic extra-articular procedure, Clin. Orthop. **172**:102-106, 1983.
14. Crock, H.V.: The blood supply of the lower limb bones in man, Edinburgh, 1967, E & S Livingstone.

15. Curtis, R.J., Delee, J.C., and Drez, D.J., Jr.: Reconstruction of the anterior cruciate ligament with freeze dried fascia lata allografts in dogs: a preliminary report, Am. J. Sports Med. **13**:408-414, 1985.
16. Davies, D.V., and Edwards, D.A.W.: The blood supply of the synovial membrane and intra-articular structures, Ann. R. Coll. Surg. Engl. **2**:142-156, 1948.
17. Forster, I.W., Ralis, Z.A., McKibbin, B., et al.: Biological reaction to carbon fiber implants: the formation and structure of carbon-induced "neotendon," Clin. Orthop. **131**:299-307, 1978.
18. Gray, H.: The anatomy of the human body. In Goss, C.M., editor: The anatomy of the human body, Philadelphia, 1975, Lea & Febiger.
19. Grood, E.S.: Personal communication, May, 1985.
20. Jenkins, D.H.R.: The repair of cruciate ligaments with flexible carbon fiber, J. Bone Joint Surg. (Br.) **62**:520-522, 1978.
21. Kaderly, R., Butler, D.L., and Noyes, F.R.: A new vascular anatomic technique: vascular casts of the human and cynamolgus monkey knee joints, Trans. Ortho. Res. Soc. **8**:382, 1983.
22. Kennedy, J.C., Weinberg, H.W., and Wilson, A.S.: The anatomy and function of the anterior cruciate ligament as determined by clinical and morphological studies. J. Bone Joint Surg. (Am.) **56**:223, 1974.
23. Kennedy, J.C., Roth, J.H., Mendenhall, H.V., et al.: Intra-articular replacement in the anterior cruciate deficient knee, Am. J. Sports Med. **8**:1-8, 1980.
24. MacNab, I. and DeHaas, W.G.: The role of periosteal blood supply in the healing of fractures of the tibia, Clin. Orthop. **105**:27-33, 1974.
25. Marshall, J.L., Arnoczky, S.P., Rubin, R.M., et al.: Microvasculature of the cruciate ligaments, Phys. Sports Med. **7**:87-91, 1979.
26. Meyers, J.F., Grana, W.A., and Lesker, P.A.: Reconstruction of the anterior cruciate ligament in the dog, Am. J. Sports Med. **7**:85-90, 1979.
27. O'Donoghue, D.H.: A method for replacement of the anterior cruciate ligament of the knee: report of twenty cases, J. Bone Joint Surg. (Am.) **45**:905-924, 1963.
28. O'Donoghue, D.H., Rockwood, C.A., Jr., Frank, G.R., et al.: Repair of the anterior cruciate ligament in dogs, J. Bone Joint Surg. **48**:503-519, 1966.
29. Paulos, L.E., Butler, D.L., Noyes, F.R., et al.: Intra-articular cruciate reconstruction. II. Replacement with vascularized patellar tendon. Clin. Orthop. **172**:78-84, 1983.
30. Scapinelli, R.: Studies on the vasculature of the human knee joint, Acta. Anat. **70**:305-331, 1968.
31. Shino, K., Kawaski, T., Hirose, H., et al.: Replacement of the anterior cruciate ligament by an allogenic tendon graft: an experimental study in the dog, J. Bone Joint Surg. (Br.) **66**:672-681, 1984.
32. Wladmirow, B.: Arterial sources of blood supply of the knee joint in man, Acta. Med. **47**:1-10, 1968.
33. Wood, G.W.: Synthetics in anterior cruciate ligament reconstruction: a review, Orthop. Clin. North Am. **16**:227-235, 1985.

4

Biomechanics of the anterior cruciate ligament

BEN GRAF

The anterior cruciate ligament is the primary restraint to anterior displacement of the tibia,[4] but its function is much more than that of a simple check rein. Along with the posterior cruciate ligament, the anterior cruciate ligament determines the blend of gliding and sliding between the tibia and femur that characterizes normal knee kinematics. As a result, anterior cruciate ligament deficiency not only produces episodic instability but consistently altered joint mechanics as well. This alteration may in turn contribute to degenerative changes often seen in patients with long-standing anterior cruciate ligament insufficiency. The goal of reconstruction, therefore, should be to prevent symptomatic instability, restore normal knee kinematics, and prevent premature degenerative joint disease.

Functional anatomy

As discussed in Chapter 1, the knee is analogous to a tent, where the articular surfaces represent the poles and the ligaments the ropes. The poles can be loaded only in compression and the ropes only in tension, but together they provide a resilient and stable structure.

Articular cartilage, with its extremely low coefficient of friction, can only be effectively loaded in compression. Tensile forces only distract the joint, and forces not perpendicular to the plane of the articular surface generate shear forces and produce translational movements. Therefore, although the shapes of the femoral condyles and tibial plateau are important in determining ligament tension, the articular surfaces themselves ineffectively resist translation.[19]

Ligaments, by contrast, cannot support compressive loads but resist tensile forces very well. When "tensioned" by the compressive loading of articular cartilage, the anterior and posterior cruciate ligament prevent the anterior and posterior displacement of the tibia respectively. Individually the cruciate ligaments act as check reins, but together they precisely define the motion of the knee.

The shape of the lateral and medial femoral condyles is intimately related to the function of the cruciate ligaments. Indeed, as shown later, the curvature of the condyles can be approximated by the four-bar linkage used to model the behavior of the ligaments. The two condyles are asymmetric; the lateral femoral condyle is a bit wider and the medial femoral condyle provides a longer surface for articulation with the tibia.[13,14] Both condyles, however, exhibit a changing radius of curvature that reflects the changing position of the instant center of rotation when the knee is flexed[11] (Fig. 4-1).

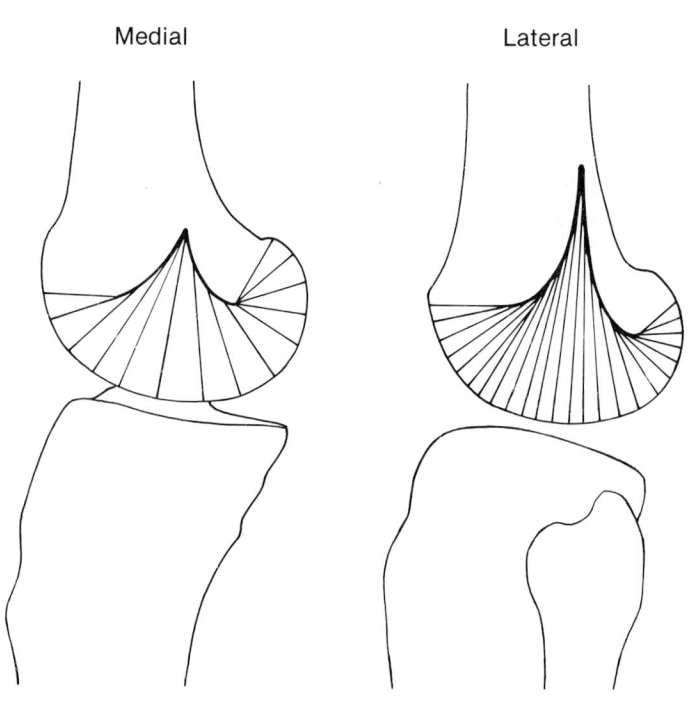

Fig. 4-1 *The radii of curvature for the medial and lateral femoral condyles are slightly different. The medial tibial plateau is concave, while the lateral is convex (Adapted from Gschwend, N.: Design criteria, present indications, and implantation techniques for artificial knee joints. In Schaldach, M., and Hohmann, D., editors: Advances in artificial hip and knee joint technology, New York, 1976, Springer-Verlag.)*

The weight-bearing surface of medial femoral condyle extends farther anteriorly than does that of the lateral femoral condyle. The medial femoral condyle contains an extra annular sector of articular surface that extends nearly to the midline, whereas the weight-bearing surface of the lateral femoral condyle ends in a depression called the *sulcus terminalis* (Fig. 4-2). When the knee is fully extended, the lateral tibial plateau reaches the anterior end of the weight-bearing surface of the lateral femoral condyle and impinges at the sulcus terminalis. But the medial femoral condyle, with its longer articular surface, allows additional gliding to occur in the medial compartment. This movement accommodates the normal 15 degrees of external tibial rotation that accompanies terminal extension.[16]

The lateral and medial tibial plateaus are also asymmetric. The medial tibial plateau is concave and corresponds to the medial femoral condyle more closely than does the convex lateral tibial plateau.[13,14] The tibial plateaus are separated by an intercondylar region

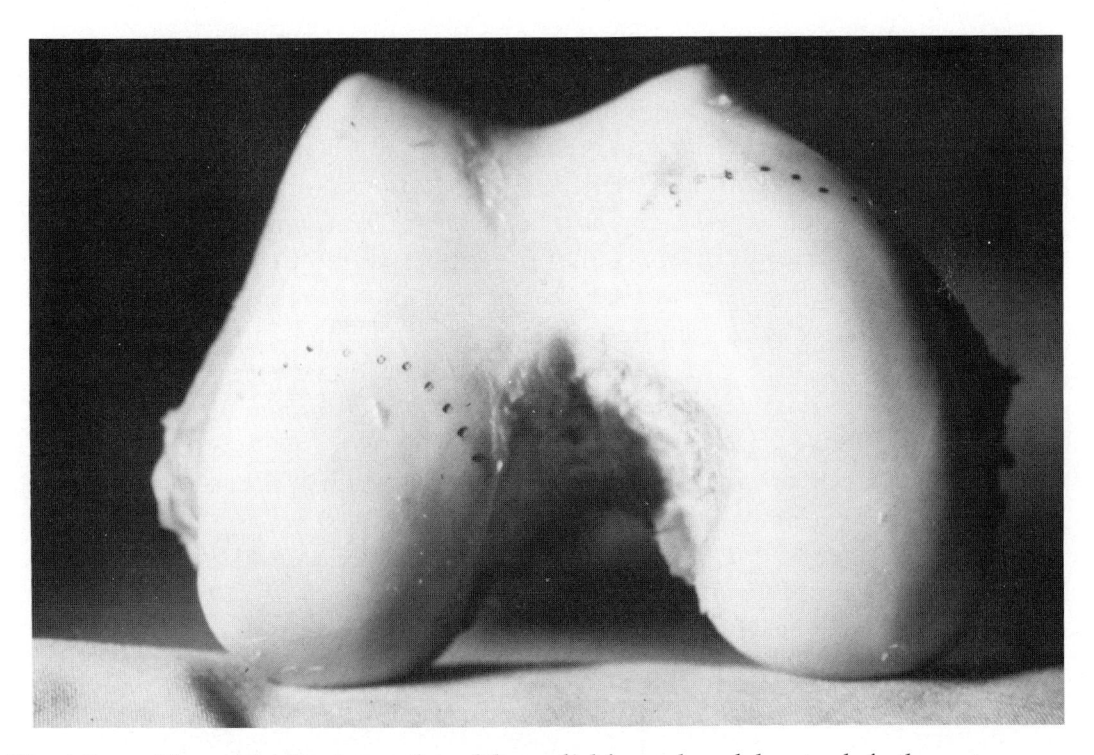

Fig. 4-2 *The weight-bearing surface of the medial femoral condyle extends farther anteriorly than does that of the lateral femoral condyle.*

containing two tibial spines—the anteriorly located medial spine and the posteriorly located lateral spine.[6] These structures prevent medial or lateral subluxation of the tibia and form a central pivot for internal and external rotation.

The menisci improve congruence between the femoral condyles and the tibial plateaus, and they are important weight-bearing structures. The medial meniscus also stabilizes the anterior cruciate deficient knee. When the cruciate ligament is severed in the laboratory, the anterior displacement of the tibia can be further increased by medial menisectomy.[15] The combination of anterior cruciate ligament deficiency and the loss of the medial meniscus is more frequently associated with early degenerative changes than is either lesion alone.[3]

The anterior cruciate ligament arises from the medial aspect of the lateral femoral condyle and inserts anterior to the medial tibial spine. Girgis and Marshall[9] found the average length of the anterior cruciate ligament to be 38 mm, whereas Gillquist[18] reported a length of 31 ± 3 mm. The femoral attachment is an oval area approximately 18 × 11 mm; the tibial attachment is also oval, approximately 17 × 11 mm. When the knee is flexed 90 degrees a twisted-fiber orientation is visible (Fig. 4-3) Anterior cruciate ligament fibers with anterior tibial insertions have femoral origins high and posterior in the intercondylar notch. Fibers with more posterior tibial insertions have femoral origins more anterior and lower in the intercondylar notch. Although the exact fiber orientation and tension remain to be determined, the anterior cruciate ligament clearly consists of a continuum of fibers that are taut in different positions of the knee.[2,22] I have found that the most isometric fibers are those lying in what is generally described as the anteromedial bundle of the anterior cruciate ligament. Several authors have reported that these fibers are taut nearly throughout the range of knee motion.[1,9] The bulk of the ligament, however, has a lower and functionally more posterior origin and as a result is taut when the knee is extended but is relatively lax when the knee is flexed.[9]

The posterior cruciate ligament arises from the lateral aspect of the medial femoral condyle and inserts near the midline of the posterior tibia. Unlike the anterior cruciate ligament insertion, which is arrayed anteriorly to posteriorly, the posterior cruciate ligament insertion contains fibers layered medially to laterally. The most isometric fibers arise high and relatively posterior on the medial fem-

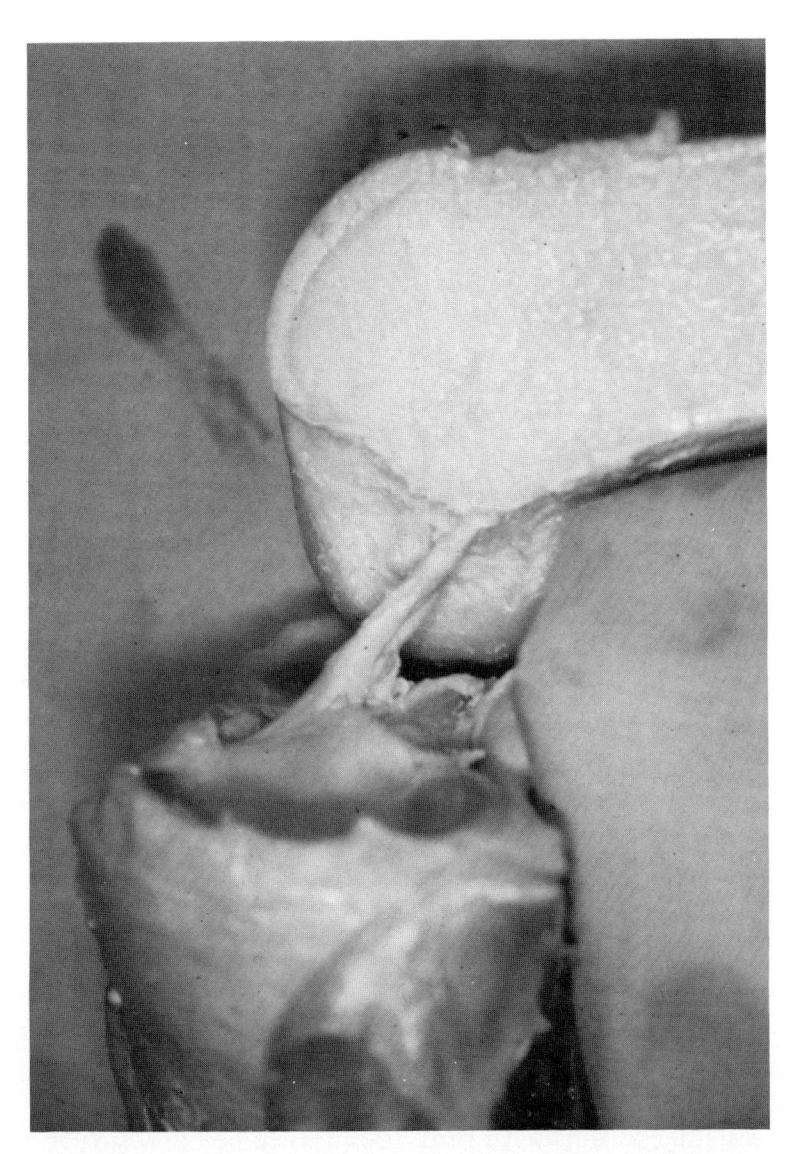

Fig. 4-3 *In the flexed knee, the fibers of the anterior cruciate ligament spiral so that anterior insertions are linked to posterior origins and so that posterior insertions are linked to anterior origins.*

oral condyle. The bulk of the ligament has a more anterior origin and is taut only when the knee is flexed.

Characteristics of knee motions

A two-dimensional analysis of knee motion, although certainly an oversimplification, provides a basis for understanding the complex biomechanics of this joint. At first glance one might consider the knee a hinge joint like the elbow. Hinge joints are characterized by a constant center of rotation and a pure gliding motion between the articular surfaces.

These characteristics can be demonstrated by calculating the center of rotation for a joint such as shown in Fig. 4-4, *A*. In this example, the femur is considered stationary, and the position of tibial points A and B are followed through a short arc of motion. Lines are drawn between corresponding tibial points for two different positions of the knee. Next, perpendicular bisectors of lines AA' and BB' are constructed. The intersection (I) of these two lines represents the instant center of rotation for the short arc of tibial motion under consideration.[7] A similar analysis can be carried out when the tibia is considered stationary and a pair of femoral points is examined (Fig. 4-4, *B*).

By definition, the motion of any point on the moving segment must be perpendicular to a line between it and the instant center of rotation. Continuing our analysis of the simple hinge joint, the point of contact between the two segments has been labeled C (Fig. 4-4, *C*). Motion occurring at point C can be described by a velocity vector perpendicular to the line segment IC. Notice that this vector is also parallel to the articular surfaces at the point of contact. Therefore no compression or tensile forces are generated during joint motion. Also notice that the "tibial" contact point does not change with the position of the joint. This constancy is characteristic of pure gliding motion.

Now consider a joint with pure rolling motion (Fig. 4-5, *A* and *B*). In this case the instant center of rotation lies on the articular surface at the point of contact. As the joint is flexed, the location of the contact point moves posteriorly on the distal segment. Since both the instant center of rotation and the contact point occupy the same location, no line segment joining them can be drawn and no velocity vector can be constructed. This condition is expected because, with pure rolling, there is no motion between the adjacent

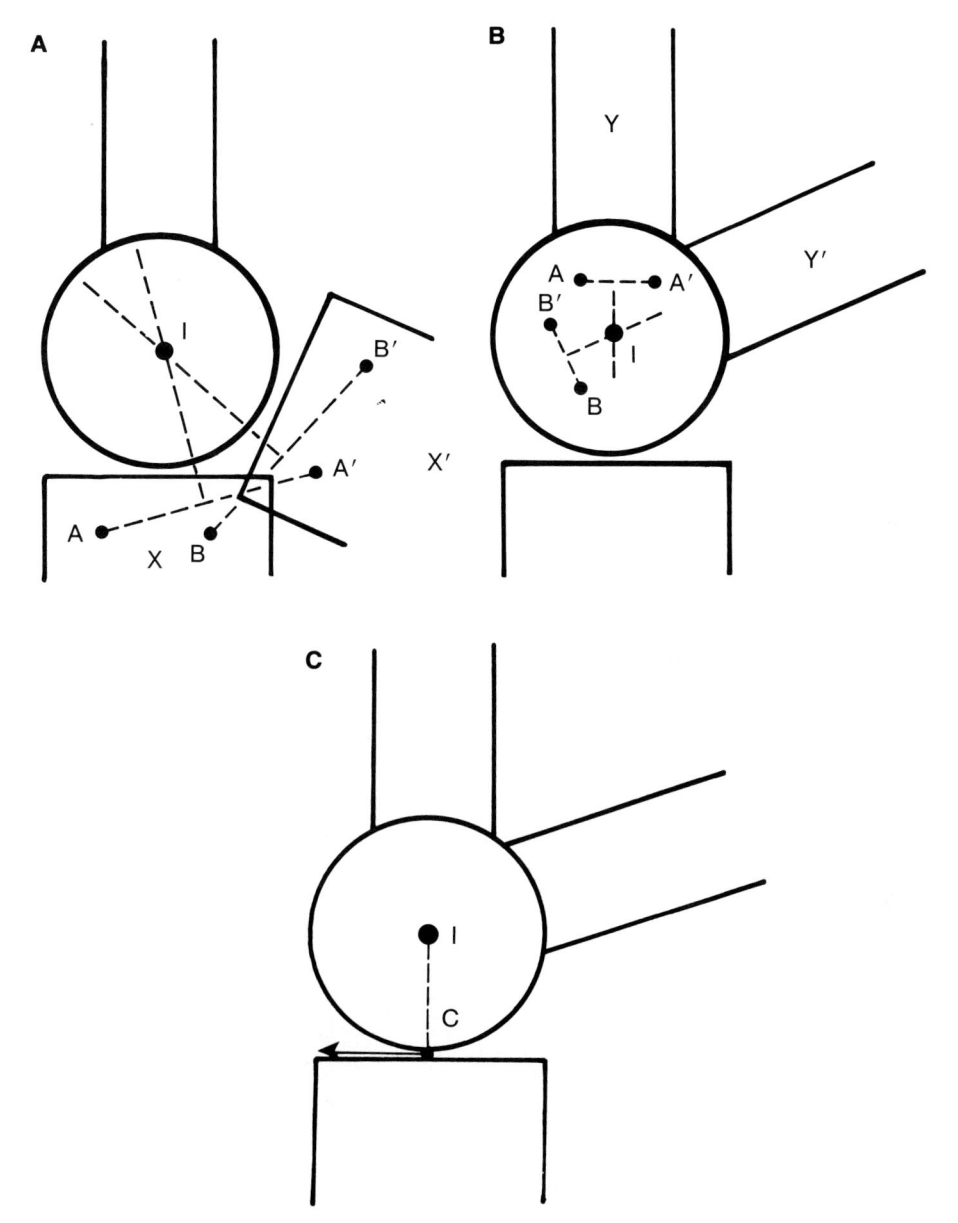

Biomechanics of the anterior cruciate ligament

Fig. 4-4 *Determination of the instant center of rotation for pure gliding motion when the femur is fixed, **A**, and when the tibia is fixed, **B**. The surface velocity vector is perpendicular to line IC (**C**).*

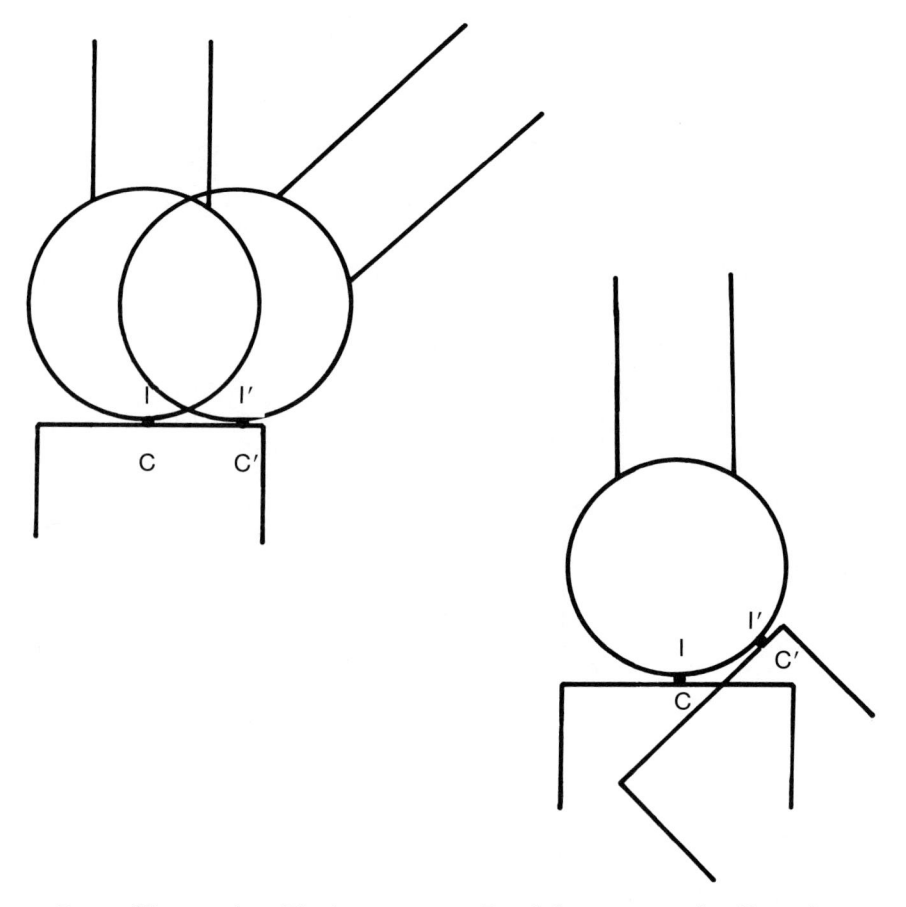

Fig. 4-5 *Pure rolling motion. The instant center I and the contact point C are the same.*

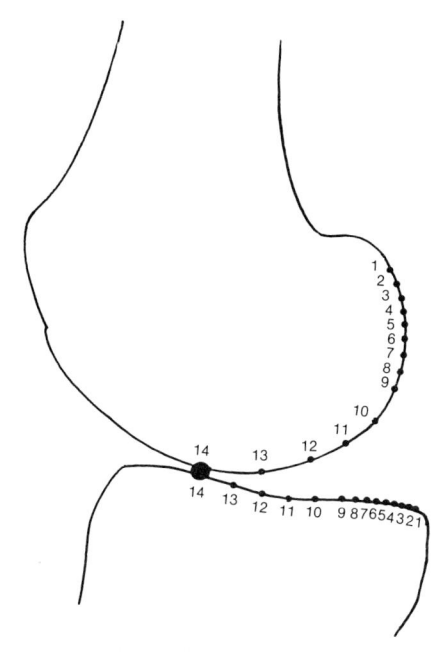

Fig. 4-6 *Corresponding femoral and tibial contact points are not the same distance apart, demonstrating the normal blend of rolling and gliding. (Adapted from Mueller, W.: The knee: form, function, and ligament reconstruction, New York, 1983, Springer-Verlag.)*

articular surfaces. Rather, their relative positions are fixed, as would occur with a pair of gears with meshed teeth.

Both gliding and rolling motions occur between the articular surfaces of the tibia and femur. As the knee is flexed, the contact point moves posteriorly on the tibia, illustrating the rolling component of normal knee motion. When femoral and tibial contact points are plotted, it is apparent that the distances between corresponding points are not the same (Fig. 4-6). The femoral points are clearly more widely spaced than the tibial points. For this condition to occur there must also be gliding motion between the tibia and femur. The ratio of rolling to gliding varies, being about 1:2 in early flexion and 1:4 in late flexion.[16] Because the radius of curvature of the distal femur changes, the location of the instant center of rotation depends on the position of the knee. Normal knees, however, show surface velocity vectors that are always perpendicular to the articular surface at the point of contact (Gerber and Matter[8] and Tamea and Henning[20]).

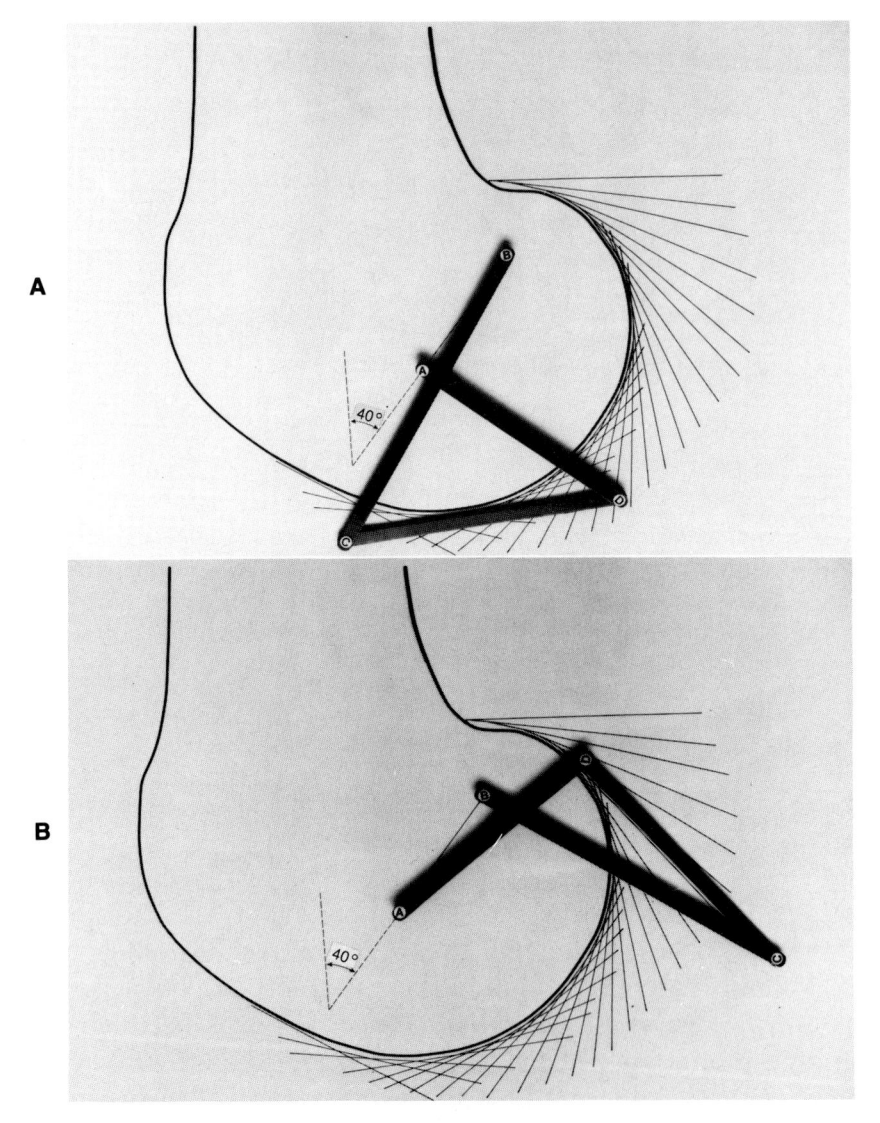

Fig. 4-7 *A* and *B*, The shape of the femoral condyle can be recreated by the four-bar linkage model. (Adapted from Mueller, W.: The knee: form, function, and ligament reconstruction, New York, 1983, Springer-Verlag.)

Four-bar linkage

The crossed four-bar linkage has been used by many authors to illustrate the motion of the human knee.[12,16,21] In this model (Fig. 4-7), four joints are connected by four rigid segments. Two crossed segments, AD and BC, represent the posterior and anterior cruciate ligament respectively. Uncrossed segment AB establishes a fixed distance between the origins of the anterior and posterior cruciate ligaments, whereas segment CD similarly establishes a distance between cruciate insertion points. If "femoral" segment AB is fixed, lines can be traced along the "tibial" surface of segment CD for varying positions of the linkage. As seen in Fig. 4-7, such a tracing results in a curve similar to the profile of a femoral condyle. The ability to approximate the curve of the femoral condyle with a simple model of the cruciate ligaments emphasizes the interrelationship between ligament function and bony anatomy. Because the cruciate ligaments appear early in prenatal development, the shape of the femoral condyles may at least partially result from early intrauterine motion within the constraints provided by the cruciate ligaments.[21] The orientation of the segment connecting the cruciate origins in relation to the long axis of the femur is an important determinant of the range of joint motion. Only when line segment AB forms an angle of 40 degrees with the long axis of the femur analogous to the normal roof of the intercondylar notch will a normal range of motion result. With this orientation, hyperextension is blocked when the anterior cruciate ligament comes to lie along the intercondylar roof yet full flexion is allowed.

The four-bar linkage not only illustrates the full range of motion, but it also demonstrates the normal combination of gliding and sliding between the tibia and femur (Fig. 4-8). With flexion, the femur moves posteriorly on the tibia, and in extension, the anterior cruciate ligament lies parallel to the intercondylar roof. For any position of the knee, the point at which "cruciate" segments AD and BC cross represents the instant center of rotation. When the path of the instant center of rotation is plotted (Fig. 4-9, *A* and *B*), we can see that it moves posteriorly with increasing knee flexion. This curve is similar, but not identical, to that obtained by Gerber.[8] Finally, if the instant center of rotation is used to construct a surface-velocity vector, it is, as expected, parallel to the joint surface for all positions of the knee.

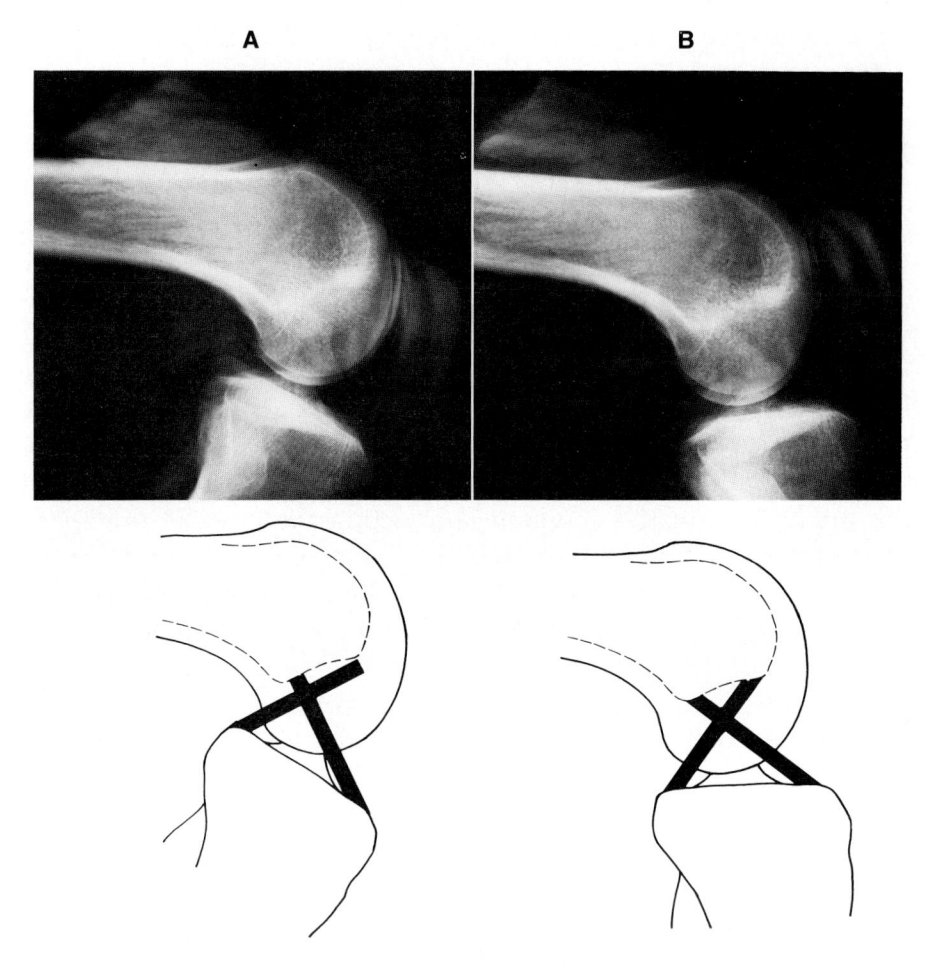

Fig. 4-8 *A* through *D*, The four-bar linkage model mimics the motion of the normal knee. With flexion, the femur moves more posteriorly on the tibia yet the bars representing the cruciate ligaments do not change in length.

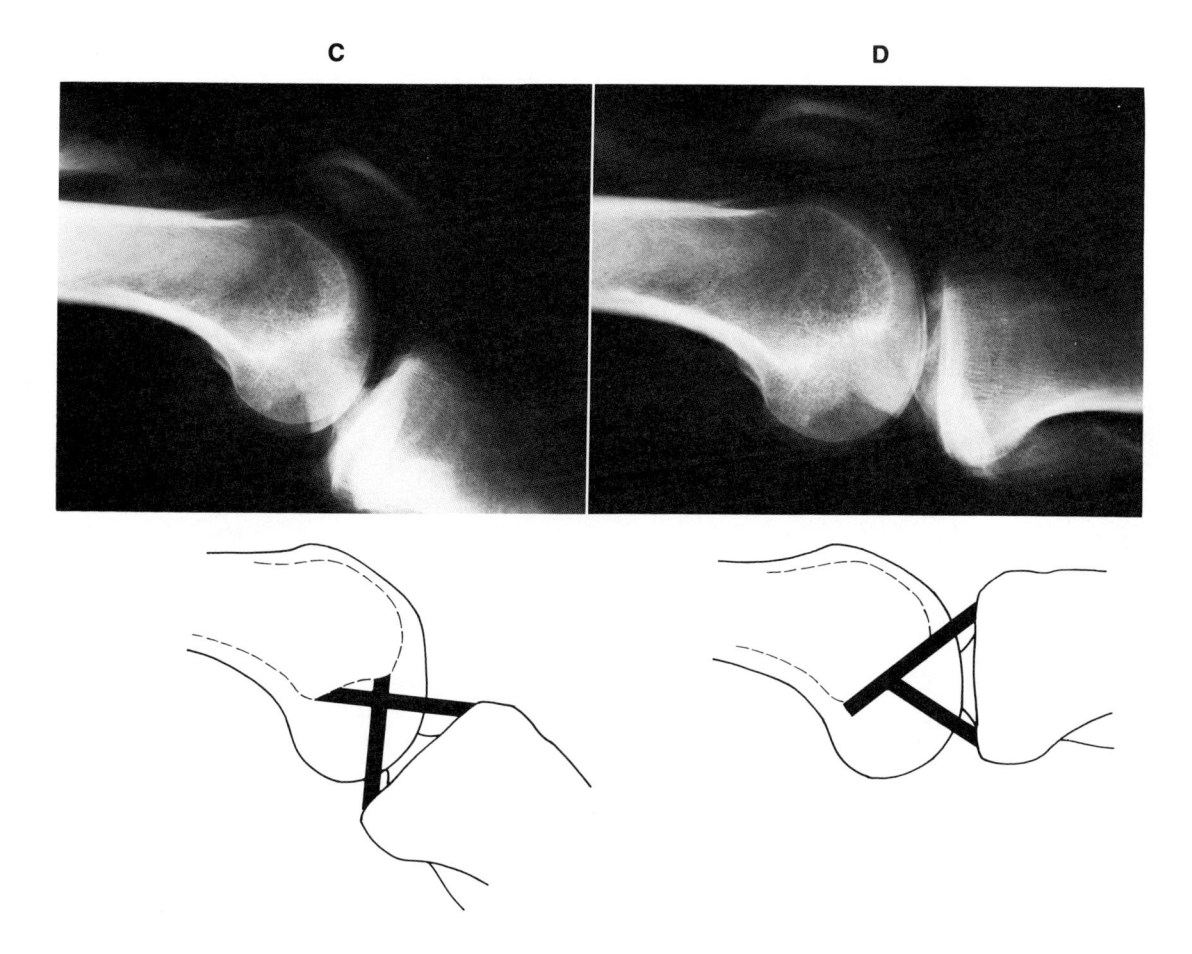

Biomechanics of the anterior cruciate ligament 67

C   D

Fig. 4-8, cont'd. *For legend see opposite page.*

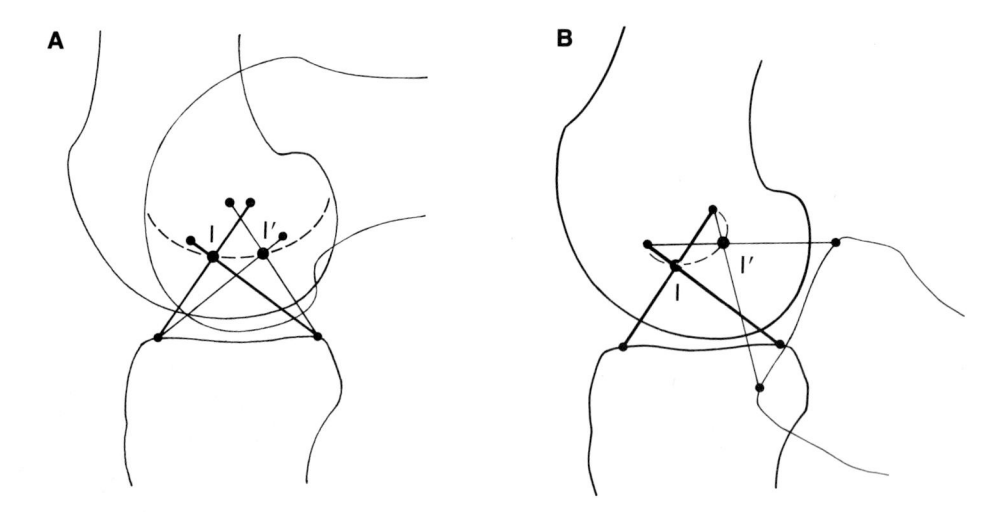

Fig. 4-9 *The point where the "cruciate segments" cross is the instant center of rotation. Its path is shown with the tibia fixed,* **A,** *and with the femur fixed,* **B.**

Automatic rotation

During the final 20 degrees of extension, there is a 15 degree automatic external rotation of the tibia. This movement has been called the "screwing-home mechanism." The anterior extension of the surface of the medial femoral condyle, as noted earlier, is significant in allowing this external rotation; it is likely that the cruciate ligaments also importantly affect this movement. Mueller has shown that the axis for this rotation lies near the insertion of the most lateral fibers of the posterior cruciate ligament.[16] These fibers may in fact guide the external rotation of the tibia. The anterior cruciate ligament is taut in extension; internal rotation further tightens it, whereas external rotation relaxes it.[1] Therefore, as the knee nears terminal extension and as the bulk of the anterior cruciate ligament becomes taut, externally rotating the tibia may serve to relax the ligament enough to allow the last few degrees of extension. Finally, an osseous axis for this rotation may be provided by the intercondylar eminence, although Goodfellow and O'Connor believed its role to be minor.[10]

Normal   Abnormal

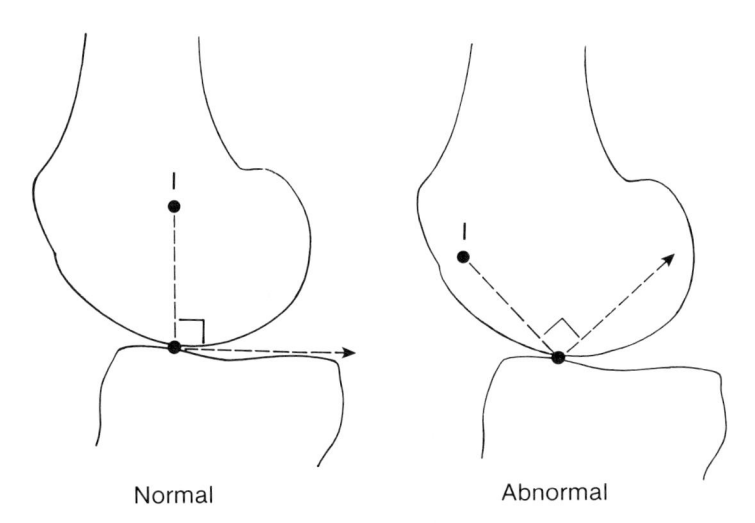

Fig. 4-10 *In the normal knee, surface velocity vectors are always parallel to the articular surface. In the cruciate deficient knee, the instant center is often abnormally located, producing nonparallel velocity vectors and compression loads on the articular surface. (Adapted from Tamea, C.D., and Henning, C.E.: Pathomechanics of the pivot shift maneuver: an instant center analysis, Am J. Sports Med. 9:31, 1981.)*

Disruption of the anterior cruciate ligament

The anterior cruciate ligament is generally accepted as the primary restraint to anterior tibial displacement. When disrupted, the anterior cruciate ligament loses 86% of its restraining force.[4] Consequently, the tibia may sublux anteriorly, producing symtoms of instability and clinical signs such as a positive Lachman test, anterior drawer test, and pivot shift maneuver. In addition to gross displacement and clinical instability, however, the loss of an anterior cruciate ligament may more subtly affect joint function. When Tamea and Henning[20] applied internal rotation and valgus forces to the tibia of a cruciate-deficient knee, lateral-knee radiographs at 10 degree increments from 0 to 90 degrees of flexion showed change in the location of the instant center of rotation. Gerber[8] found similar changes in unstressed anterior cruciate ligament deficient knees, suggesting that a pivot shift maneuver is not necessary to demonstrate the altered knee kinematics. Altered instant centers of rotation are reflected in surface velocity vectors that are no longer parallel to the joint surface (Fig. 4-10). This alteration produces abnormal compressive forces across the joint and may explain the accelerated degenerative joint disease frequently accompanying injuries to cruciate ligaments.

Reconstruction

The goals of anterior cruciate reconstruction should be to reproduce the function of the normal anterior cruciate ligament, with sufficient strength and durability through a surgical procedure entailing the lowest possible morbidity. Noyes[17] examined the strength of biological implants. He found that semitendinosus and gracilis tendons had only 70% and 49% of the initial strength of the anterior cruciate ligaments, respectively. An 18-mm wide strip of fascia lata had only 44% of the strength of the anterior cruciate ligament. However, a 14-mm wide bone-patellar-tendon-bone graft had a mean strength 159% that of the anterior cruciate ligament. When interpreting these numbers, it must be recalled that during incorporation, biological implants lose strength initially and only slowly regain it. In a study of Rhesus monkeys, Clancy[5] found that a reconstruction using the medial one third of the patellar tendon exhibited 53% of the control strength of the patellar tendon graft at 3 months, but it had 81% of the control strength at 9 months and 81% at 1 year. Properties of biological and nonbiological implants over longer periods are not known.

At the present time, no reconstructive procedure has been shown to restore normal mechanics to the anterior cruciate ligament deficient knee. Operations that can provide the check-rein function of the anterior cruciate ligament and eliminate complaints of instability may not sufficiently restore normal kinematics to prevent the progression of degenerative joint disease. Gross tests of instability, such as the anterior drawer test and Lachman test, may not be sensitive enough to predict the fate of a reconstructed cruciate-deficient knee. Only long-term clinical trials and further biomechanical analyses will provide needed comparisons of available reconstruction procedures.

REFERENCES

1. Arms, S.W., Pope, M.H., Johnson, R.J., et al.: The biomechanics of anterior cruciate ligament rehabilitation and reconstruction, Am. J. Sports Med. **12**:8, 1984.
2. Arnoczky, S.P.: Anatomy of the anterior cruciate ligament, Clin. Orthop. **172**:19, 1983.
3. Balkfors, B.: The course of knee-ligament injuries, Acta Orthop. Scand. (Suppl.) **198**:1, 1982.
4. Butler, D.L., Noyes, F.R., and Grood, E.S.: Ligamentous restraints to anterior-posterior drawer in the human knee, J. Bone Joint Surg. (Am.) **62**:259, 1980.
5. Clancy, W.G., Narechania, R.G., Rosenberg, T.D., et al.: Anterior and posterior cruciate ligament reconstruction in rhesus monkeys: a histological, microangiographic, and biomechanical analysis, J. Bone Joint Surg. (Am.) **63**:1270, 1981.
6. Danzig, L.A., Newell, J.D., Guerra, J., et al.: Osseous landmarks of the normal knee, Clin. Orthop. **156**:201, 1981.
7. Frankel, V.H., Burstein, A.H., and Brooks, D.B.: Biomechanics of internal derangement of the knee, J. Bone Joint Surg. (Am.) **53**:945, 1971.
8. Gerber, C., and Matter, P.: Biomechanical analysis of the knee after rupture of the anterior cruciate ligament and its primary repair: an instant-centre analysis of function, J. Bone Joint Surg. (Br.) **65**:391, 1983.
9. Girgis, F.G., Marshall, J.L., and Al Monajem, A.R.S.: The cruciate ligaments of the knee joint: anatomical, functional, and experimental analysis, Clin. Orthop. **106**:216, 1975.
10. Goodfellow, J. and O'Connor, J.: The mechanics of the knee and prosthesis design, J. Bone Joint Surg. (Br.) **60**:358, 1978.
11. Gschwend, N.: Design criteria, present indications, and implantation techniques for artificial knee joints. In Schaldach, M., and Hohmann, D., editors: Advances in artificial hip and knee joint technology, New York, 1976, Springer-Verlag, p. 90.
12. Kapandjii, I.A.: The physiology of the joints, Vol. II, London, 1970, Churchill Livingstone.
13. Hollinshead, W.H.: Anatomy for surgeons: the back and limbs, Philadelphia, 1982, Harper & Row.
14. Insall, J.N.: Anatomy of the knee. In Insall, J.N., editor: Surgery of the knee, New York, London and Melbourne, 1984, Churchill Livingstone, p. 1.
15. Levy, I.M., Torzilli, P.A., and Warren, R.F.: The effect of medial meniscectomy on anterior-posterior motion of the knee. J. Bone Joint Surg. (Am.) **64**:883, 1982.
16. Muller, W.: The knee: form, function, and ligament reconstruction, Berlin Heidelberg New York, 1983, Springer-Verlag.
17. Noyes, F.R., Butler, D.L., Grood, E.S., et al.: Biomechanical analysis of human ligament grafts used in knee-ligament repairs and reconstruction, J. Bone Joint Surg. (Am.) **66**:344, 1984.
18. Odenstein, M., and Gillquist, J.: Functional anatomy of the anterior cruciate ligament and a rationale for reconstruction, J. Bone Joint Surg. (Am.) **67**:257, 1985.
19. Swanson, S.A.V.: Biomechanics. In Freeman, M.A.R., editor: Arthritis of the knee, Berlin Heidelberg New York, 1980, Springer-Verlag, p. 1.
20. Tamea, C.D., and Henning, C.E.: Pathomechanics of the pivot shift maneuver: an instant center analysis, Am. J. Sports Med. **9**:31, 1981.
21. Teil, L. and Menschik, A.: Mechanik Des Kniegelenkes, Z. Orthop. **112**:481, 1974.
22. Welsh, R.P.: Knee joint structure and function, Clin. Orthop. **147**:7, 1980.

5

Clinical examination of the knee for anterior cruciate ligament laxity

FRANK O. BONNARENS

DAVID DREZ, Jr.

The necessity for a thorough examination of the patient with knee complaints has not been diminished by advances in technology. There is no question that arthrography, arthroscopy, computerized tomography, and magnetic resonance imaging can be valuable aids to the clinician in the management of patients with knee problems. However, the mainstay in proper diagnosis and treatment remains the ability to accurately evaluate patient complaints and perform a thorough examination.

The intent of this chapter is not to provide a comprehensive method of evaluating the patient with knee complaints but to focus on the history and clinical examination of the patient with a deficiency of the anterior cruciate ligament. The mechanics of the laxity examination in the anterior cruciate deficient knee are also explained.

Patients with an acute anterior cruciate ligament injury will usually have had a twisting injury accompanied by a pop and by an effusion that occurs several hours later.[1] A large number of patients will experience the knee "coming apart" or the "joint separating." Those patients with chronic, symptomatic, anterior cruciate ligament laxity experience similar episodes but without the pop or the degree of swelling present with acute injuries.

Request reprints from: David Drez, Jr., M.D., 2615 Enterprise Boulevard, Lake Charles, Louisiana, 70601.

Terminology of knee laxity

Stability is the patient's interpretation of a joint's ability to accept an applied load without allowing abnormal motion. Therefore *instability* is the patient's description of abnormal knee movement under an applied load. *Laxity* is a movement elicited during examination and is either normal or abnormal. Abnormal laxities can be graded I, II, or III: grade I is 0 to 5 mm of displacement; grade II is 5 to 10 mm of displacement; and grade III is greater than 10 mm of displacement. This defines only the magnitude (amount) of the laxity. To be useful clinically it is also necessary to assign direction to the abnormal movement. This turns the scalar measure of displacement into a vector, that is, the magnitude and direction of displacement.

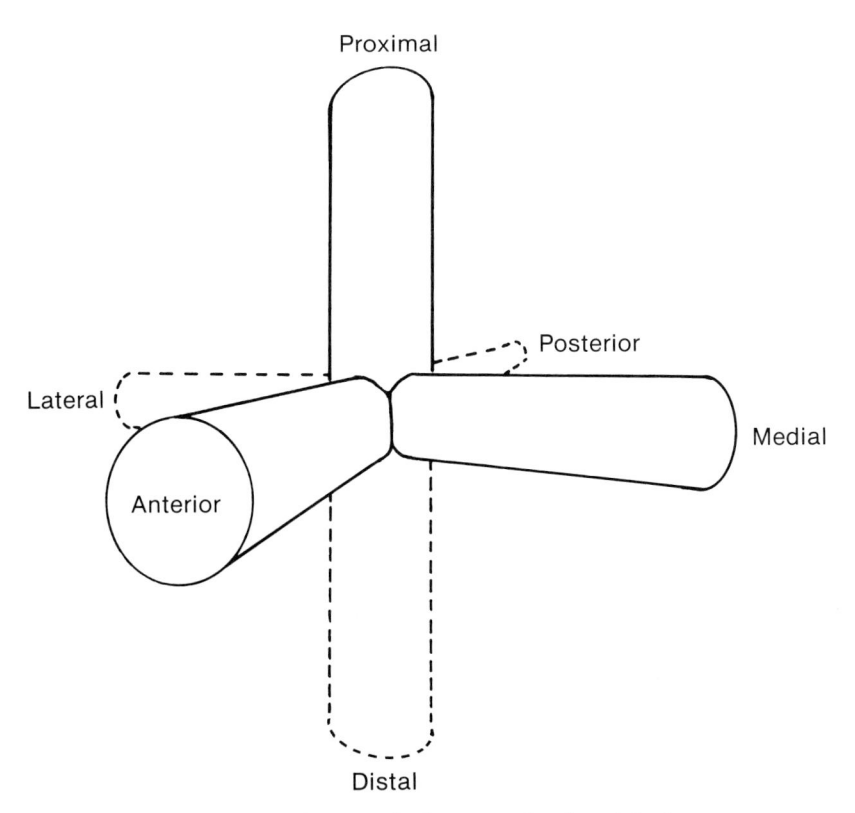

Fig. 5-1 *The translation axes for the right knee.*

The potential direction of these vectors of abnormal movement can be linear, rotational, or a combination of the two. They can be described using the six degrees of freedom. There are three linear translations and three rotations in the knee. The translations are anterior-posterior, proximal-distal (distraction-compression), and medial-lateral (Fig. 5-1). The three rotations are varus-valgus, internal-external, and flexion-extension (Fig. 5-2). A *translation* movement means that every point of the moving object simultaneously has the same velocity and direction of motion. *Rotation* is the pivoting or turning of an object about an axis. *Translocation* is a change in position; this may be a combination of translation and rotation.

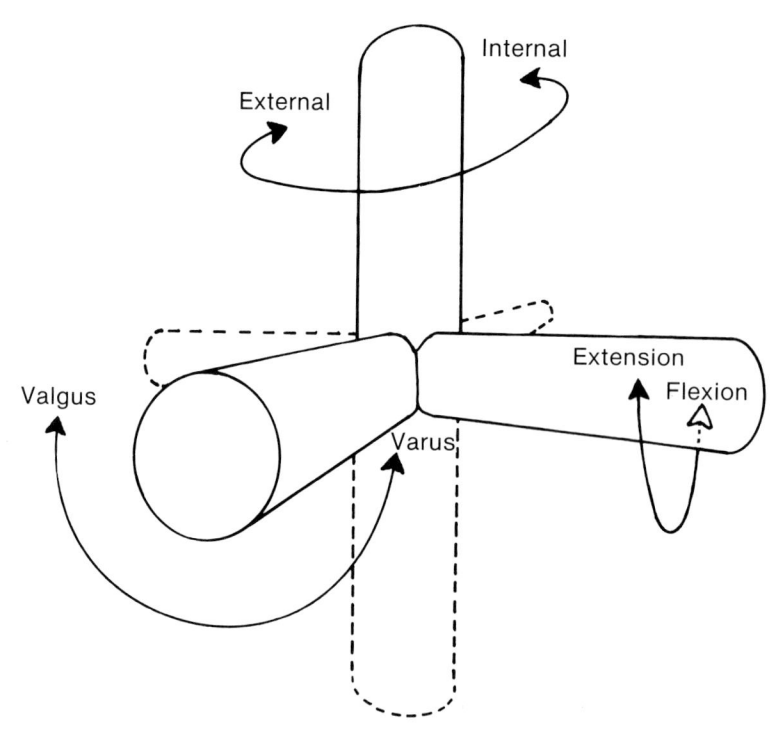

Fig. 5-2   *The rotation axes for the right knee.*

Tests demonstrating translation

There are two clinical tests of the anterior cruciate ligament that test translation—the 90-degree anterior drawer test and the Lachman test. The *90-degree anterior drawer test* is performed with the patient in the supine position (Fig. 5-3). The hip is flexed approximately 45 degrees, the knee is flexed 90 degrees, and the patient's tibia is in neutral rotation with the foot flat on the table. The examiner's hands are then placed with the fingers over the patient's hamstrings and gastrocnemius heads; the thumbs are placed on the tibial plateaus and the joint line. The ulnar border of the examiner's arm on the medial side is placed against the anterior aspect of the patient's leg. A smooth, steady pull is then made in an anterior direction. This is repeated with the leg in internal and then external rotation. The resulting displacements are recorded.

The *Lachman test* is performed with the patient's knee in approximately 20 degrees of flexion.[17] The examiner uses one hand to stabilize the patient's femur by grasping the distal thigh just proximal to the patella (Fig. 5-4). With the other hand the examiner grasps the tibia just distal to the tibial tubercle. Firm pressure is then applied to the posterior aspect of the tibia in an effort to produce an anterior translation. The amount of anterior translation is recorded. If the test is positive it means that the tibia underwent an anterior subluxation. It does not represent reduction of a posteriorly displaced tibia.

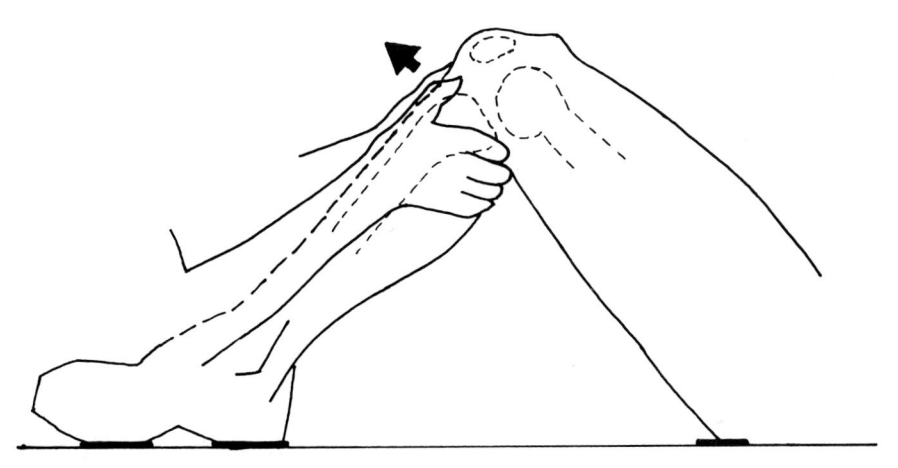

Fig. 5-3   *The 90-degree anterior drawer test. The test is positive if the tibia subluxes anteriorly.*

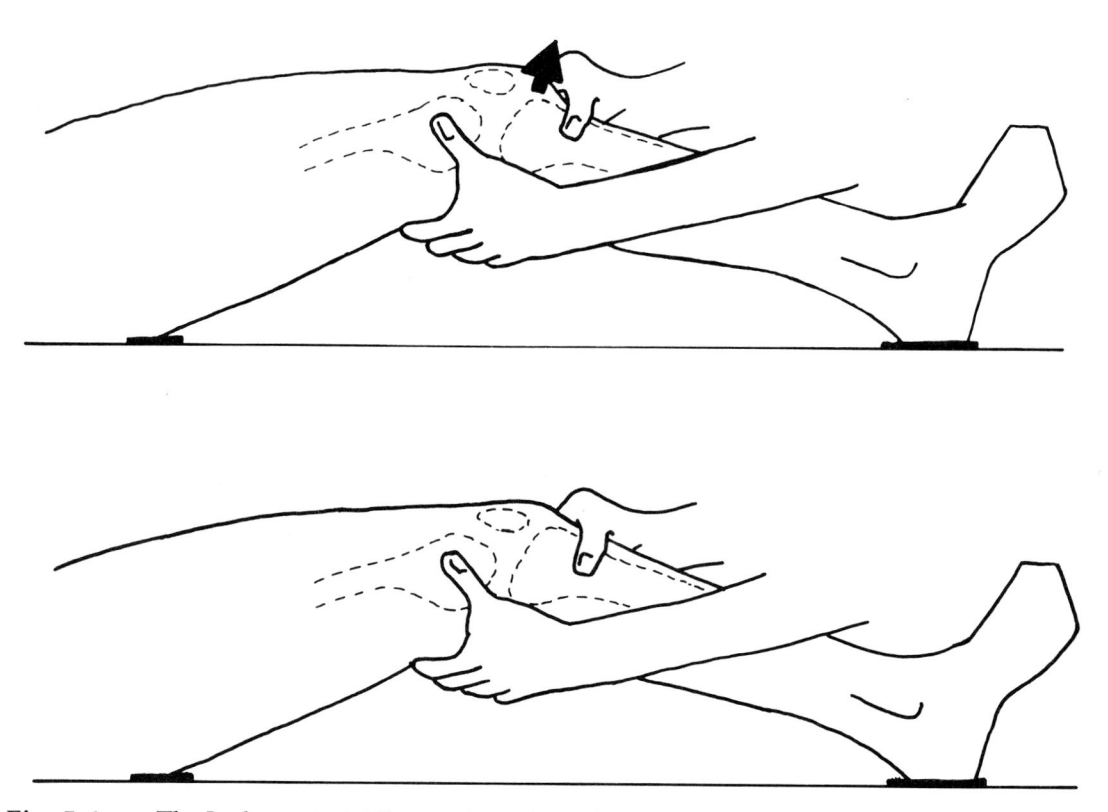

Fig. 5-4 *The Lachman test. The test is positive if the tibia subluxes anteriorly.*

Tests demonstrating anterolateral rotatory laxity

The *pivot shift test* of MacIntosh and Galway, the *Losee test*, the *flexion-rotation drawer test*, and the *Slocum test* show anterolateral rotatory laxity. Anterolateral rotatory laxity is a combination of anterior-posterior translation and internal-external rotation. The *pivot-shift test* of MacIntosh and Galway requires a relaxed patient.[5] The examiner uses one hand to grasp the patient's ankle (Fig. 5-5) and places the other hand with the heel over the lateral head of the gastrocnemius heads and with the palm behind the fibula. The patient's knee is fully extended and internally rotated with the examiner's hand near the ankle. A valgus strain is applied as the knee

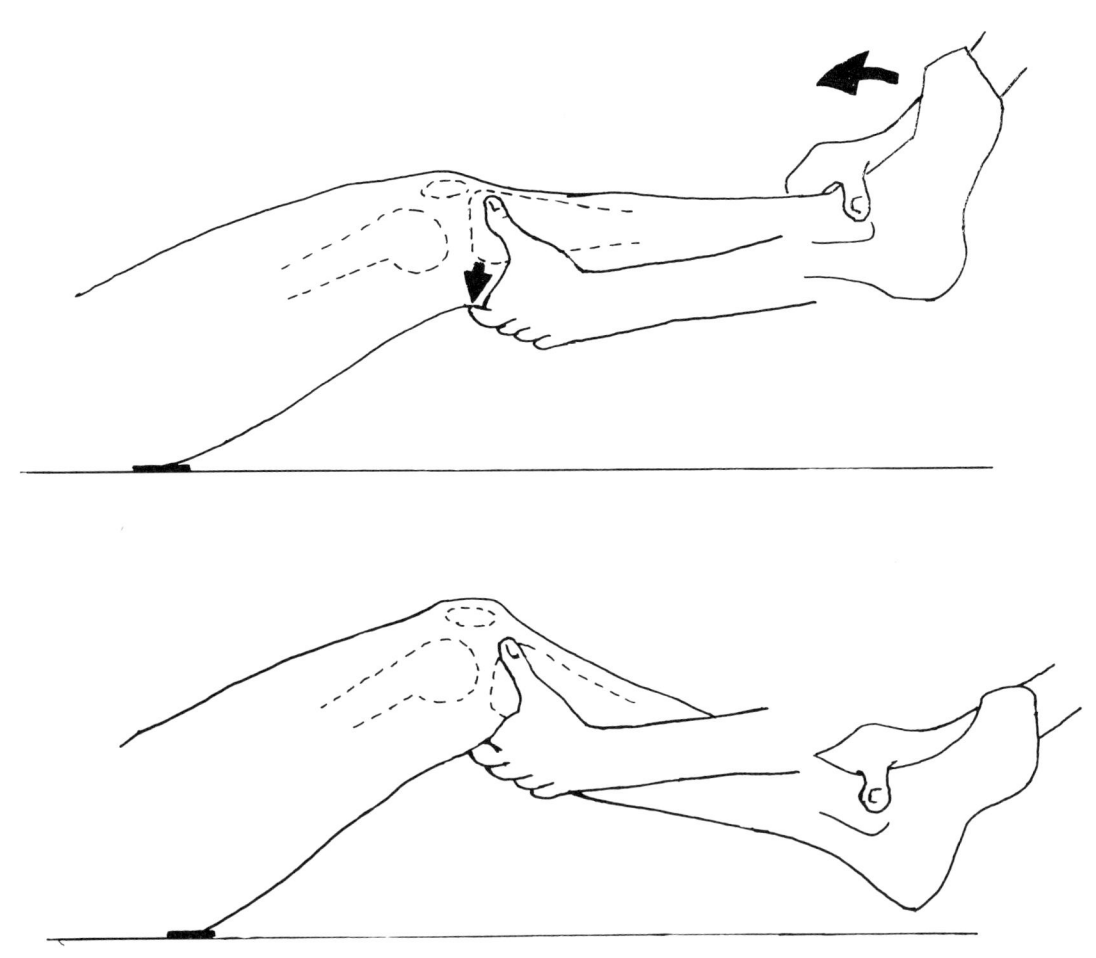

Clinical examination of the knee for anterior cruciate ligament laxity 77

Fig. 5-5 *The pivot-shift test. The tibia is held in internal rotation. The test is positive if the tibia assumes the reduced position during flexion.*

is slowly flexed. The tibial plateau subluxes forward initially. If the test is positive, the subluxation will reduce, often in a dramatic fashion. If the test is grossly positive, the tibia impinges on the femur, inhibiting reduction. Care must be taken not to produce an osteochondral fracture. The result is graded by estimating the amount of tibial motion that occurs.

The *Losee test* is performed with the patient in the supine position.[9,10] The patient's foot is supported in one hand of the examiner with the leg slightly externally rotated and braced against the examiner's abdomen (Fig. 5-6). The knee is then placed in 30 degrees of flexion. The tibial subluxation is reduced in this position. The

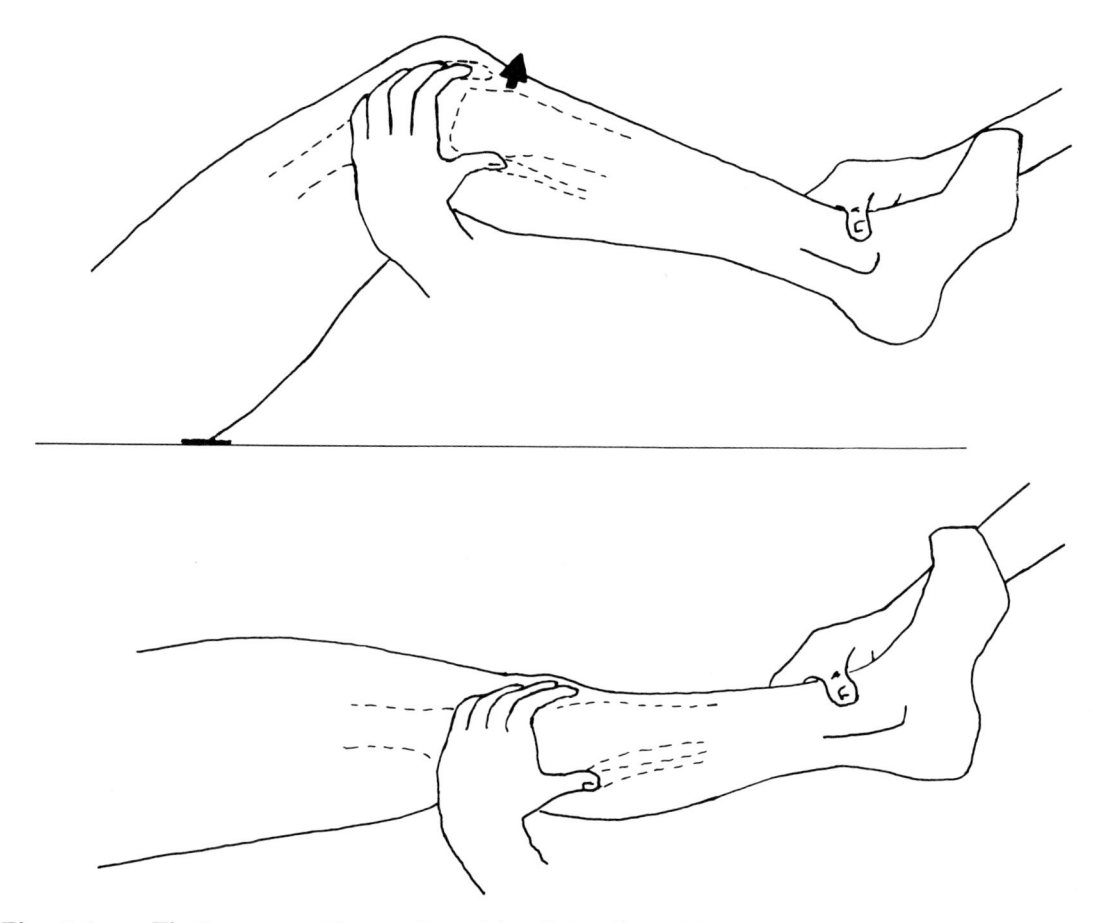

Fig. 5-6 *The Losee test. The test is positive if the tibia subluxes anteriorly as the knee is extended.*

examiner's other hand is then placed palm down with the fingers over the patient's patella and with the thumb posterior to the fibular head. A valgus strain is then applied by using the abdomen of the examiner. The knee is then slowly extended and the leg is allowed to go into internal rotation. The fibular head is pushed anteriorly with the examiner's thumb, and the fingers push the femur posteriorly. If the test is positive, the tibial plateau subluxes anteriorly just short of full extension and the patient recognizes this as his symptom. The result is graded by estimating the amount of tibial motion that occurs.

The *flexion-rotation drawer test* combines the pivot-shift test and the Lachman test[13] (Fig. 5-7). The patient's leg is positioned with the

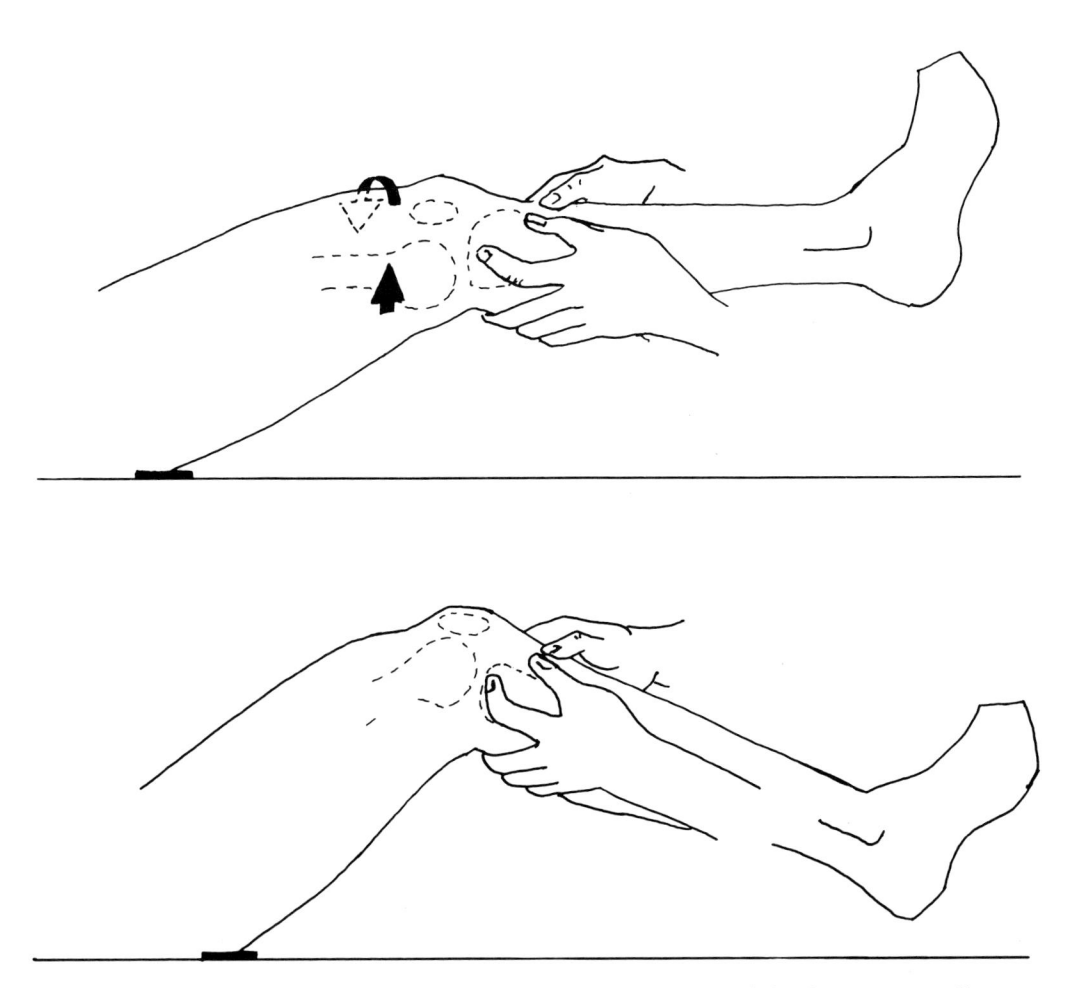

Clinical examination of the knee for anterior cruciate ligament laxity 79

Fig. 5-7 *The flexion rotation drawer test. The test is positive if the femur internally rotates as it assumes the reduced position.*

knee in 20 degrees of flexion. The examiner's index finger of one hand is placed along the patient's lateral joint line, and the other fingers support the lateral calf. The examiner's index finger of the opposite hand is placed along the medial joint line with the other fingers also supporting the calf. Both thumbs of the examiner are placed along the anterior tibia, and the patient's ankle rests gently on the examiner's side. In this position, if the tibia is held firmly, the femur will translate posteriorly and externally rotate. This is equivalent to the anterior subluxation of the tibia in the previous two tests. The patient's knee is then gently flexed as the examiner's thumbs push the tibia posteriorly. The test is positive if the femur internally rotates as it assumes the reduced position. The femur will sublux if

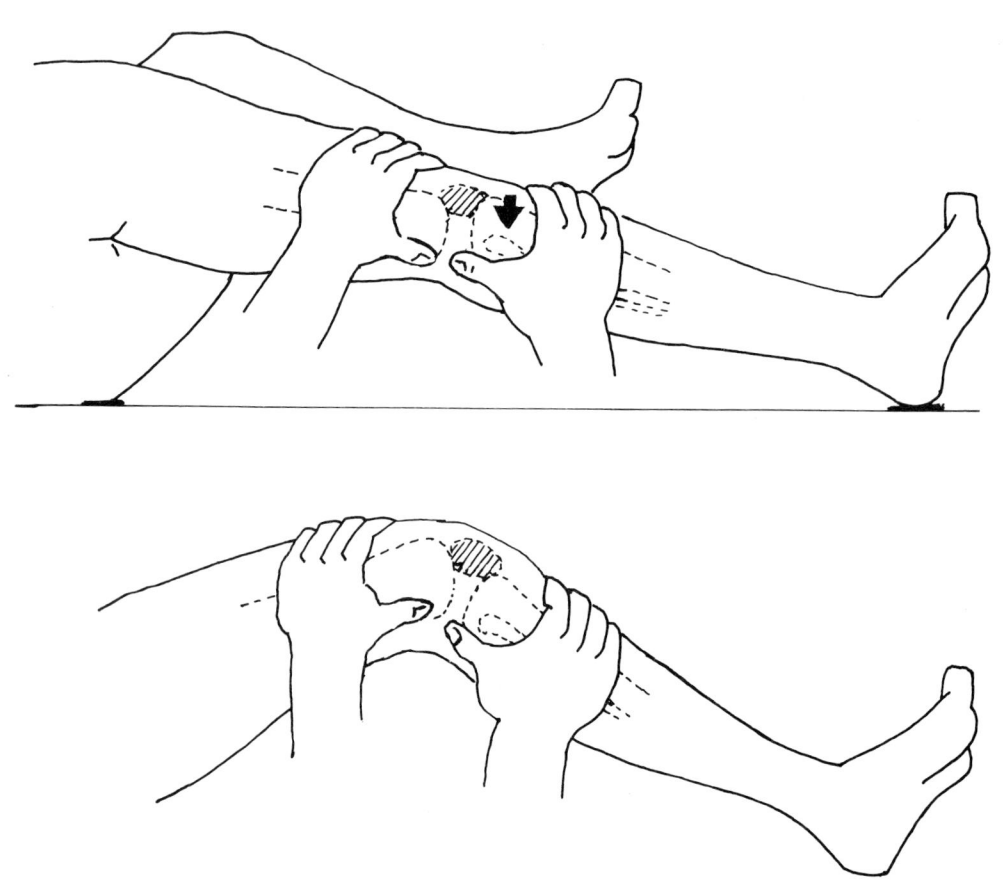

Fig. 5-8 *The Slocum test. The test is positive if the tibia assumes the reduced position as the knee is flexed.*

the knee is gently extended and the tibia is flipped anteriorly. The drawer component is similar to and will be positive for the same reasons as the Lachman test even with small laxities. The rotational component can be accentuated with axial compression to demonstrate the pivot-shift phenomenon.

The *Slocum test* has the advantage over the previous three tests of allowing complete quadriceps relaxation and greater ease of performance on large or muscular patients.[14,15] (Fig. 5-8). The patient lies with the normal side in a lateral decubitus position and with the lower hip and knee flexed enough to stay clear of the upper leg. The knee being tested is superior. The upper hip and pelvis are then rotated posteriorly until the weight is borne by the heel of the upper leg with the knee free of the table. The knee is then placed in 10 degrees of flexion. It will sag into valgus, and the tibia will rotate internally and translate anteriorly. The examiner's hands are positioned on the lateral side with the examiner posterior. The hand of the examiner nearest the foot is placed with the thumb behind the fibula and the index finger along the joint line. The examiner's other hand grasps the distal femur with the thumb over the lateral femoral condyle. While applying equal pressure with both hands the patient's knee is gently pushed into flexion. When the knee is flexed past about 25 degrees the anteriorly subluxed tibia will reduce by moving posteriorly and by rotating externally, if anterolateral rotatory laxity is present. This reduction is usually palpable but may be subtle with lesser laxities.

Mechanics of the knee

To fully comprehend why these tests are meaningful an understanding of the mechanics of the knee is required. As the knee flexes and extends, the articular surfaces undergo a combination of rolling and gliding movements[11] (Fig. 5-9). These movements are controlled by a combination of the forces of the muscle-tendon units, the ligamentous constraints, and the bony geometry.

The ligaments of the knee guide the motion of the joint. For each joint position and for each direction of motion certain ligaments will provide most of the restraint against abnormal movement. These are designated as the *primary restraints*.[3] The primary restraints protect the *secondary restraints* from excessive force. The terms primary and secondary do not mean one is more important than the other. It is a comment on the relative contribution to joint restraint and is dependent on both joint position and the direction of the applied forces. The primary and secondary restraints act in concert to guide the motion of the knee.

The forces applied during clinical examination average between 50 and 100 newtons (N).[12] Forces during the activities of daily living are commonly as high as 500 N.[6] Seen in this light, a positive clinical test shows a significant loss of primary restraint function. As a result of the low forces applied during clinical testing, a false-positive result may occur due to intact secondary restraints.

The anterior cruciate ligament is the primary restraint to anterior translation of the tibia.[3] To produce an anterior translation of 5 mm with a normal knee flexed 90 degrees requires 440 N. If the anterior cruciate ligament is transected, a 90 N force is required to displace the tibia anteriorly 5 mm at 90 degrees of flexion as a result of the

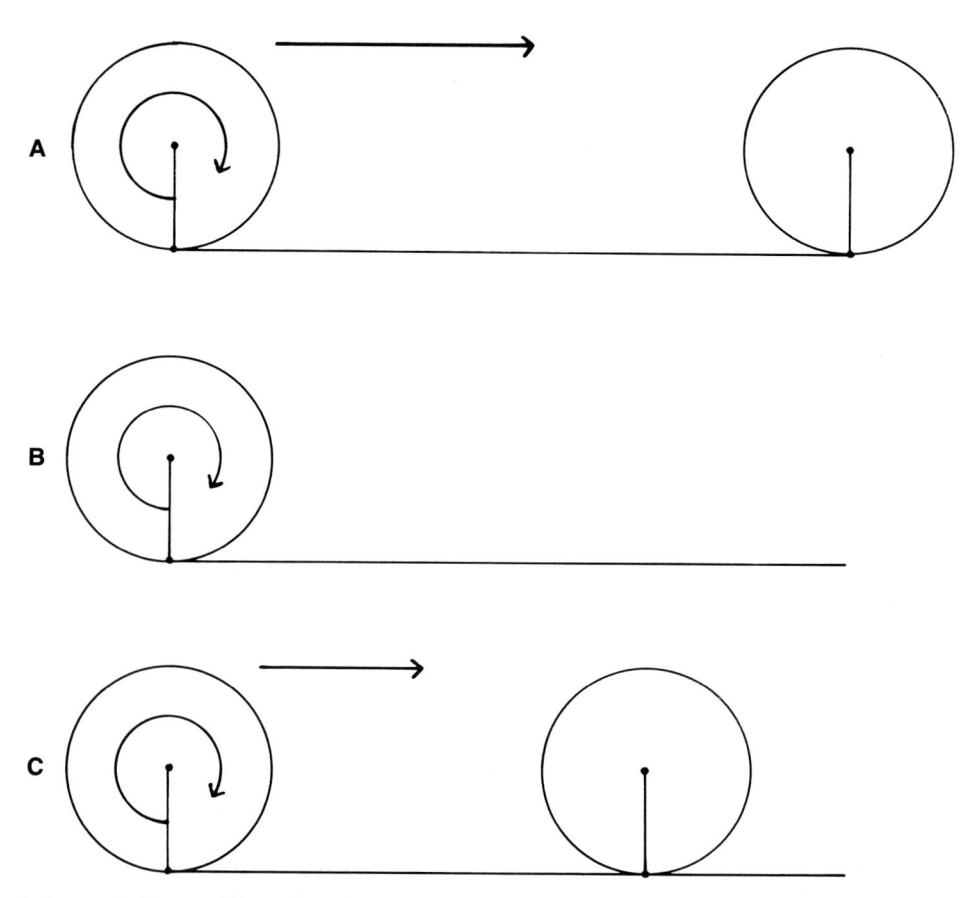

Fig. 5-9 *A, Pure rolling: the wheel travels a distance equal to its circumference. B, Pure gliding: the wheel does not change position as it turns. C, Rolling and gliding: the wheel travels a distance less than its circumference but proportionate to its rolling component. That is, 50% rolling would cause a travel distance of 50% of the circumference of the wheel.*

secondary restraints. At 30-degree flexion the forces are 330 N and 90 N respectively. As specified earlier, the forces during clinical testing are just sufficient to produce 5 mm anterior displacement with the anterior cruciate ligament transected and the secondary restraints intact. It has been stated that the Lachman test is more sensitive than the anterior drawer test.[8] The reasons stated are that the knee is held in a position more comfortable for the patient, that the mechanical advantage of the hamstrings is negated, and that the contact area on the lateral tibial plateau is slightly convex in this position. These three factors interact to reduce the coefficient of static friction, thus making the Lachman test easier to perform with clinical forces.

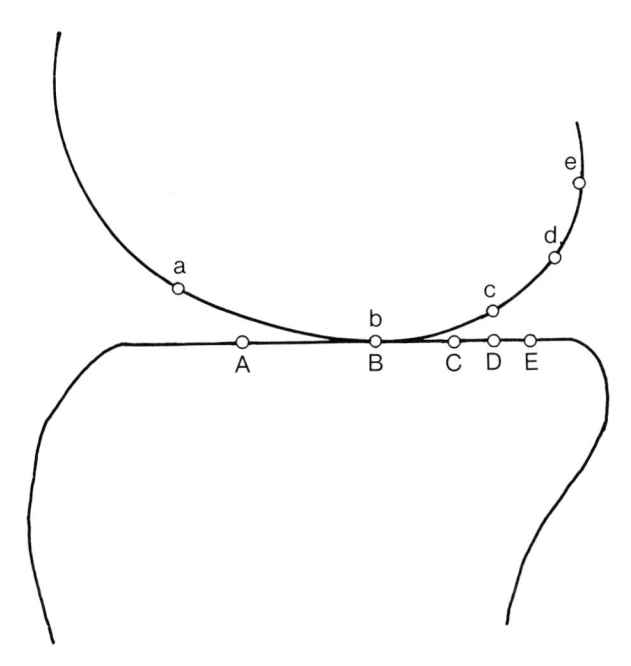

Fig. 5-10 *The ratio of points AB:ab is equal to 1:2. The ratio of points DE:de is equal to 1:4. This is the result of the combined rolling and gliding during flexion-extension.*

If the tibia is placed in internal rotation with the knee flexed 90 degrees, the iliotibial band is the primary restraint with both clinical and functional forces.[2] If the knee is then placed in external rotation, the medial collateral ligament is the primary restraint with clinical forces but the anterior cruciate ligament is the primary restraint with functional forces.

To understand the pivot-shift phenomenon it is necessary to appreciate the kinematics of the normal and the anterior cruciate deficient knee. As the normal knee is flexed, the joint surfaces undergo a combination of sliding and rolling movements. The precise ratio varies with joint position but starts with a rolling to gliding ratio of 1:2 and ends in full flexion with a ratio of 1:4[11] (Fig. 5-10). This implies that sliding predominates in all joint positions. This relationship is determined by the joint geometry and the ligaments. The cruciate ligaments are the dominant ligamentous restraints controlling this ratio.

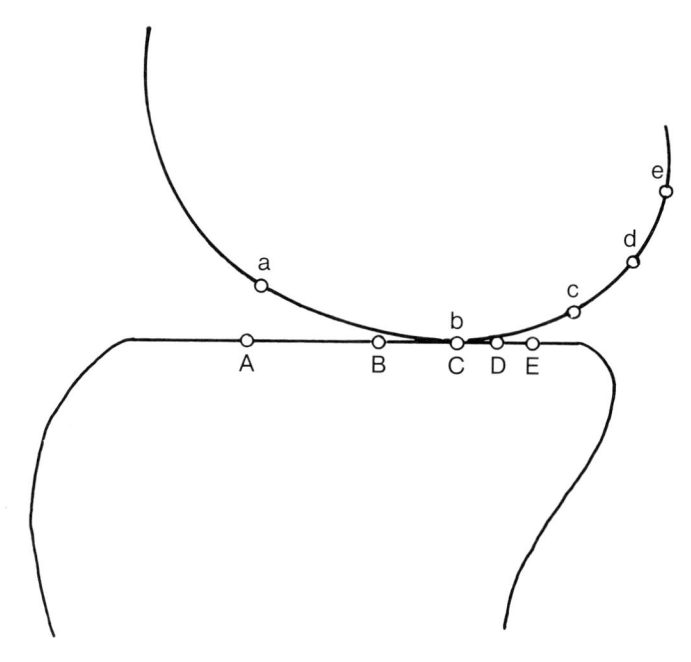

Fig. 5-11 *The increased rolling in anterior cruciate ligament deficient knee causes the tibia to sublux anteriorly.*

In the anterior cruciate deficient knee rolling movement predominates during early flexion.[16] This causes the tibia to sublux anteriorly (Fig. 5-11). The greater radius of curvature of the lateral femoral condyle and the convexity of the lateral tibial plateau contribute to the relatively greater amount of anterior displacement of the lateral tibial plateau (internal rotation) (Fig. 5-12).[7] It is important to remember that both the medial and lateral sides sublux anteriorly.

The iliotibial band plays a central role in the pivot-shift phenomenon. In the normal knee the iliotibial band functions as a knee extensor when the knee is extended because its mean line of force is anterior to the flexion axis of the knee (Fig. 5-13). When the knee is fully flexed, the iliotibial band's mean line of force is posterior to the flexion axis of the knee and it functions as a knee flexor. There is a critical point between 20 and 30 degrees of flexion when the mean line of force intersects with the central axis. Flexion past this point converts the extensor function of the iliotibial band to flexion. If the knee ligaments are intact, this is a smooth transition.

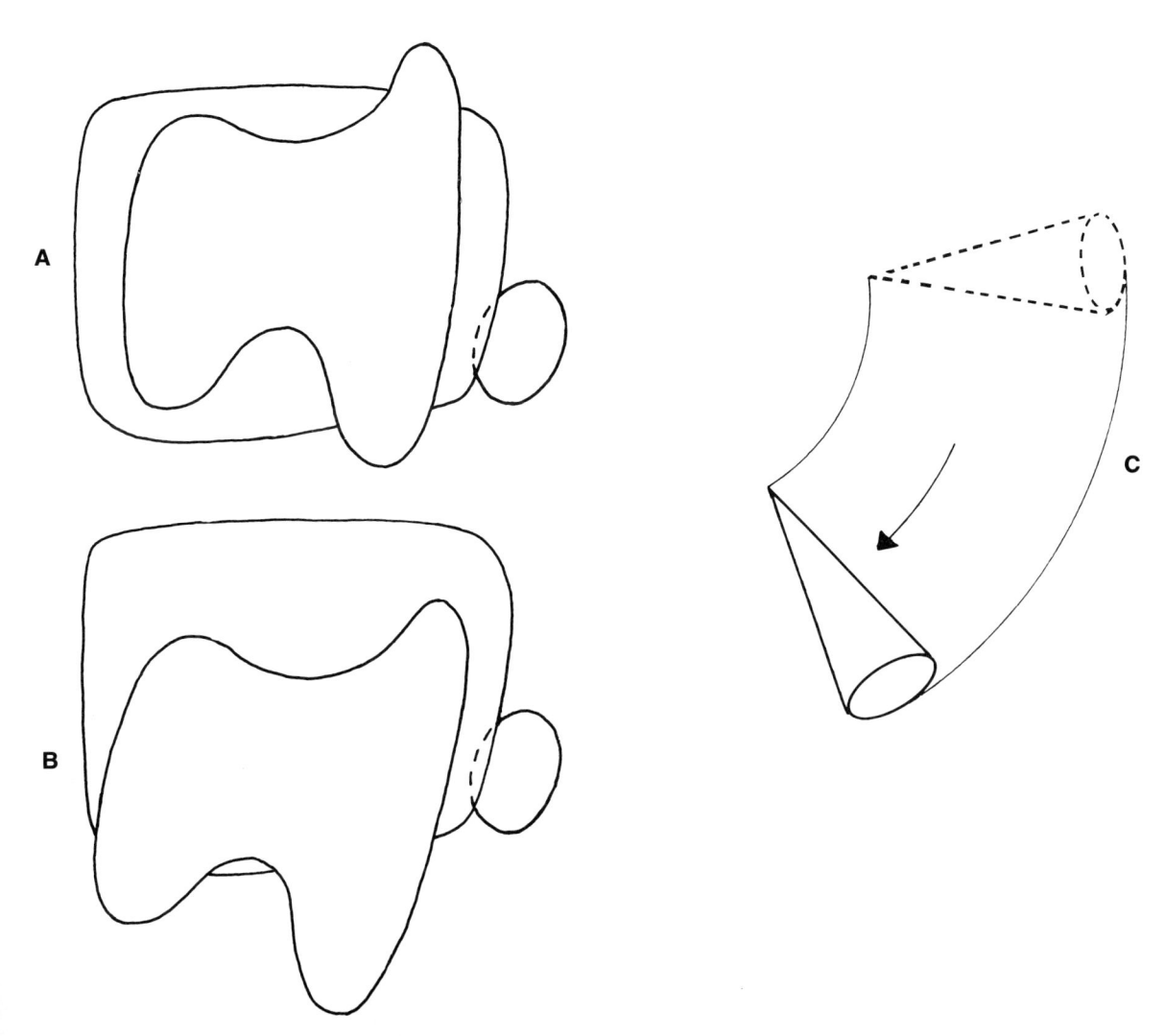

Fig. 5-12 The example is distorted for emphasis. **A** and **B**, The lateral femoral condyles greater radius of curvature contributes to the internal rotation of the tibia as it subluxes anteriorly. **C**, An ice cream cone is a familiar example of this phenomenon.

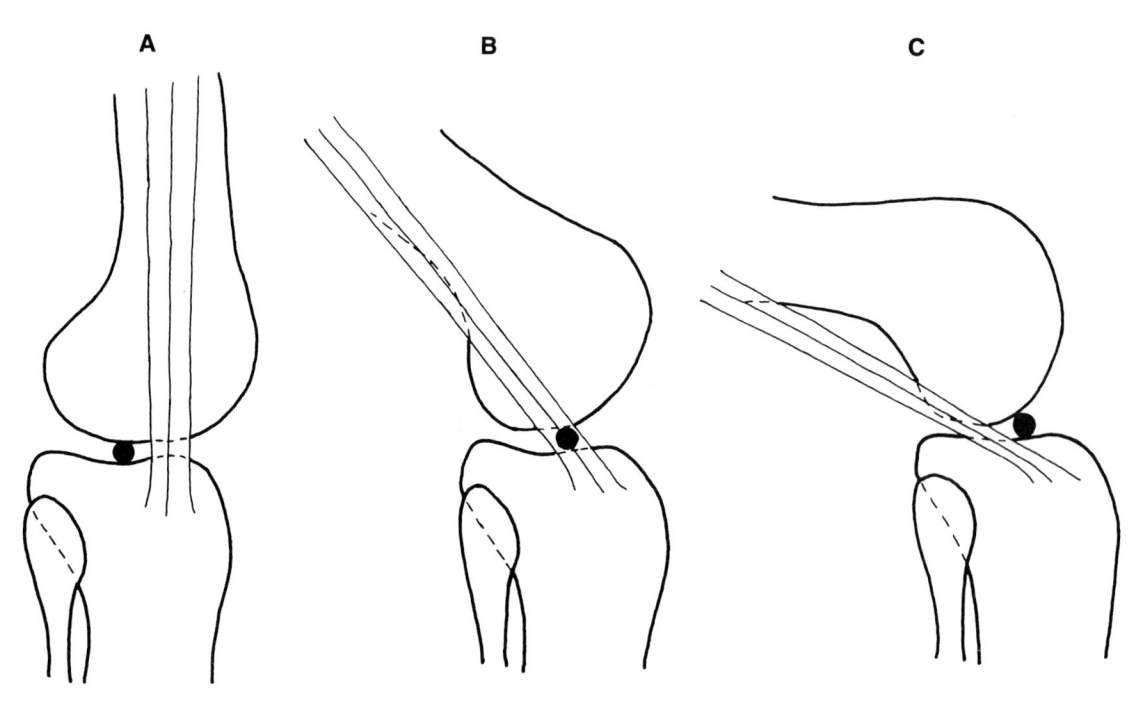

Fig. 5-13 *The normal knee.* ***A,*** *The iliotibial band (ITB) is anterior to the transverse flexon axis in extension.* ***B,*** *The ITB intersects with the transverse flexion axis at 20 degrees of flexion.* ***C,*** *The ITB is posterior to the transverse flexion axis at greater than 20 degrees of flexion.*

Loss of the anterior cruciate ligament is a necessary condition for production of the pivot shift phenomenon.[4] As the anterior cruciate deficient knee is flexed from full extension, the femur rolls on the tibial plateau. This produces an anterior translation of the tibia (Fig. 5-14). Tension on the iliotibial band is increased because it is abnormally lengthened during this phase. When the knee flexion angle passes the critical point, the iliotibial band suddenly becomes a knee flexor and the direction of the force pulls the tibia posteriorly into the reduced position. It continues to hold the tibia in the reduced position for the remainder of knee flexion.

The iliotibial band is functioning as a dynamic restraint against anterior laxity. The sudden reduction is the "pivot shift." It is accentuated by lateral and posterior-lateral capsular laxity.[7] Internal rotation will increase the reduction phenomenon because it increased the original subluxation; for this same reason, external rotation may eliminate the pivot shift because of decreased subluxation.

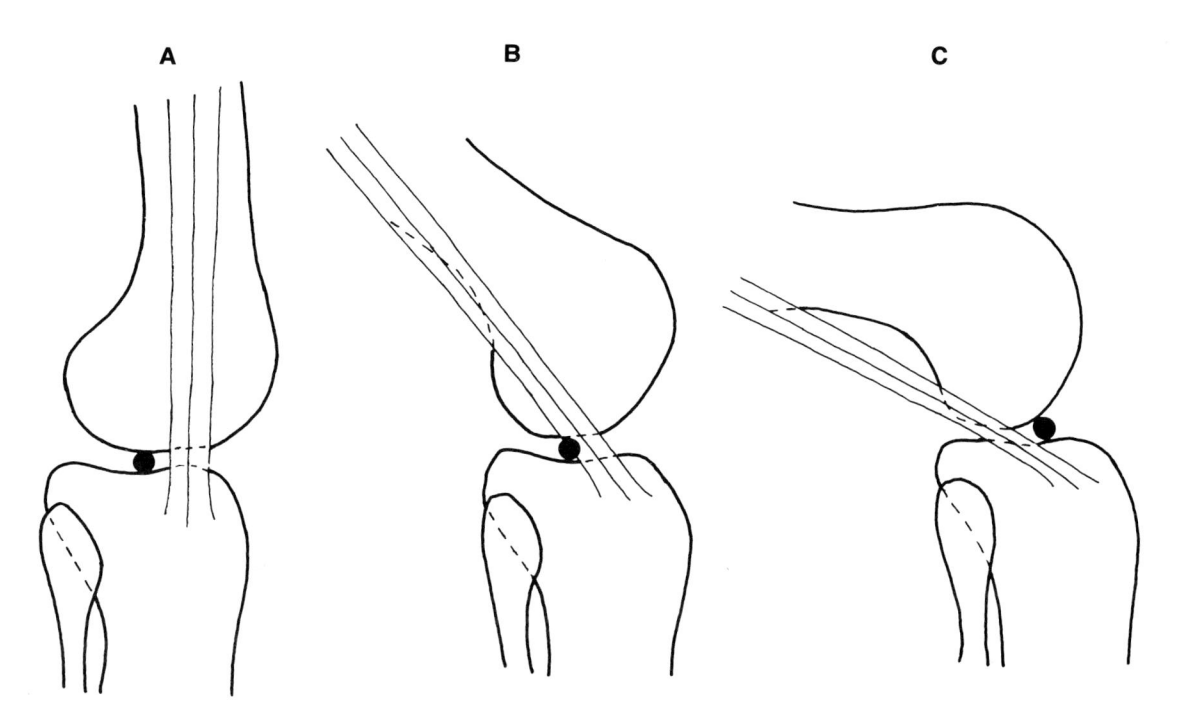

Fig. 5-14 *The anterior cruciate ligament deficient knee. **A**, The iliotibial band (ITB) is anterior to the transverse flexion axis in extension. **B**, The ITB is still anterior to the transverse flexion axis at 20 degrees of flexion. **C**, The ITB becomes posterior to the transverse flexion axis at the greater flexion angle than in the normal knee. When this occurs the anterior subluxation and internal rotation are reduced.*

True pivot-shift test versus the reversed pivot-shift test

Before we conclude our discussion of the clinical examination, it is essential that we distinguish a true pivot-shift test from a reversed pivot-shift test. The *reversed pivot-shift test* is done with the patient in the supine position[20] (Fig. 5-15). The examiner places one hand around the patient's ankle and the patient's foot is placed against the examiner's pelvis. The other hand of the examiner is used to support the lateral side of the calf with the palm on the proximal fibula. The knee is then flexed to 70 degrees. The tibia is externally rotated and a valgus strain is applied. The patient's leg is slowly extended while a small axial load is applied. If the test is positive, the lateral tibial plateau will suddenly move forward and internally rotate when the knee approaches about 20 degrees of flexion. The knee is now in a reduced position. This is the opposite of what happens in the true pivot-shift test where the tibia subluxes in extension and reduces in flexion.

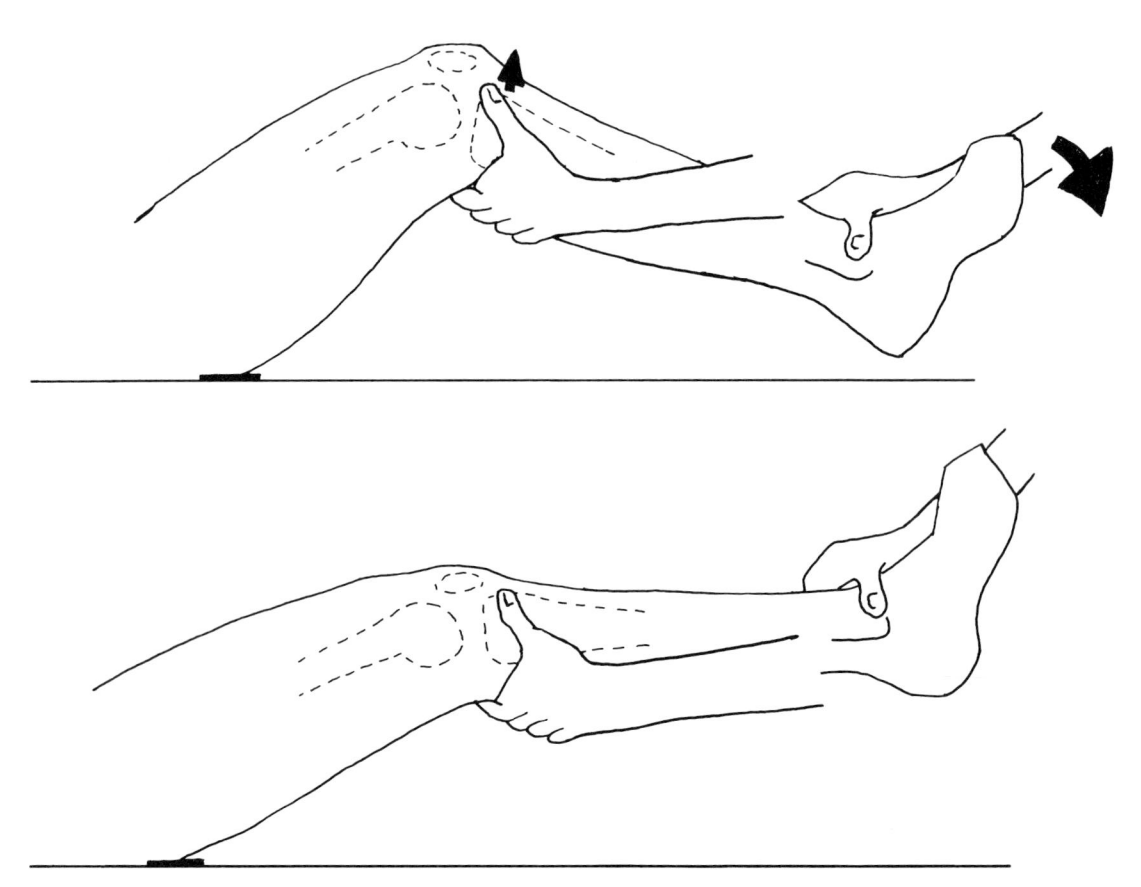

Fig. 5-15 *The reverse pivot-shift test. The tibia is held in external rotation. The test is positive if the tibia assumes a reduced position as the knee is extended.*

The specific anatomical lesion in the reversed pivot-shift test is in the popliteus muscle and tendon with its expansion to the arcuate ligament.[7] With the loss of posterior-lateral stability the femur rolls excessively on the tibia as the knee is extended. This results in a posterior subluxation of the tibia. It also produces external rotation for the same reasons that produced internal rotation during the true pivot-shift test. When the knee extends past 20 degrees the lateral gastrocnemius muscle and posterior capsule are tightened, forcing the tibia into the reduced position with a snap. The forward translation of the lateral tibial plateau produces internal rotation of the tibia. For the remainder of extension the rolling to sliding ratios are normal. Internal rotation abolished this phenomenon because the tibia is held in the reduced position. Posterior cruciate deficiency will accentuate the test because it allows additional posterior subluxation before reduction.

REFERENCES

1. Arnold, J.A., et al.: Natural history of anterior cruciate tears, Am. J. Sports Med. **7:** 305-313, 1979.
2. Butler, D.L., Noyes, F.R., and Grood, E.S.: Ligamentous restraints in the human knee: anterior-posterior stability, Orthop. Trans. **2:**161-162, 1978.
3. Butler, D.L., Noyes, F.R., and Grood, E.S.: Ligamentous restraints to anterior-posterior drawer in the human knee, J. Bone Joint Surg. (Am.) **62:**259-270, 1980.
4. Fetto, J.F., and Marshall, J.L.: Injury to the anterior cruciate ligament producing the pivot shift sign, J. Bone Joint Surg. (Am.) **61:**710-714, 1979.
5. Galway, H.R., and MacIntosh, D.L.: The lateral pivot shift: a symptom and sign of anterior cruciate ligament insufficiency, Clin. Orthop. **147:**45-50, 1980.
6. Grood, E.S., and Noyes, F.R.: Cruciate ligament prosthesis: strength, creep, and fatigue properties, J. Bone Joint Surg. (Am.) **58:**1083-1088, 1976.
7. Jakob, R.P., Hassler, H., and Staeubli, H.: Observations on rotatory instability of the lateral compartment of the knee, Acta Orthop. Scand. (Suppl. 191), **152:**1-32, 1981.
8. Jonsson, T., et al.: Clinical diagnosis of ruptures of the anterior cruciate ligament, Am. J. Sports Med. **10:**100-102, 1982.
9. Losee, R.E.: Concepts of the pivot shift, Clin. Orthop. **172:**45-51, 1983.
10. Losee, R.E., Johnson, T.R., and Southwick, W.O.: Anterior subluxation of the lateral tibial plateau, J. Bone Joint Surg. (Am.) **60:** 1015-1030, 1978.
11. Müller, W.: The knee: form, function and ligament reconstruction, Berlin, 1982, Springer-Verlag.
12. Noyes, F.R., Grood, E.S., Butler, D.L., et al.: Clinical laxity tests and functional stability of the knee: biomechanical concepts, Clin. Orthop. **146:**84-89, 1980.
13. Noyes, F.R., Grood, E.S., Suntag, W.J., et al.: The three dimensional laxity of the anterior cruciate deficient knee as determined by clinical laxity tests, Iowa Orthop. J. **3:**32-44, 1982.
14. Slocum, D.B., and Larson, R.L.: Rotatory instability of the knee, J. Bone Joint Surg. (Am.) **50:**211-225, 1968.
15. Slocum, D.B., James, S.L., Larson, R.L., et al.: Clinical test for anterolateral rotatory instability of the knee, Clin. Orthop. **118:** 63-69, 1976.
16. Tamea, C.D., and Henning, C.E.: Pathomechanics of the pivot shift maneuver, Am. J. Sports Med. **9:**31-37, 1981.
17. Torg, J.S., Conrad, W., and Kalen, V.: Clinical diagnosis of anterior cruciate ligament instability in the athlete, Sports Med. **4:**84-93, 1976.

6

Quantitative examination for anterior cruciate laxity

KEITH L. MARKOLF

There are a number of distinct advantages in performing instrumented knee testing to quantify the knee laxity examination. For example:
1. The manual clinical examination tends to be subjective in nature, since unknown forces are applied to the lower limb and since tibial-femoral motions are visually estimated.
2. Stiffness of the knee can be sensed clinically as a "soft" or "firm" resistance to applied force but cannot be quantified unless the load deformation response curve of the knee is recorded and the slope of the curve calculated.
3. Stiffness and laxity as calculated from the anteroposterior force versus displacement curve of the knee can be used to detect the presence or absence of the anterior cruciate ligament in a noninvasive manner.
4. The effectiveness of anterior cruciate ligament substitution with autogenous tissue, allografts, or synthetic ligaments can be accurately assessed by preoperative and postoperative comparisons of stiffness and laxity values computed from the force versus displacement curves.

The UCLA portable instrumented clinical testing apparatus

A clinical testing apparatus capable of recording anteroposterior force versus displacement response curves of the tibia with respect to the femur has been under development at the UCLA biomechanics laboratory since 1976.[3] Our newest portable version of this research device is shown in Fig. 6-1. In using this device, the examiner has the patient sit on the floor against a reclining back support with his knee flexed to 20 degrees. The femur is clamped to the base of the device by a framework containing sand-filled leather

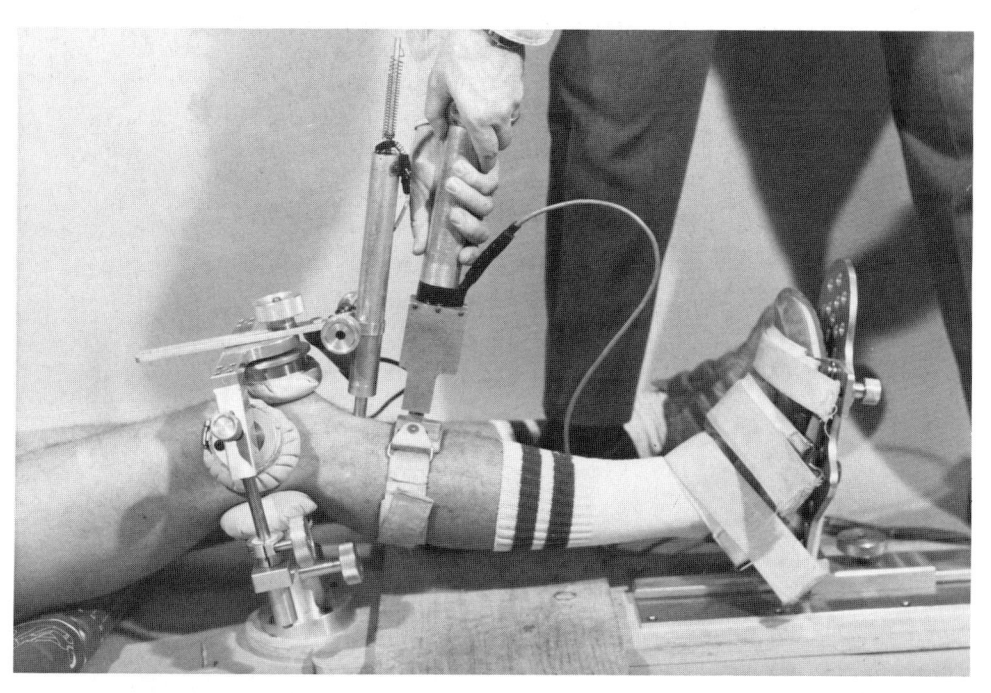

Fig. 6-1 *The UCLA portable instrumented clinical knee testing apparatus records a continuous force versus displacement response curve on an x-y recorder. The femur is clamped by a framework containing sand pads while 200 N of force is applied to the tibia with a load cell connected to a strap encircling the calf. Displacement of the tibial tubercle is measured by a transducer connected to a spring-loaded plunger.*

pouches that fix the femoral condyles and patella. Care is taken to ensure that the joint line is anterior to the posterior sand pads so that posterior tibial displacement will not be blocked. The foot is strapped to a movable plate that allows testing in positions of internal and external tibial rotation. An anteroposterior force of 200 N (45 lbs) is applied to the tibia through an instrumented load cell connected to a small anterior pad strapped to the tibia. Tibial displacement is measured by a spring-loaded plunger that contacts the tibial tubercle and connects to a displacement transducer. Accurate test curves require that the femur be "grounded" to the test base. Before recording a test curve, the examiner grasps the interface between the sand pad and the peripheral margins of the patella with the fingers to detect possible patellar movement as tibial force is applied. Three or four preliminary test curves are then recorded to check for repeatability and muscle guarding. If muscle guarding is present, it can be detected easily by irregularities in the response curve.

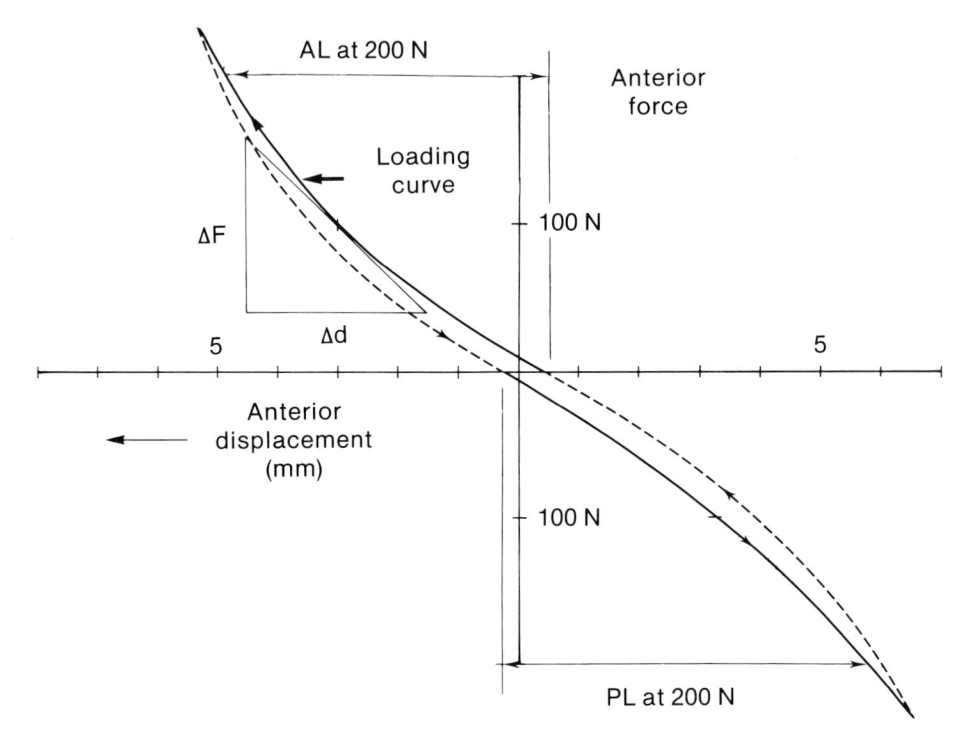

Fig. 6-2 *A sample force versus displacement test curve. Anterior laxity (AL) is measured as the horizontal distance along the loading curve between 0 and 200 N of applied anterior tibial force. Anterior stiffness is calculated from the slope of the anterior loading curve at 100 N of applied force.*

A typical force versus displacement curve is shown in Fig. 6-2. Although a full hysteresis loop is recorded, only the anterior and posterior loading curves are used for analysis. Anterior laxity is defined as the tibial displacement measured along the anterior loading curve. Anterior laxity is computed at 200 N of applied anterior force. Anterior stiffness, which is calculated at 100 N of applied force, is defined as the slope of the anterior loading curve.

Laxity and stiffness of normal knees

One would expect laxity and stiffness to be equal for both knees in a normal individual, and on the average this is true. However, laxity and left-right differences in laxity are normally distributed and follow a Gaussian or bell-shaped probability distribution (Fig. 6-3). As a result of testing normal subjects with this device, we have

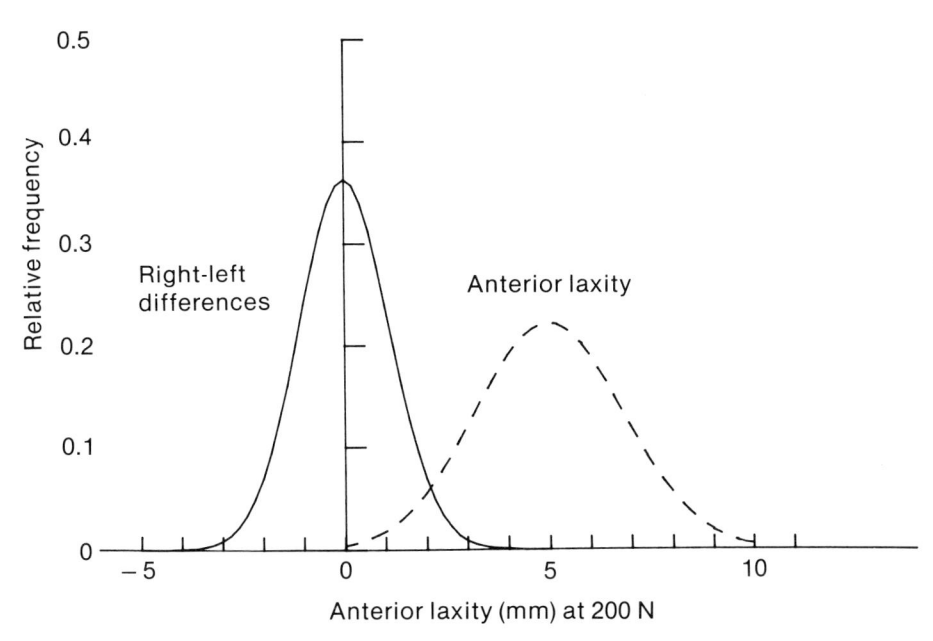

Fig. 6-3 *Normal knee variation. Gaussian probability distributions for anterior laxity (dashed line) and right-left differences in anterior laxity (solid line) for normal, uninjured individuals.*

established 95% confidence intervals for the "normal" ranges of laxity and stiffness and for right-left differences in laxity and stiffness. A convenient way of displaying right-left scatter is shown in Fig. 6-4, A, where right laxity is plotted versus left laxity. If laxities were identical for both knees, all points would lie on a 45-degree line. However, because of normal side to side variation, the points are spread on either side of this line. The dashed 45-degree lines define the limits of the normal range for right-left scatter, that is, 95% of the points will lie within the bounds of the dashed 45-degree lines (2 mm side to side laxity difference). Also shown is the cut-off limit for the upper boundary of anterior laxity, illustrating that at 200 N, 95% of normal knees will have an anterior laxity less than 7.5 mm. The mean anterior laxity of a normal knee as measured with our device is approximately 5 mm.

Fig. 6-4, B shows a normal scattergram for anterior stiffness at 100 N. This figure illustrates that 95% of normal uninjured individuals will have an anterior stiffness greater than 30 N/mm and a side to side difference less than 20 N/mm.

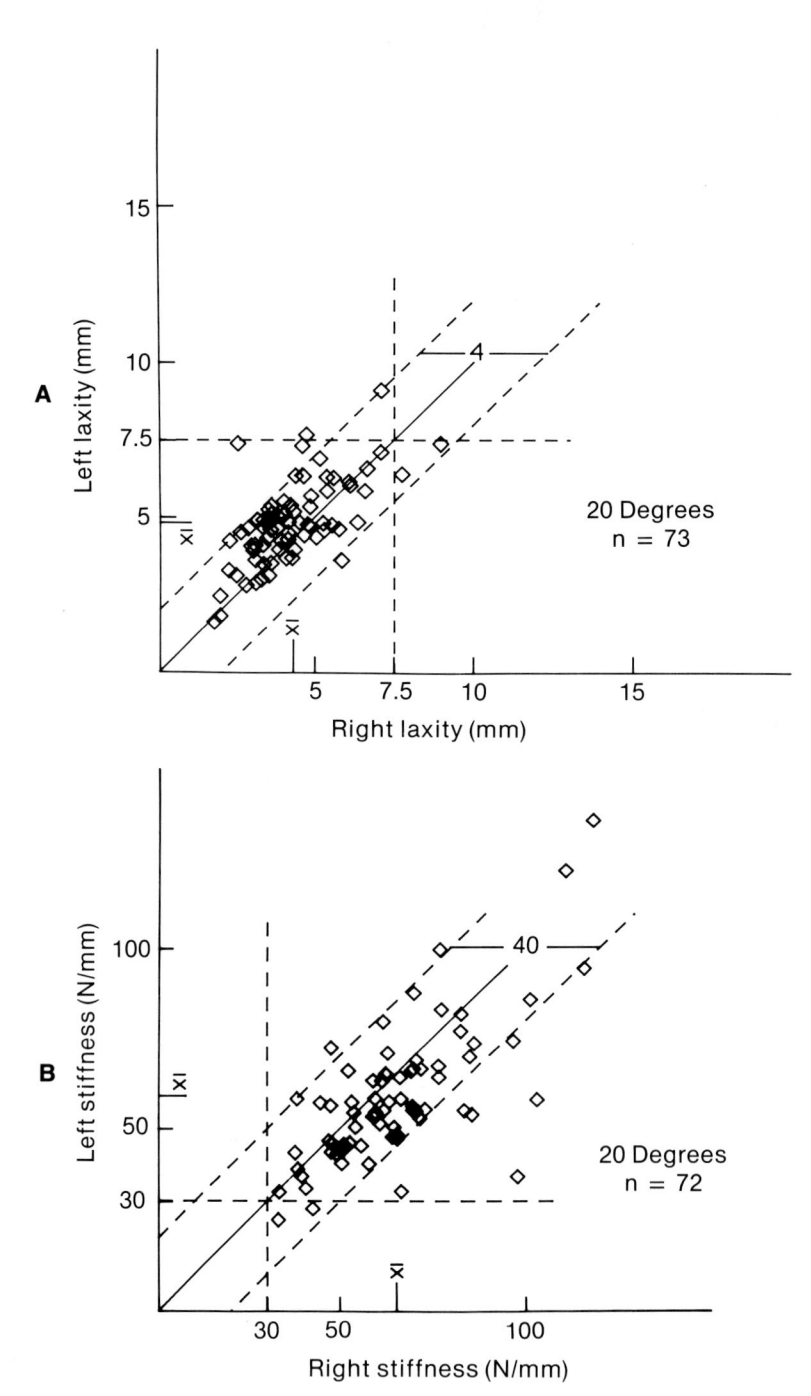

Fig. 6-4 *For legend see opposite page.*

Laxity and stiffness of anterior cruciate deficient knees

As measured with the UCLA clinical testing apparatus, an anterior cruciate deficient knee has an anterior laxity of approximately 10 mm. The scattergram of anterior laxity for a group of 99 patients with documented absence of the anterior cruciate ligament in one knee and an uninjured opposite extremity is shown in Fig. 6-5, *A*. Most patients, but not all, have an injured knee laxity greater than 7.5 mm and a right-left difference greater than 2 mm. One might question how some anterior cruciate deficient knees can still lie within the normal range. It must be remembered that everyone has a "tight" knee and a "loose" knee. If an individual with a large right-left difference (before injury) should happen to injure the "tight" knee, the laxity increase resulting from loss of the anterior cruciate ligament may not be enough to bring the right-left difference outside of the normal range. Similarly, Fig. 6-5, *B* shows that not all anterior cruciate deficient patients have an anterior stiffness less than 30 N/mm and an injured-normal difference less than 40 N/mm.

The 99 "pooled" anterior cruciate deficient patients shown in Fig. 6-5, *A* and *B* represent all of the anterior cruciate deficient patients we have tested at UCLA. Over half of these patients were tested with our "dental chair" prototype of this apparatus.[4] In studying those patients tested only with the new portable version, which has more reliable femoral clamping, we were able to correctly classify 90% to 95% of the anterior cruciate deficient patients as testing outside the normal range.

Fig. 6-4 *A, Right versus left scattergram of anterior laxity for a group of normal knees at 200 N. The locations (x) on the horizontal and vertical axes represent the mean values of laxity for the right and left knees. The vertical and horizontal dashed lines are 95% confidence cut-off levels that bound the normal range of anterior laxity. The 45-degree dashed lines bound the 95% confidence intervals for side to side differences in anterior laxity for a normal population. Ninety-five percent of normal knees will have an anterior laxity less than 7.5 mm and a side to side difference in anterior laxity less than 2 mm. B, Right versus left scattergram of anterior stiffness for a group of normal knees at 100 N. Ninety-five percent of normal knees will have an anterior stiffness greater than 30 N/mm and a side to side difference in anterior stiffness less than 20 N/mm.*

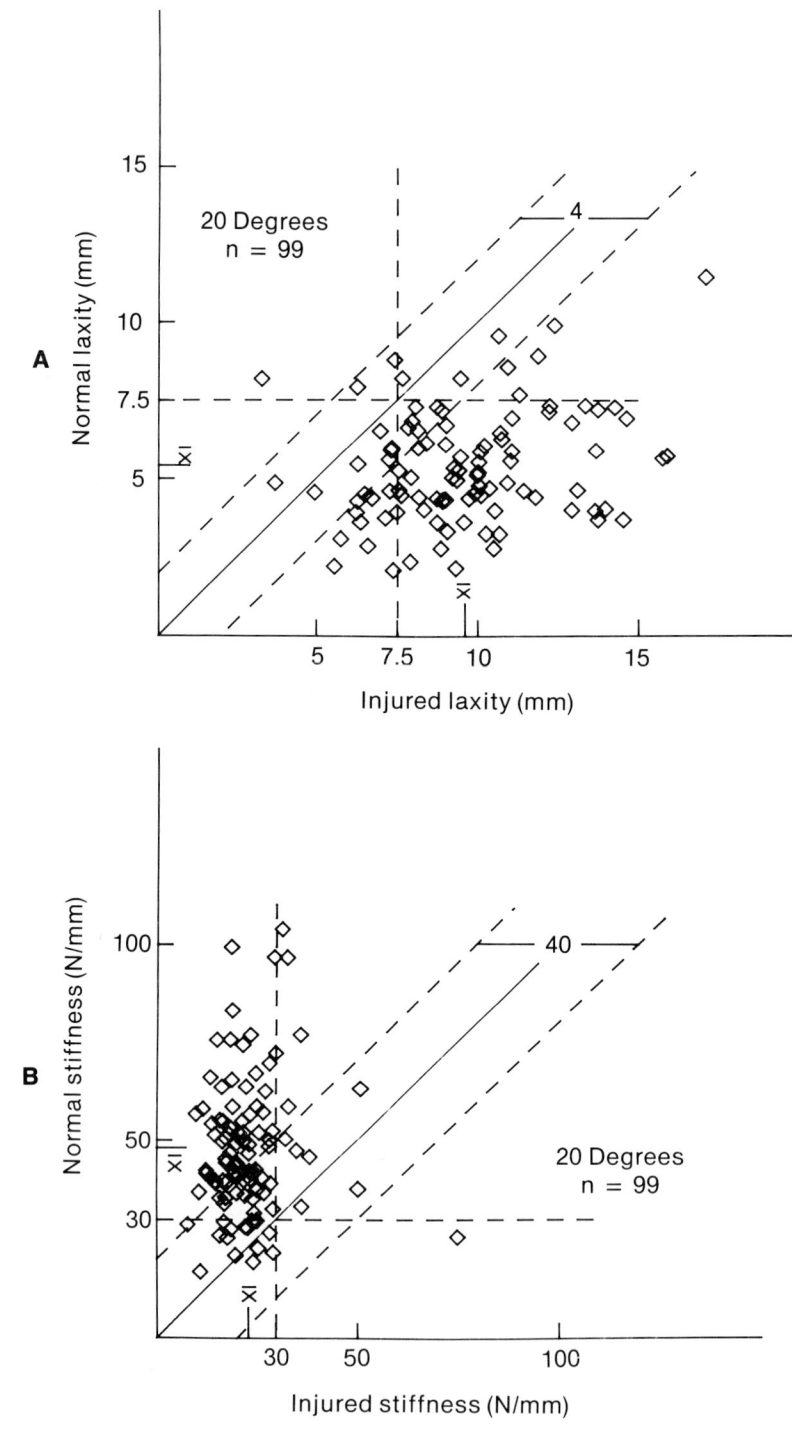

Fig. 6-5 *A, Injured versus normal scattergram of anterior laxity at 200 N for a group of patients with documented absence of the anterior cruciate ligament in one knee and a normal opposite extremity. Note that a number of anterior cruciate deficient knees lie within the normal range. B, Injured versus normal scattergram of anterior stiffness at 100 N for the same group of anterior cruciate deficient knees depicted in A. Again a considerable number of patients lie within the normal range.*

Anteroposterior testing of anterior cruciate deficient patients undergoing intra-articular reconstructions

Our first study of anterior cruciate deficient patients[2] consisted of eleven individuals with intra-articular anterior cruciate ligament reconstructions using the medial or lateral one third of the patellar tendon plus extra-articular procedures and a second group of seven patients with extra-articular procedures alone. All patients were tested preoperatively and 3 years postoperatively. The major finding of this study is illustrated in Fig. 6-6, A and B. Mean anteroposterior force versus displacement test curves at 20 degrees are presented for both patient groups. At 3 years, the mean anterior loading curve for the injured knees of the substitution group was not significantly different from that of the uninjured knees; in the group without substitution, the anterior curve for the injured knees was unchanged by the extra-articular procedures. In terms of actual laxity measurements, the anterior cruciate ligament substitution group had a mean preoperative laxity value of 12.2 mm and an injured-normal laxity difference of 6.3 mm. These values were improved by surgery to 5.7 mm and 1.5 mm respectively at 3 years follow-up. In contrast, the group without substitution showed no significant changes in laxity at 3 years. A return to normal anterior stiffness was also observed at 3 years for the group receiving substitution, while stiffness was unchanged in the group receiving extra-articular procedures only. However, it was interesting that the activity scores, the decreased feelings of giving way, and the elimination of the pivot shift were comparable for both groups of patients, suggesting that improvements in dynamic function may have been attributed to the extra-articular procedure.

More recently, we have tested two groups of patients postoperatively who had documented absence of the anterior cruciate ligament.[1] The first group consisted of 76 patients who had an intra-articular substitution of an absent anterior cruciate ligament using the torn meniscus. The second group consisted of 34 patients who underwent partial meniscectomy, had no anterior cruciate ligament substitution, and were simply followed along. Fig. 6-7, A and B show scattergrams for laxity and stiffness of the substitution group; it is apparent that a great many patients are outside the normal ranges for both groups. However, there were small but significant differences in stiffness and laxity between the groups. The substitution group had an average of 1.4 mm less side to side difference in

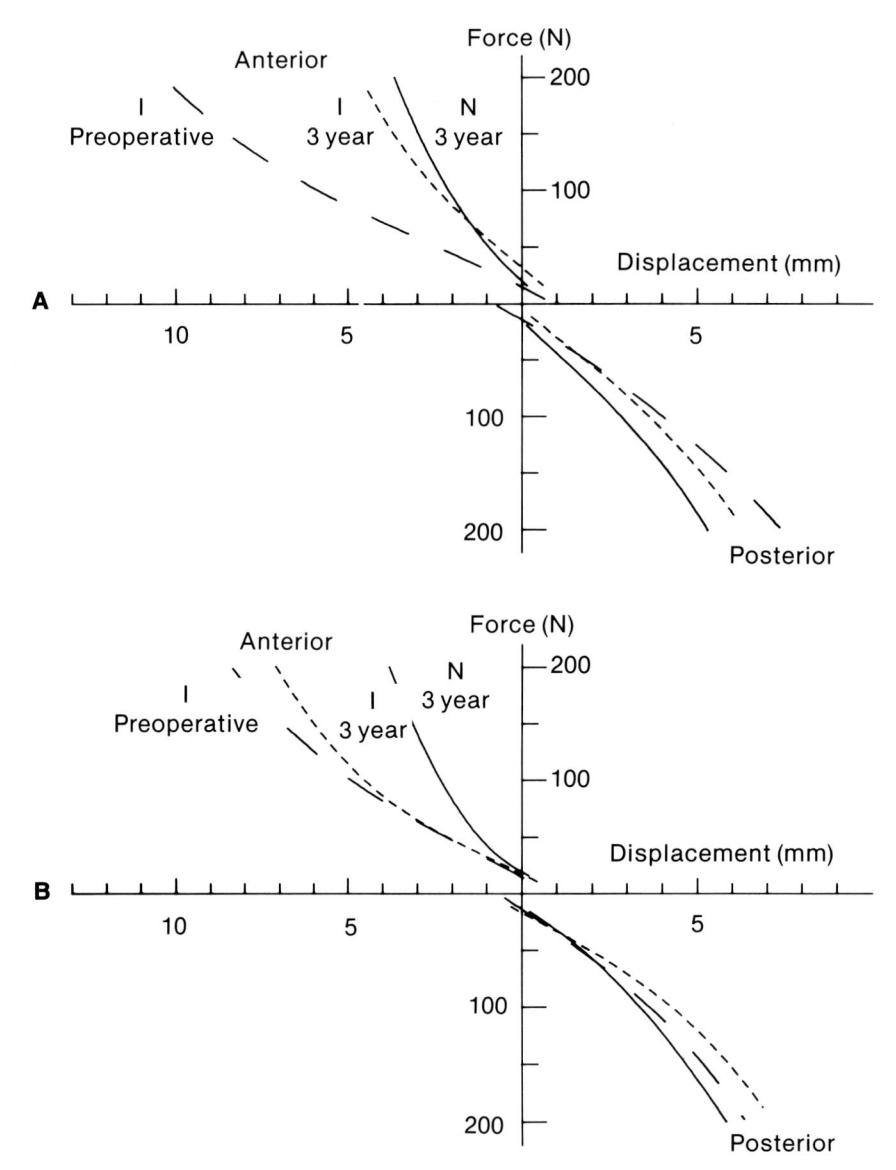

Fig. 6-6 *A, Preoperative and 3-year postoperative mean anteroposterior force versus displacement curves for knees having an intra-articular anterior cruciate ligament substitution with a portion of the patellar tendon (20-degree flexion). The 3-year postoperative curve for the injured knee is not statistically different from that of the normal knee. B, Preoperative and 3-year postoperative mean curves for patients not receiving an anterior cruciate ligament substitution (20-degree flexion). The curve for the injured knee is unchanged 3 years after surgery.*

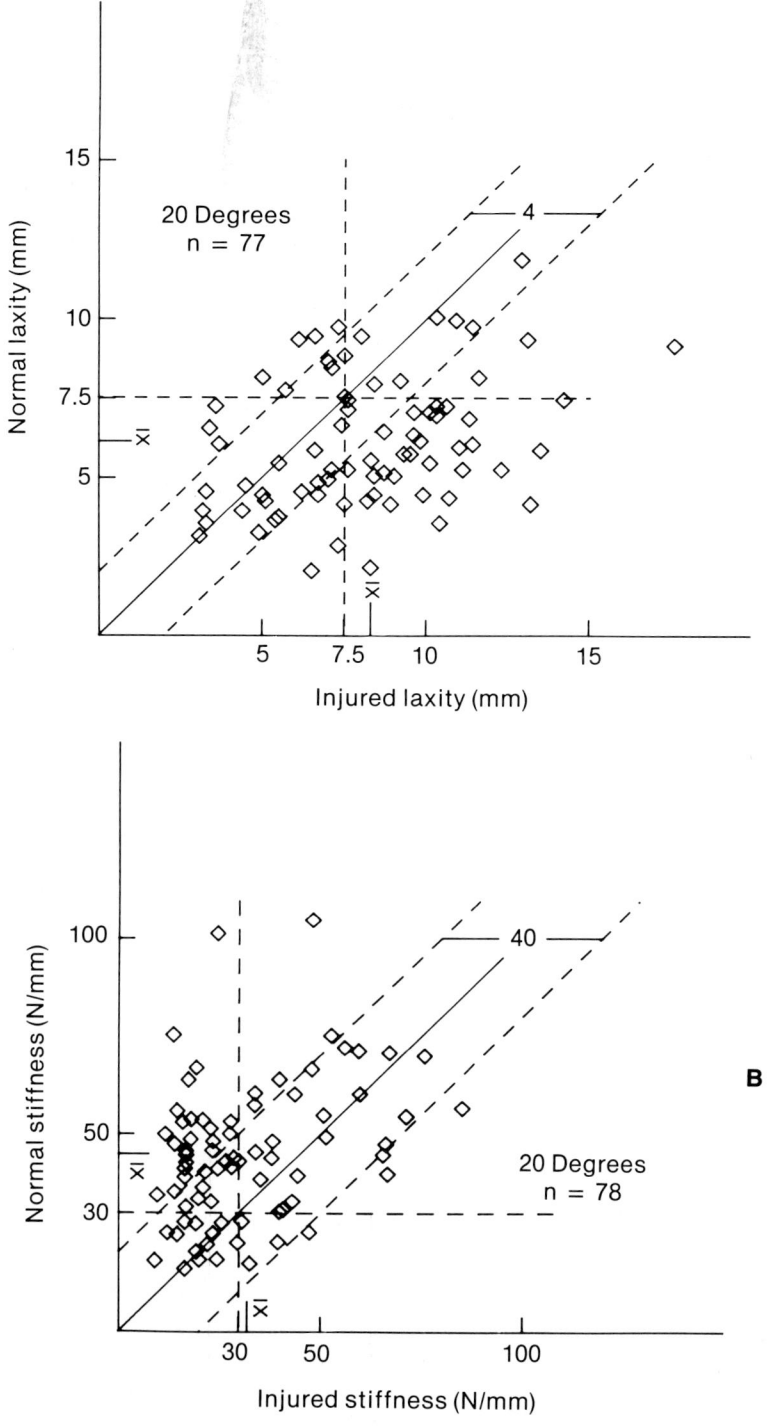

Fig. 6-7 *A, Three-year postoperative injured versus normal scattergram of anterior laxity at 200 N for patients receiving an intra-articular anterior cruciate ligament substitution using the torn meniscus. Note that seven patients were over-corrected by the surgical procedure and lie to the left of the 45-degree line. B, Scattergram of anterior stiffness at 100 N for the meniscal substitution patients in A. Four patients lie to the right of the 45-degree dashed line, indicating that their injured knees are now stiffer than their normal knees and that they are beyond the normal right-left limit.*

laxity. Of the substituted patients, 51% still had an injured knee laxity that was at least 2 mm greater than the uninjured knee; this can be contrasted to 76% of the partial meniscectomy patients who exceeded this upper limit of the normal range. At 20 degrees, anterior stiffness of the injured knees of the substitution patients was 26% greater than the injured knees of the partial meniscectomy group; 42% of the substituted patients had an injured knee stiffness within the normal range, while only 18% of the partial meniscectomy patients fell within normal limits.

The major conclusion reached in this study was that the meniscal substitution procedure clearly did not restore to normal the stiffness and laxity of a great many patients. Clinically however, there were clear differences in Lysholm scores: the meniscal substitution group had 84% good-excellent results, 12% fair, and 4% poor, while the group without substitution had only 47% good-excellent results, 23% fair, and 21% poor.

Summary

Our studies to date have produced what seem to be contradictory findings. In the one instance there were large differences in static stability as measured by the UCLA portable instrumented clinical knee testing apparatus and no differences in patient function. In the second, there were smaller group differences in stiffness and laxity but greater differences in clinical function. These results serve to emphasize the fact that the role of biomechanical stability testing has yet to be clearly defined. The stiffness and laxity information gained from these tests provide additional information for the evaluation of results of a surgical procedure. Biomechanical test results cannot be considered in isolation since they are meant to supplement but not replace a thorough clinical examination and patient history. More patient studies with instrumented testing devices are needed before final conclusions can be drawn as to their usefulness.

REFERENCES

1. Ferkel, R., Goodfellow, D., Markolf, K., et al.: The ACL deficient knee: substitute or follow along? Proceedings of the 30th Annual Meeting of the Orthopaedic Research Society, **9**:132, 1984.
2. Kochan, A., Markolf, K., and More, R.: Anterior-posterior stiffness and laxity of the knee following major ligamentous reconstruction, J. Bone Joint Surg. (Am.) **66**:1460-1465, 1984.
3. Markolf, K., Graff-Radford, A., and Amstutz, H.: In vivo knee stability: a quantitative assessment using an instrumented clinical testing apparatus, J. Bone Joint Surg. (Am.) **60**:664-674, 1978.
4. Markolf, K., Kochan, A., and Amstutz, H.: Measurement of knee stiffness and laxity in patients with documented absence of the anterior cruciate ligament, J. Bone Joint Surg. (Am.) **66**:242-253, 1984.

7
Isometric placement of substitutes for the anterior cruciate ligament

BEN GRAF

The reproducible placement of substitutes for the anterior cruciate ligament is essential if predictable results are to be obtained. Melhorn and Henning have shown that in some instances, postoperative laxity can be correlated with errors in placement.[6] They found that isometrically placed grafts resulted in the most stable knees. Over-the-top placement consistently produced a negative Lachman test but a positive anterior drawer test; a too anterior femoral origin produced a positive Lachman test and a negative anterior drawer test. Our own study, which compares all combinations of twelve femoral and three tibial sites for attaching anterior cruciate ligaments in ten cadaveric knees, supports the observations of Melhorn and Henning. We agree that the isometric placement of current substitutes for anterior cruciate ligaments is desirable, and we have developed a technique that can help surgeons attain this goal.

The normal anterior cruciate ligament

Before proposing the isometric placement of ligament substitutes, we first examine the behavior of the normal anterior cruciate ligament. Although the kinematics of the knee can be modeled with a four-bar linkage that uses isometrically placed segments of fixed length to represent cruciate ligaments, the function of real cruciate ligaments is much more complicated. The anterior and posterior cruciate ligaments are three-dimensional structures with broad attachments and a continuum of fibers. These fibers are of different lengths, have different attachment sites, and are under different tensions. Although the fibers that are often described as making up the anteromedial bundle of the anterior cruciate ligament, are nearly isometric,[1] most of the anterior cruciate ligament is lax when the knee is flexed and only becomes taut as the knee is fully extended.[2,4]

There are reasons why not all fibers of the anterior cruciate ligament are isometrically placed. We have found that areas for isometric attachment are quite small, and it would not be possible for a large ligament such as the anterior cruciate ligament to insert entirely in such a restricted area. Also, the orientation of nonisometric fibers differs from that of isometric fibers. When the knee is extended, for example, the nonisometric fibers with low and posterior femoral origins are more horizontal than the vertically oriented isometric fibers. The nonisometric fibers therefore may be better positioned to resist anterior tibial displacement. More complete data on fiber-specific strain are needed for a fuller understanding of the functions of the individual cruciate fibers.

Although many cruciate fibers are not isometric, isometric placement is desirable because current substitutes for cruciate ligaments have not duplicated the complex orientation of normal anterior cruciate ligaments. Fibers are generally of equal length, arranged parallel to one another, and under tensions not determined for each individual fiber but for the ligament as a whole. Even though complex substitutes with several independently located and tensioned bundles of fibers may better reproduce the functions of the anterior cruciate ligament, current substitutes are best when placed isometrically. Such placement maximizes the number of fibers that can be taut throughout the range of motion and allows for early knee motion without generating high ligament strains. In our laboratory study we found that osseous tunnels only 5 mm apart produce significantly different strains in a cruciate substitute.[5] This result emphasizes the importance of accurate placement. A too anterior placement of the anterior cruciate ligament origin or insertion results in a ligament that is taut in flexion but lax in extension. Posterior placement, as in the over-the-top femoral position, causes the ligament to be taut in extension but lax in flexion. Only isometric placement provides stability throughout the range of motion.

Determining isometric sites for anterior cruciate ligament insertion

Instruments and outline of technique

To evaluate potential points of ligament insertion, Kirschner (K) wires are passed from the lateral femoral metaphysis to the proposed anterior cruciate ligament origin and from the medial tibial metaphysis to the proposed tibial insertion. A suture is passed through the holes left by the K-wires and proximally secured with a clamp or

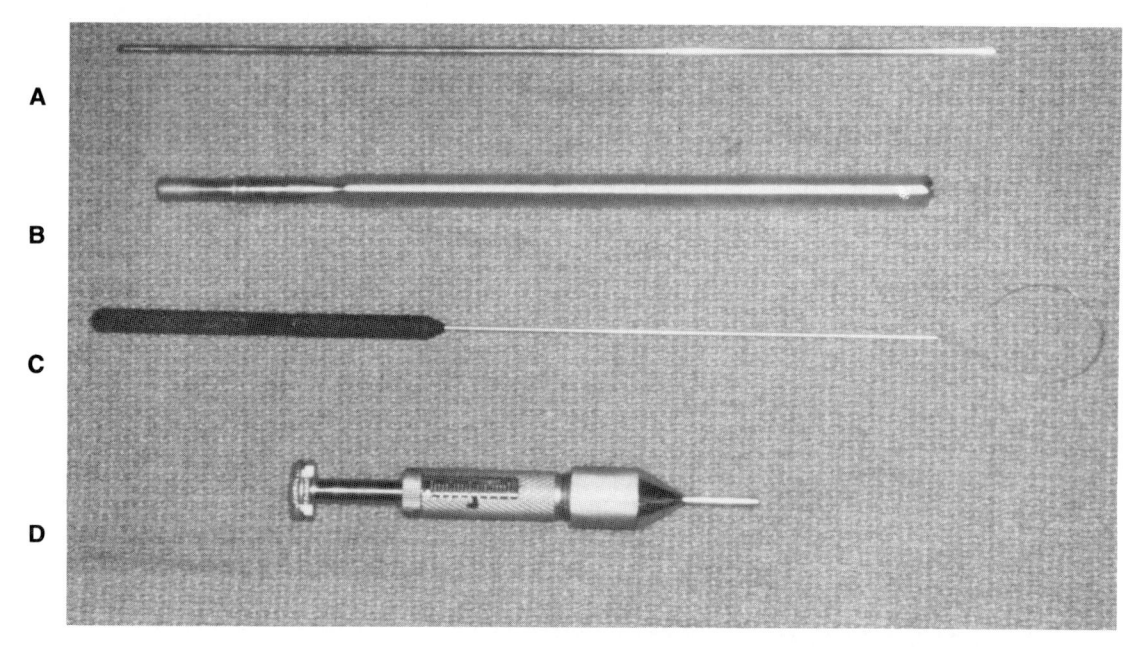

Fig. 7-1 *Instruments used to determine isometric sites for anterior cruciate ligament insertion. **A**, 3/32" or 2 mm K-wire, **B**, cannulated reamer, **C**, Hewson suture passer, and **D**, strain gauge.*

button. The distal end of the suture is then passed through a spring-loaded strain gauge, and the excursion of the suture is recorded as the knee is put through a range of motion. When a small excursion indicating nearly isometric placement is obtained, the K-wires are placed back in the holes and used as guides for drilling the osseous tunnels.

The instruments required for this technique are a set of cannulated reamers or drills, K-wires, an instrument to pass the suture through the 2-mm holes left by the K-wires, and a spring-loaded strain gauge for measuring the excursion of the suture (Fig. 7-1). We have found a Hewson-type suture passer quite useful. Our spring-loaded gauge applies approximately 1 kilogram of force to the suture and reads the excursion in millimeters. The nose of the instrument is designed to slip into the tibial hole left by the K-wire and is hollow to allow the suture to pass through the device (Fig. 7-2). This

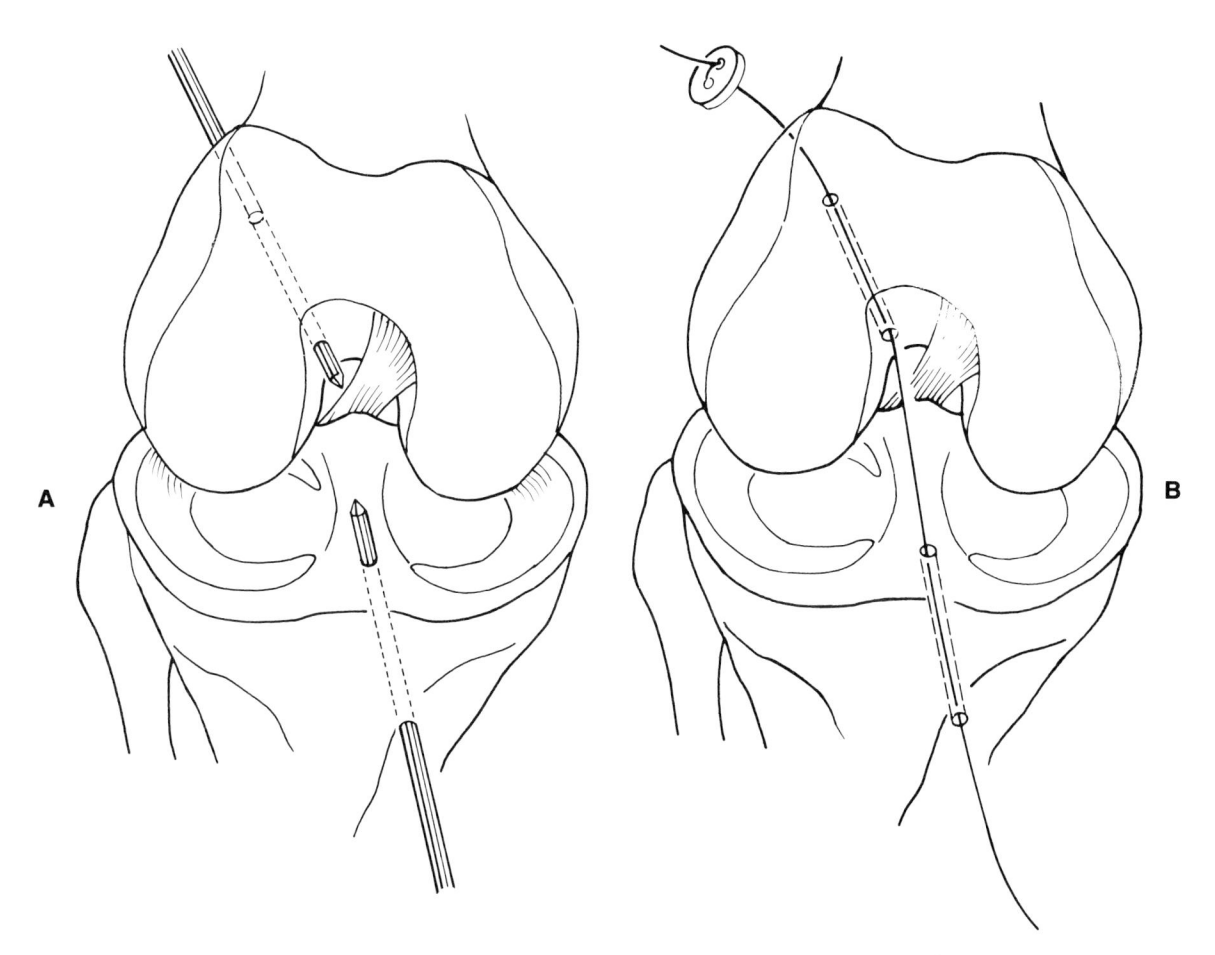

Fig. 7-2 *Technique for measuring excursion. **A**, K-wires are placed according to anatomical landmarks. With the knee in full extension, the tibial K-wires should contact the roof of the intercondylar notch. **B**, A suture is passed through the K-wire holes.*

Continued.

suture is then anchored to the plunger, and the spring is engaged. After the device is zeroed with the knee flexed 30 degrees, readings are made at 0, 30, 60, and 90 degrees. Positive excursion corresponds to a lengthening of the intra-articular portion of the suture, and negative excursion corresponds to a shortening of the intra-articular portion of the suture. The maximal excursion throughout the range of motion is also recorded. Frequently, the position of one or both K-wires must be changed to accommodate isometric placement. A drill guide that allows the placement of parallel K-wires 3, 5, or 7 mm apart is useful for this task.

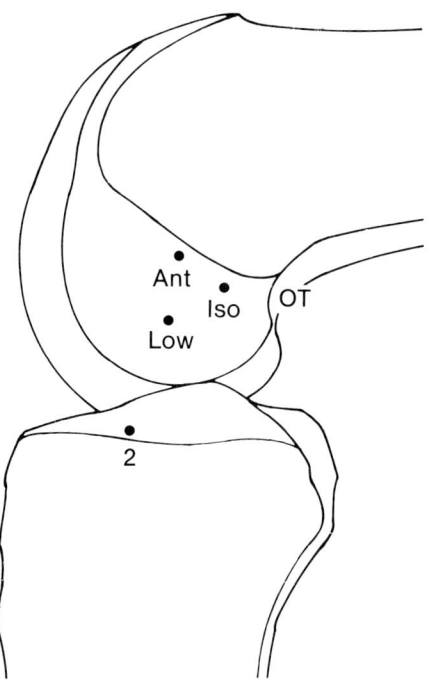

Fig. 7-3 *The pattern of excursion identifies a point as anterior, posterior, or low. A value of ≤1.5 mm defines a nearly isometric pair of points.*

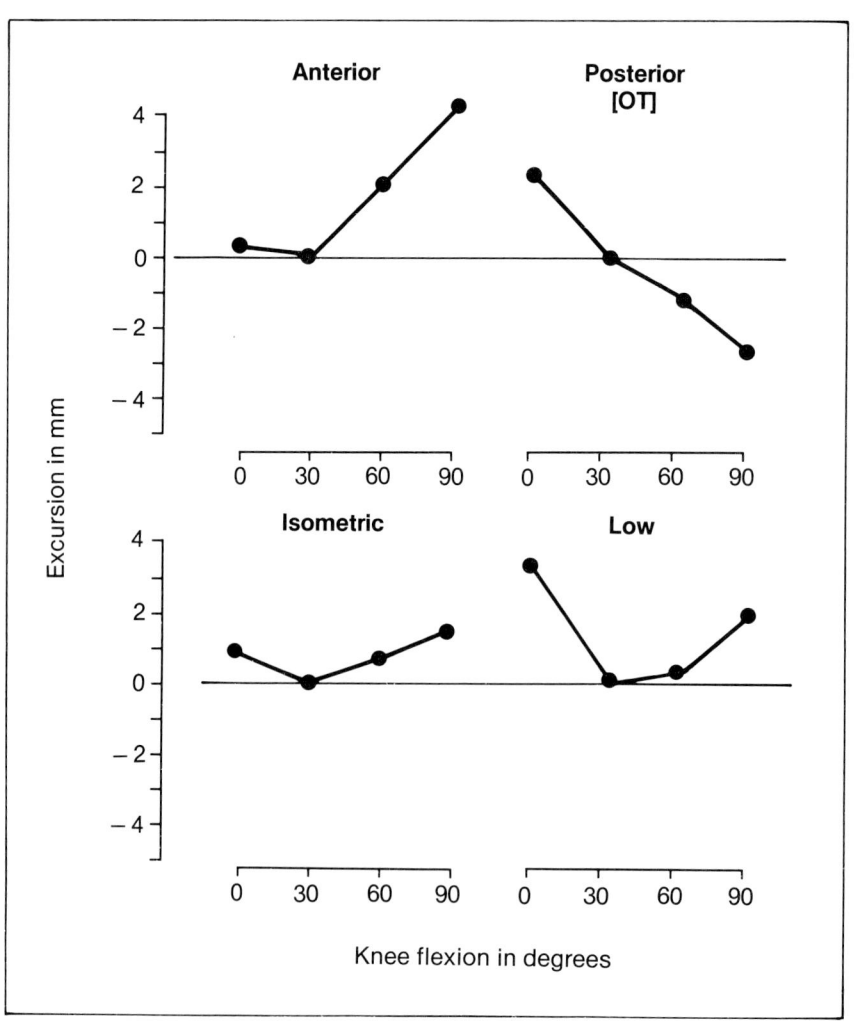

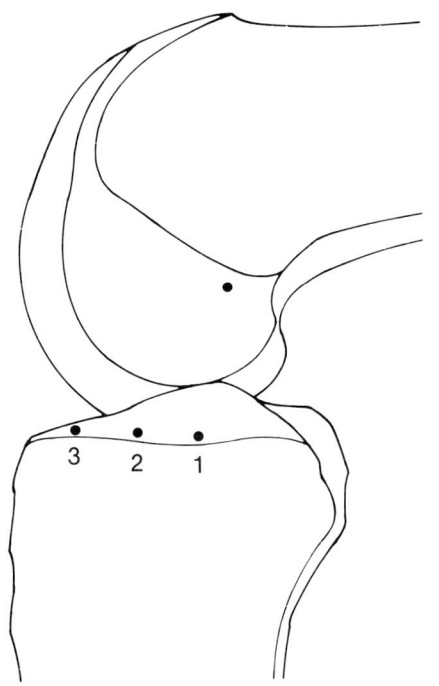

Fig. 7-4 *The location of the tibial point is also important. Like femoral points, an anterior tibial point (T_3) has a more positive excursion at 90 degrees flexion than a posterior tibial point (T_1). Similarly, a posterior point has a more positive excursion at 0 degrees than an anterior tibial point.*

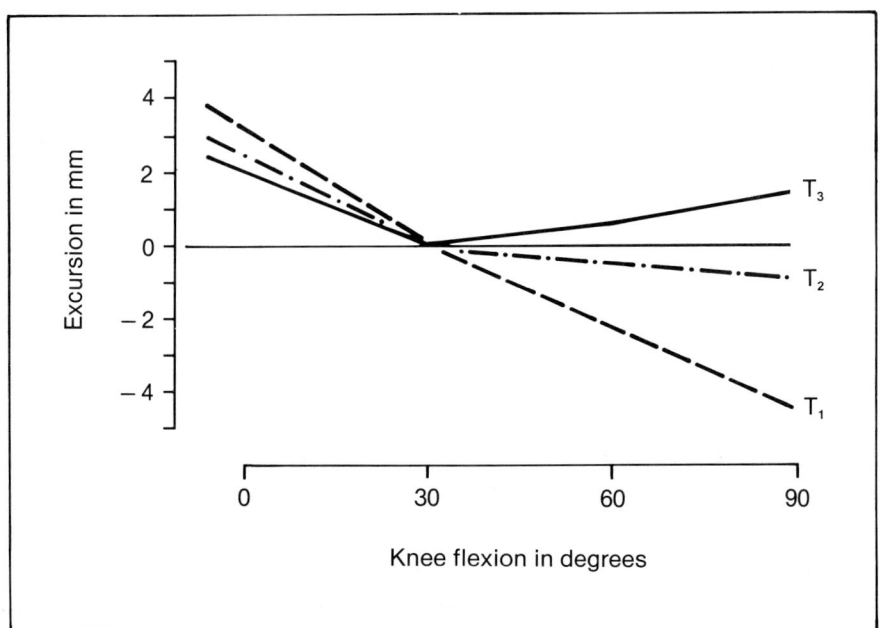

data cannot distinguish between errors in tibial and femoral placement, anatomical relationships can provide such distinction. In full extension, the isometric fibers of the anterior cruciate ligament run parallel to and nearly in contact with the intercondylar roof. The suture used for strain measurements should be oriented in the same way. If the suture impinges on the roof, the tibial point is probably too anteriorally located, and if the suture is vertical and far from the roof, the point is probably too far posteriorly located. Once tibial placement has been confirmed as anatomically reasonable, the femoral point location is changed as indicated by the excursion. Once the 1.5-mm criterion is met, the points are accepted.

Tunnel placement

When isometric attachment points have been identified, tunnels must be placed so that the graft they contain is centered on these points. Depending on the nature of the graft and on the size of the tunnel, this placement may mean that the tunnel is centered about the isometrically positioned K-wire; this is certainly the case for substitutes that completely fill the osseous tunnel. Often, however, this centering does not occur. Bone-patellar tendon-bone composites frequently consist of a strip of patellar tendon that is wider than it is thick and that in no way fills the relatively large tunnels required to contain the bone block. When the block is flush with the distal end of the femoral tunnel, it may approximately center the patellar tendon (Fig. 7-5, *A*). However, when the block is recessed, as it generally is because bone-patellar tendon-bone grafts are longer than the cruciate ligament they are substituting for, the tendon will lie along the edge of the tunnel and not at its center (Fig. 7-5, *B*). This orientation is particularly important for the femoral tunnel.[7] Under such circumstances, the tunnel must be eccentrically placed relative to the isometric point so that the circumference of the tunnel (not its center) lies at the isometric point (Fig. 7-6).

Our study of cadavers also suggests that the orientation of the fibers in the tunnel may be important. The data predict that a graft with twisted fibers linking points within the femoral and tibial tunnels, anterior-to-posterior and posterior-to-anterior, would have significantly decreased ligament strain compared to a parallel fiber arrangement (Fig. 7-7). Further study is required to confirm this hypothesis. Additional work may help tailor placement to the characteristics of the substitute. Regardless of the implant, the determination of a site for isometric attachment provides an important functional landmark that allows for precise and reproducible placement.

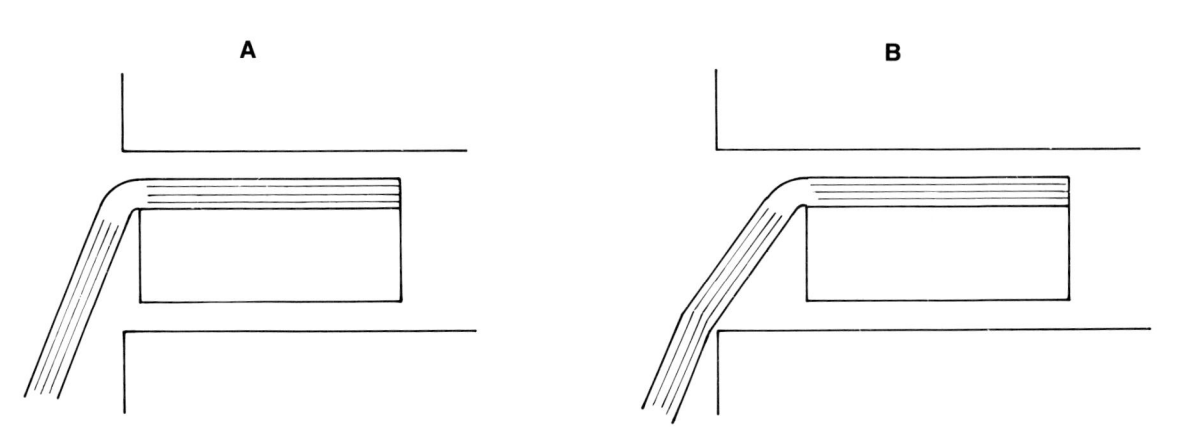

Fig. 7-5 *A,* A flush bone block centers the tendon in the tunnel. *B,* A recessed bone block allows the tendon to lie at the edge of the tunnel.

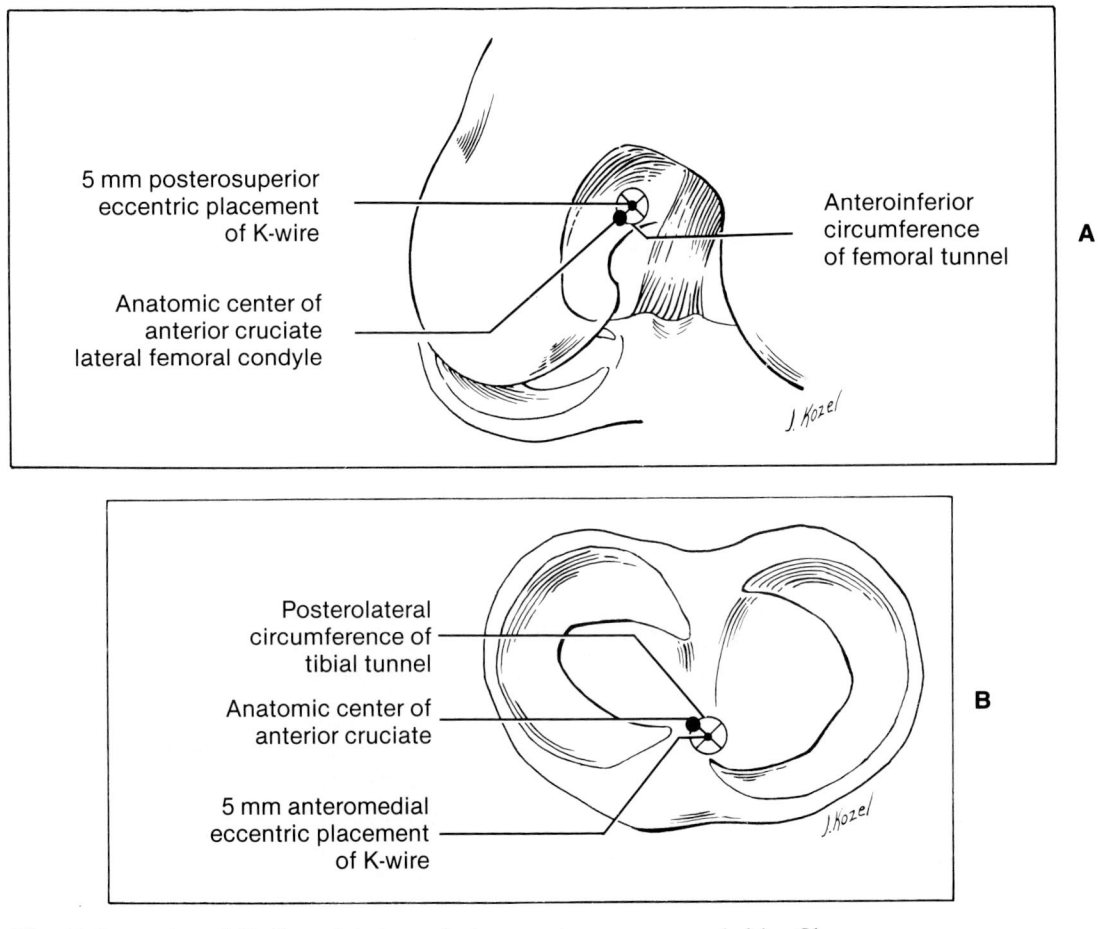

Fig. 7-6 *A* and *B,* Eccentric tunnel placement as recommended by Clancy.

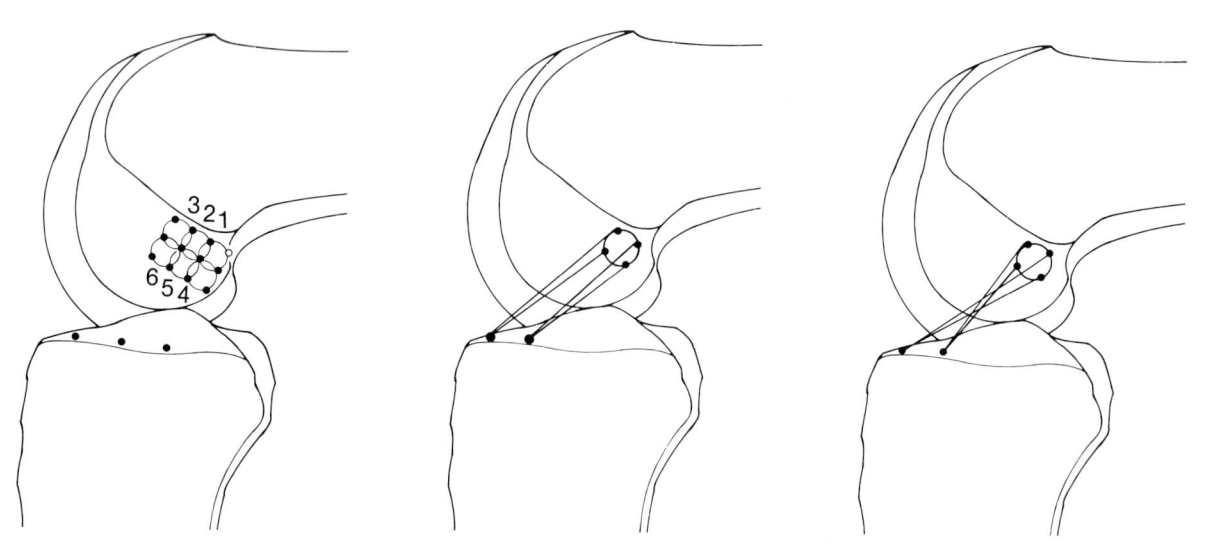

Tunnel	Anterior cruciate ligament strain	
	Average/peak	Average/peak
1	3.95/5.8	3.3/4.6
2	2.9/4.6	2.3/3.4
3	3.7/5.8	3.6/4.8
4	5.3/7.0	5.0/6.5
5	4.2/6.1	3.8/5.6
6	3.9/5.6	3.8/5.2

Fig. 7-7 *A study of ten cadaveric knees suggests that tunnels only 5 mm apart have significantly different strains. Grafts with twisted fibers linking femoral and tibial points anterior to posterior and posterior to anterior may have smaller strains than parallel fiber grafts.*

Summary

Although no substitutes completely reproduce the function of the anterior cruciate ligament, Arms et al.[1] have shown that the strain of isometrically placed anterior cruciate ligament substitutes can closely mimic the strain pattern of the anteromedial fibers of normal ligaments. Such mimicry was clearly not the case for non-isometrically placed substitutes. By determining the isometricity of pairs of possible attachment sites before drilling osseous tunnels, it should be possible to obtain nearly isometric placement of grafts in all cases.

REFERENCES

1. Arms, S.W., Pope, M.H., Johnson, R.J., et al.: The biomechanics of anterior cruciate ligament rehabilitation and reconstruction, Am. J. Sports Med. **12:**8-18, 1984.
2. Arnoczky, S.P.: Anatomy of the anterior cruciate ligament, CORR **172:**19-25, 1983.
3. Clancy, W.G., Narechania, R.G., Rosenber, T.D., et al.: Anterior and posterior cruciate ligament reconstruction in Rhesus monkeys, J. Bone Joint Surg. (Am.) **63:**1270-1284, 1981.
4. Girgis, F.G., Marshall, J.L., and Al Monajem, A.R.S.: The cruciate ligament of the knee joint: anatomical, functional, and experimental analysis, CORR, **106:**216-231, 1975.
5. Graf, B., Simon, T., and Jackson, D.: Isometric placement of cruciate ligament substitutes: a new technique. Unpublished.
6. Melhorn, M.J., and Henning, C.: Unpublished.
7. Odensten, M., and Gillquist, J.: Functional anatomy of the anterior cruciate ligament and a rationale for reconstruction, J. Bone Joint Surg. (Am.) **67:**257-262, 1985.

8
Fixation of soft tissue

DALE M. DANIEL

DANIEL B. ROBERTSON

DAVID L. FLOOD

EDMUND N. BIDEN

Among the multiple factors that influence the success of surgery to repair or reconstruct the anterior cruciate ligament are the methods of soft-tissue fixation. The ideal fixation technique will secure the soft tissue without compromising its vascularity or healing. Fixation techniques need to be evaluated for both their initial strength and their effect on tissue healing. To date there are few reports on the study of soft-tissue fixation. In this chapter, soft-tissue repair and fixation techniques will be divided into four sections: (1) soft tissue to soft tissue, (2) soft tissue to bone, (3) bone to bone, and (4) artificial ligament to soft tissue.

Suturing soft tissue to soft tissue

The goal of a midsubstance repair of a ligament is to decrease the healing gap between the ligament ends and to reestablish normal ligament tension. In a canine model of collateral ligament transection, Clayton et al.[2,3] noted diminution of separation in ligament ends and therefore significantly decreased scar formation with repair. Suturing of sharply divided ligaments led to what might be called primary ligament healing with no visual break in the continuity of the original tissue at the suture line. Unsutured ligaments always healed with a separation and with slightly more scar tissue. However, the suturing process itself adds to ligament trauma. In an unreported study using a rabbit medial collateral ligament model we demonstrated increased ligament inflammation and a decrease in ligament strength following suturing of a sharply sectioned ligament as opposed to the sectioned, unsutured ligament. In the rabbit model there was little separation of the ends of the sharply sectioned medial collateral ligament. Significant reduction in tensile strength and stiffness have been reported as a result of simply suturing an undivided tendon.[5]

Repair has been shown particularly important in the cruciate ligament, since without suturing to oppose the ligament ends there is no potential for ligament healing.[12,13] The midsubstance repair of the anterior cruciate ligament is challenged by many clinicians on the basis of the failure of healing caused by the "hostile" environment of the synovial space. Advocates of primary anterior cruciate ligament repair[4,8] have recommended a suture technique that includes passing several sutures through different portions of the proximal ligament end and bringing these sutures out drill holes in the tibia. Several loops of the suture material are passed through the distal ligament remnant and passed through drill holes in the femur, or one end of the suture is brought out through a drill hole and the other end is passed over the lateral femoral condyle (Fig. 8-1). It is recommended that fat pad or synovium be attached to the ligament as a source of improved vascularity.

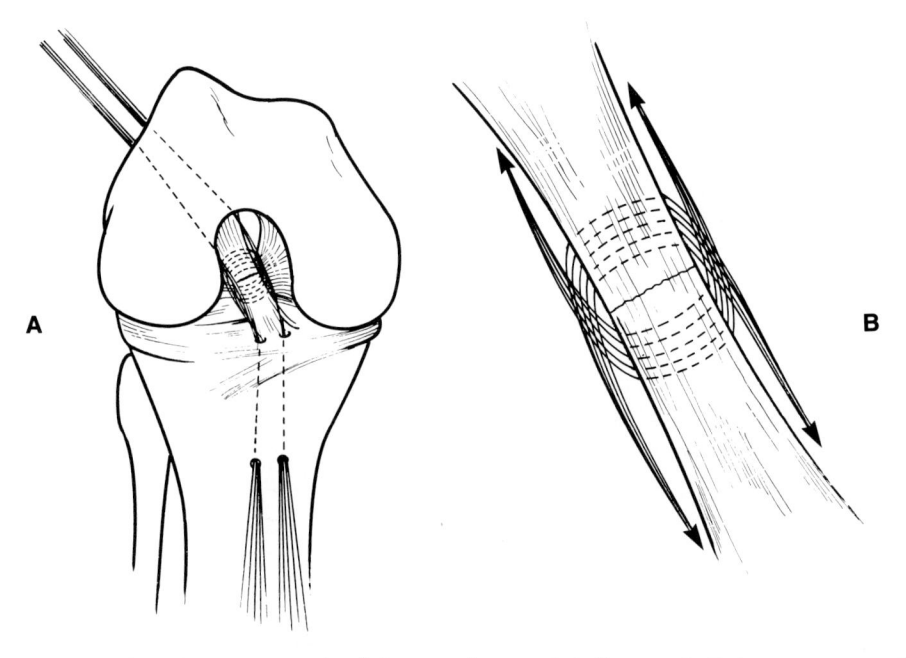

Fig. 8-1 *A and B, Primary repair of the anterior cruciate ligament. Sutures are passed through different portions of the ligament to distribute tension.*

Numerous studies on the soft tissue to soft tissue suturing technique are reported in the literature.[6,9,10,14] Urbaniak et al.[15] reported an analysis of various suture techniques in the tendon. Techniques studied that would be applicable to ligament repair were the multiple interrupted suture, the Mason-Allen suture, the Bunnel suture, and the Kessler "grasping" suture (Fig. 8-2). In using a flexor tendon model in dogs it was found that the Mason-Allen, the Bunnel, and the Kessler suture techniques had similar initial strength (39 newtons [N]). Urbaniak et al. performed an in vivo study to compare the strength of the Kessler and Bunnel suture techniques during healing. At 5 days following repair the Kessler repair tendon strength was 18 N versus 6 N for the Bunnel technique. Urbaniak et al. commented that the strength of all repairs reached a minimum from 3 to 12 days; they also stated that an anastomosis that is located where the pull of the suture is parallel to the collagen bundles will fail at lower loads than in those techniques where the longitudinal shearing force is converted to a compressive force either by the suture or by the tendon itself. The Kessler grasping suture provided the strongest repair.

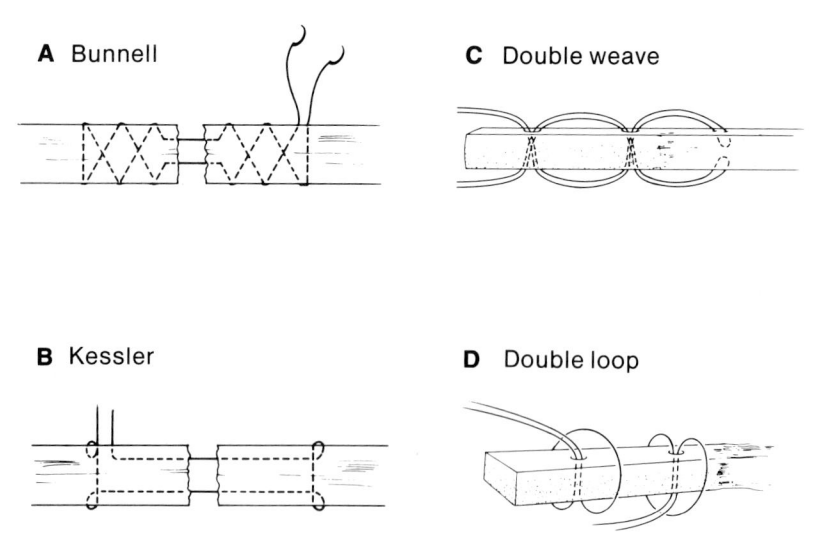

Fig. 8-2 *Suture fixation techniques for use with soft tissue (A and B) or bone tendon preparation (C and D).*

Soft tissue to bone fixation

Intra-articular reconstruction of the anterior cruciate ligament frequently involves passing tissue through a hole or trough in the tibia and in the femur. The ligament course as it enters and exits the bone channel is of importance. The bone channel should be as nearly tangent to the intra-articular course of the ligament as is possible, and any change in direction should be gradual. Bone edges should be chamfered (Fig. 8-3). Passing soft tissue over sharp bone edges results in points of high stress and results in failure of the soft tissue, especially when a knee motion program is initiated prior to ligament healing.[1]

We performed a series of studies using cadaveric tissue to compare the holding power of soft tissue by sutures, staples, a screw with a plastic spiked washer, and a screw with a metallic soft-tissue plate. Four methods of suture fixation were studied using a #2 Mersilene or #0 Dexon suture. The Bunnell and the modified Kessler suture techniques were used to secure the soft tissue (see Fig. 8-2). In initial studies the sutures were passed through drill holes in the bone and securely tied over a bone ridge. The sutures were frequently pulled through the holes in the bone or were sawed through by the sharp edge of the bone channel. In later experiments we tied the suture around a cancellous screw that served as a fixation post. We have subsequently used the fixation post technique in

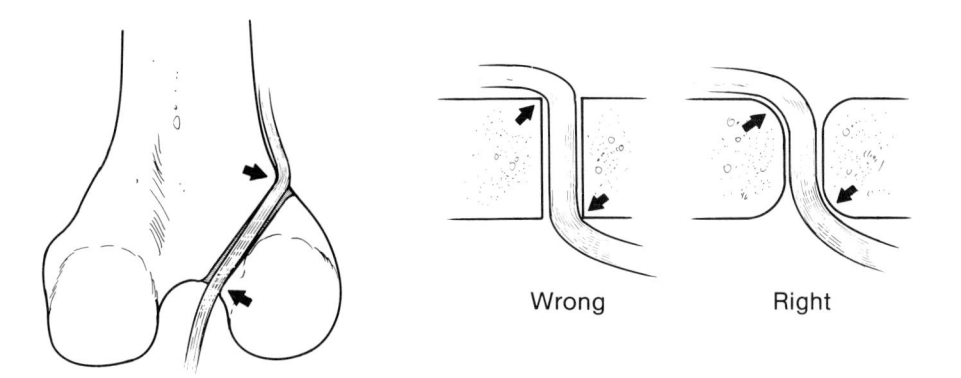

Fig. 8-3 *A change in direction as the graft exits a bone hole results in points of increased stress on the ligament. To decrease the points of stress the holes should be placed as tangent to the course of the intra-articular ligament as possible and the bone edges should be chamfered.*

ligament surgery. The screw selected as a fixation post should have a smooth neck so that it does not cut the suture. Care should be taken not to leave the screw head prominent under the skin where it will be a source of irritation (Fig. 8-4).

Three staples were also studied. The Stone staples (Richards Company) used were the 1.2 cm staple with a single central hole and the 1.5 cm staple with five holes. The length of the legs of the staple were 1.8 cm and 2.5 cm respectively. The central fixation screw was not used with the Stone staple. The barbed staple (3M Company) was 1.75 cm across the top with the two legs measuring 2.8 cm. In addition to the barbs on each leg the staple had multiple small tangs from the undersurface of the top to fix the soft tissue. Staples were inserted using instrumentation supplied with the staples.

A 6.5 mm cancellous screw was used with a circular plastic washer that was 14 mm in diameter with multiple spikes on its undersurface or with a rectangular spiked soft-tissue plate (Synthes Company). The plate was bent with the supplied instruments so

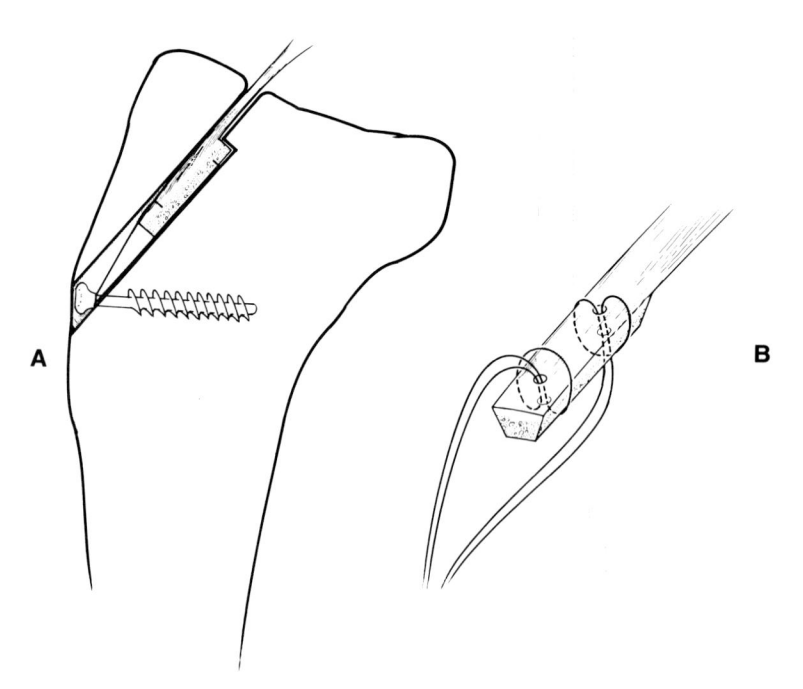

Fig. 8-4 *A, A screw with a smooth neck serves as a fixation post around which the sutures are tied. This diagram demonstrates the technique of a step cut tibial channel, which captures the tendon bone preparation. **B**, Suture fixation of a bone tendon preparation by the double loop technique.*

Fixation of soft tissue

that it conformed to the underlying bone contour. The tissue was then secured under the spiked portion of the plate or washer. In each case a 3.2 mm drill bit was used to drill a hole in the bone and a screw was then secured with a hexagonal head screw driver. Fig. 8-5 illustrates the screw fixation devices tested.

The tissues that were tested were classified into three types. Type A tissue was broad and thin and included medial and lateral capsule, medial collateral ligament, and iliotibial track. Type B tissue was narrow and cord-like and included lateral collateral ligament and hamstring tendons. Type C tissue was the thick quadriceps tendon and patellar tendon structures. The bone used in the study was the distal femur, which was also harvested from the cadaveric tissue. The testing apparatus cyclically loaded the tissue at the rate of 2 cycles per minute. Loads were increased in 13 N increments every 5 cycles until the tissue failed. A total of 137 trials were performed. A minimum of five trials were performed for each fixation technique and for each tissue type.

The Stone staple was the poorest fixation technique tested. The

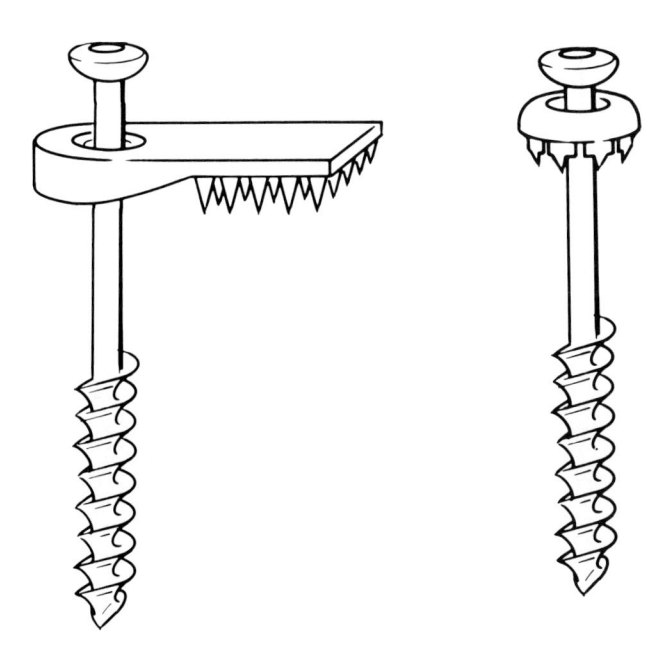

Fig. 8-5   *Soft-tissue fixation devices secured with a screw.*

Stone staple allowed the tissue to be pulled out from beneath the staple. The staple would pull out of the bone. Fixation by the Stone staple was improved when the legs of the staple passed through the tissue.

In the suture techniques, with cyclical loading at low loads, the suture consistently pulled away from the fixation site 2 to 4 mm. This resulted from tightening of the suture in the tissue, stretching of the suture and tightening of the suture knots. Failure usually occurred as a result of tearing of the suture through the tissue; on occasion breaking of the suture resulted in failure.

The barbed staple failed as a result of the tearing of tissue beneath the leading edge of the staple. The barbed staple did not pull out of the bone as did the Stone staple. When stapling type B or C tissue, a double-back staple technique reportedly gives improved fixation[16] (Fig. 8-6). However, this technique was not included in our studies.

The screw with a spiked plastic washer and the screw with a soft-tissue fixation plate proved to be the most secure fixation devices (Table 8-1). Better fixation was provided by placing the screw directly through the tissue by way of a small incision as opposed to placing the device adjacent to the tissue. Tissue fixation with only one side of the washer would pull out. If the tissue is too narrow to place the device through it, the tissue should be completely wrapped around the screw in a clockwise fashion beneath the washer before it is tightened down (Fig. 8-7). The screw with the soft-tissue plate provided fixation similar in overall performance to that of the spiked plastic washer. The rectangular metallic device

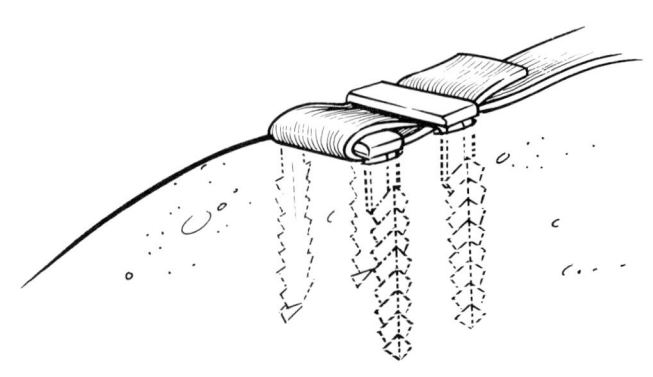

Fig. 8-6 *Double-back staple fixation technique.*

Fixation of soft tissue 121

TABLE 8-1 / Mean failure load for soft-tissue fixation devices

	MEAN FAILURE LOAD (NEWTONS)		
	Tissue type		
FIXATION DEVICE	A	B	C
Screw			
Washer	211	180	225
Plate	266	238	202
Staple			
Stone	121	22	40
Barbed	76	13	81
Suture	99	72	202*

*Sutures passed through attached bone.

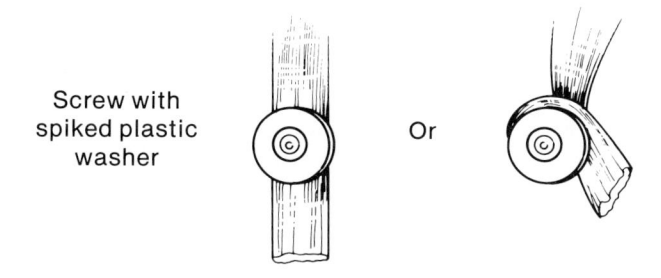

Fig. 8-7 *Preferred methods of fixation of soft tissue with a screw and spiked washer.*

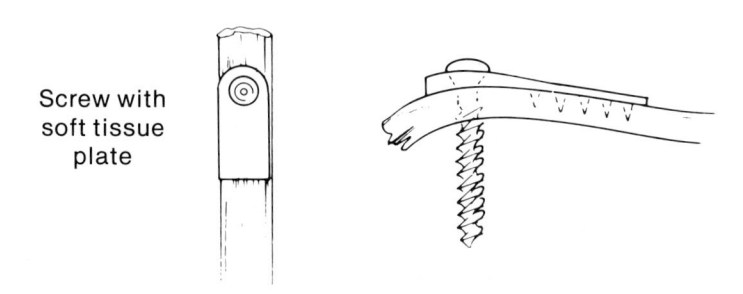

Fig. 8-8 *Preferred method of fixation of soft tissue with a screw and soft-tissue fixation plate.*

TABLE 8-2 / Canine medial collateral ligament study

FIXATION DEVICE	N	FAILURE LOAD (N)*
Normal knee	2	694 ± 18
Repaired ligament		
No fixation	6	283 ± 6
Washer	6	327 ± 32
Plate	5	292 ± 50
Staple	5	176 ± 23

*Mean ± standard error. N, Newton.

should be placed in line with the anticipated tension on the tissues. Optimal fixation is obtained by passing the screw through the tissue with the plate aligned appropriately. If the tissue is fixed at the side of the screw, higher loads will cause the device to turn and the fixation will be compromised. The plate should be bent to the contour of the underlying bone (Fig. 8-8).

In describing the advantages of the spiked plastic washer for soft-tissue fixation, Muller[11] stated that the peripheral arrangement of the teeth firmly grasp the ligament over a broad area and that because of the design and spacing of the teeth the microcirculation to the tissue was not greatly altered. We performed an in vivo study of ligament fixation to compare the use of barbed staples to the spiked washer and spiked fixation plate. Thirteen dogs were used in the study; the animals were sacrificed 6 weeks after ligament sectioning and fixation. The tissue under the barbed staples appeared to have grossly necrosed, and the tissue under the spiked washers and plates appeared viable. Ligaments that were fixed with barbed staples failed at a lower load than did those fixed with the soft-tissue plate or the spiked plastic washer. Failure loads from the study are presented in Table 8-2.

Bone to bone fixation

The patellar tendon, with the attached tibial tubercle and patellar bone, is often used as an anterior cruciate ligament graft. As part of the previously described studies with cadaver tissue, we evaluated securing the patellar tendon with attached bone to a fixation post with a suture. We found two suture techniques that provided good fixation. The first technique was the "double weave technique" in which a double suture was brought through the tendon

Fixation of soft tissue

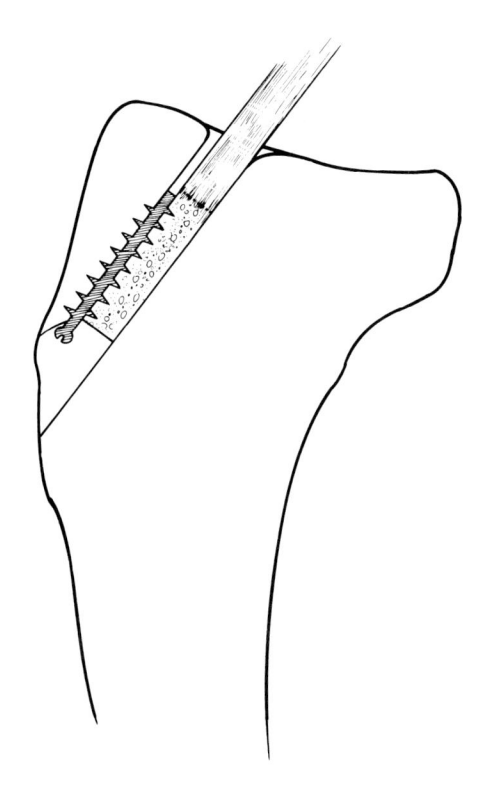

Fig. 8-9 *A 3 cm 6.5 mm cancellous screw is used to obtain an interference fit. The bone plug must fit snugly in the bone hole.*

proximal to the bone block and then woven in a figure eight fashion through two drill holes in the bone. The second technique was a double loop technique in which two separate sutures were passed through drill holes and looped over the bone to grasp the bone block (see Fig. 8-2). These two suture techniques were satisfactory in holding the bone; however, as seen with the capsular and tendinous tissues that were sutured, the specimens pulled away from the site of fixation 2 to 4 mm at low loads. In each preparation, care was taken to tie the knots down firmly with several square knots. Nevertheless, the knots tightened down further and the sutures pressed into the tissue when cyclic loading was applied.

Lambert[7] reported the use of an interference fit screw technique. In this technique the bone attached to the patellar tendon graft source is pulled into the bone hole and secured with a 6.5 mm cancellous screw. The screw engages both the wall of the drill hole and the bone plug of the graft (Fig. 8-9). The strength of this fixation technique depends on a snug fit of the graft bone into the bone hole. If the bone plug does not fit tightly in the bone hole, the screw will not securely engage both bone surfaces.

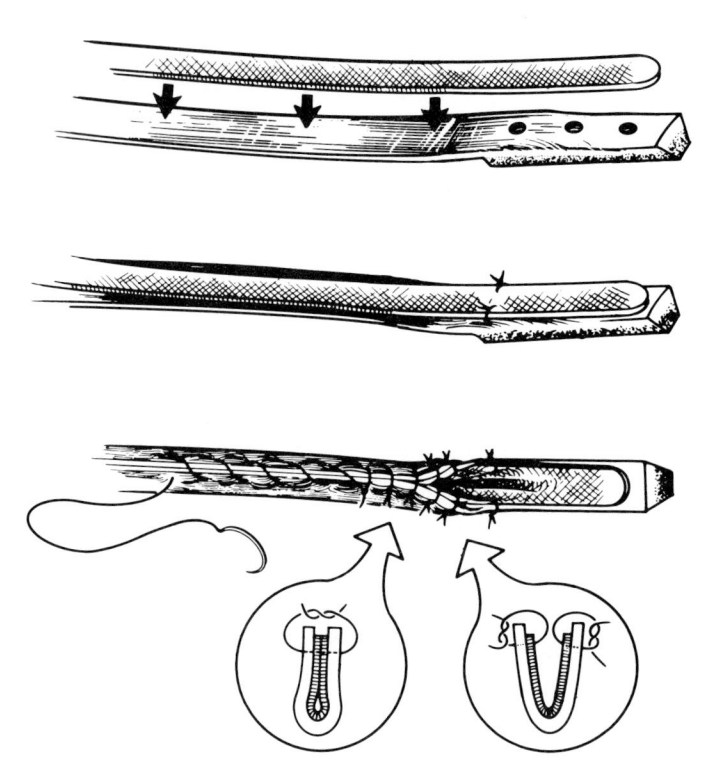

Fig. 8-10 *Polypropylene augmentation device (LAD, 3M Company) sutured to the patellar tendon graft with attached tibial tubercle bone. The sutures are placed at 1 cm intervals.*

Fixation of artificial ligaments

A proposed advantage of artificial ligaments is that they provide immediate secure joint stability and allow an early motion and activity program. The weak link in the implant is the point of fixation to bone with ligament replacement devices and to soft tissue with autogenous tissue augmentation devices. We have performed cadaver studies on a polypropylene augmentation device (Kennedy LAD [3M Company]). The LAD device was sutured to cadaveric tissue, including the patellar tendon, semitendinosus tendon, gracilous tendon, and iliotibial band. A total of 21 specimens were studied. Sutures were placed in either a running or interrupted fashion at 1 cm intervals on each side of the autogenous tissue composite. Five pairs of 00 Ethibond suture were placed in the distal 5 cm of the graft and then running or interrupted sutures were used proximally using 00 Dexon suture (Fig. 8-10). The graphs were 15 cm in length, and a total of 30 passes of suture went through the composite graft. To test the strength of the suture linkage between the LAD device and the graft tissue, the tissue was only fixed to bone at the distal end and a load was applied to the LAD at the proximal end. The length of the graft was measured while a 14 N load was applied, and the graft was then cyclically loaded with 90 N ten times. This resulted in a 4% mean elongation. After 120 cycles with a 180 N load the graft mean elongation was 8% and there was no suture failure. Between the 180 and 300 N load 13% of the sutures failed (untied, broke, or pulled out of the soft tissue). The fact that all of the failed sutures were at the distal end of the graft suggests that the load transferred from the LAD to the graft tissue is principally at the distal end.

Summary

In the surgical management of knee ligament injuries the surgeon's goal is to re-establish normal joint motion. Ligaments can be repaired or reconstructed using a number of techniques, some of which have been presented here along with documentation of their efficacy. If the joint laxity achieved with surgery is to be verified by standard clinical tests or arthrometer measurements in the operating room and if a motion program (passive or active) is to be initiated prior to soft-tissue healing, the security of the surgical fixation procedures are especially important.

REFERENCES

1. Burks, R., Daniel, D.M., Losse, G.: The effect of continuous passive motion on anterior cruciate ligament reconstruction stability, Am. J. Sports Med. **1**:323-327, 1984.
2. Clayton, M.L., and Weir, G.J.: Experimental investigations of ligamentous healing, Am. J. Surg. **98**:373, 1959.
3. Clayton, M.L., Miles, J.S., and Abdulla, M.: Experimental investigations of ligamentous healing, Clin. Orthop. **61**:146, 1968.
4. Collehan, D.L., Warren, R.F., and Wickiewicz, T.L.: Acute repairs of the anterior cruciate ligament: past and present, Orthop. Clin. North Am. **16**:111-125, 1985.
5. Hirsch, G.: Tensile properties during tendon healing, Acta Orthop. Scand. (Suppl.) **153**:7, 1974.
6. Kessler, I.: The "grasping" technique for tendon repair, Hand **5**:253-255, 1973.
7. Lambert, K.L.: Vascularized patella tendon graft with rigid internal fixation for anterior cruciate ligament insufficiency, Clin. Orthop. Vol. 172, 1983.
8. Marshall, J.R., et al.: Ligamentous injuries of the knee in skiing, Clin. Orthop. **108**: 197-198, 1975.
9. Mason, M.L.: Primary and secondary tendon suture: a discussion of the significance of the technique in tendon surgery, Surg. Gynecol. Obstet. **70**:392-402, 1940.
10. Mason, M.L., and Shearon, C.G.: Process of tendon repair: an experimental study of tendon suture and tendon graft, Arch. Surg. **25**:4, 616-691, 1932.
11. Muller, W.: The Knee, New York, 1983, Springer-Verlag New York Inc, p. 157.
12. O'Donoghue, D.H., et al.: Repair of the anterior cruciate ligament in dogs, II, J. Bone Joint Surg. (Am.) **48**:503, 1966.
13. O'Donoghue, D.H., et al: Repair and reconstruction of the anterior cruciate ligament in dogs: factors influencing long term results, J. Bone Joint Surg. (Am.) **53**:710, 1971.
14. Peacock, E., Jr.: Some technical aspects and results of flexor tendon repair, Surgery **58**: 330-342, 1965.
15. Urbaniak, J.R., Cahill, J.D., Jr., and Mortenson, R.A.: Tendon suturing methods: analysis of tensile strengths, Symposium on Tendon Surgery in the Hand, Philadelphia, Pennsylvania, March 1974.
16. Woodward, P.: Personal communication, January, 1983.

9
Factors affecting choices of anterior cruciate ligament surgery

PHILIP G. WILCOX

DOUGLAS W. JACKSON

Management choices

Management of the anterior cruciate ligament deficient knee is based on numerous factors. Each of the patient's goals and needs has several treatment options. When discussing the individualized management with the patient these options can be grouped into four basic approaches, (Fig. 9-1). These approaches include: (1) nonoperative management, (2) arthroscopic surgery for the associated injuries with or without an extra-articular stabilization, (3) arthroscopic surgery for the associated injuries with arthroscopic or limited open repair or reconstruction of the anterior cruciate ligament, and (4) traditional open surgical repair or replacement of the anterior cruciate ligament. Most patients will play an active role in deciding which approach is the best for them. Thus they must understand the natural history of the anterior cruciate deficient knee, as well as the possible benefits and risks of surgical intervention.[10]

Nonoperative management of the anterior cruciate ligament rupture includes patient education, physical therapy, and selective bracing. Many factors come into consideration if this method is to give patient satisfaction. The patient's age, activity level, and socioeconomic factors contribute to this choice. Some patients will wish to avoid surgery and decide on this approach. Many patients have a fear of surgery or are willing to "wait and see" what their result will be without surgery. Previous reports have indicated that a large percentage of patients do quite well with this type of management if they are willing to alter their lifestyle in accordance with their level of instability.[5,13,19,24] Instability is not synonymous with disability. Disability from ligament instability is often a very subjective and

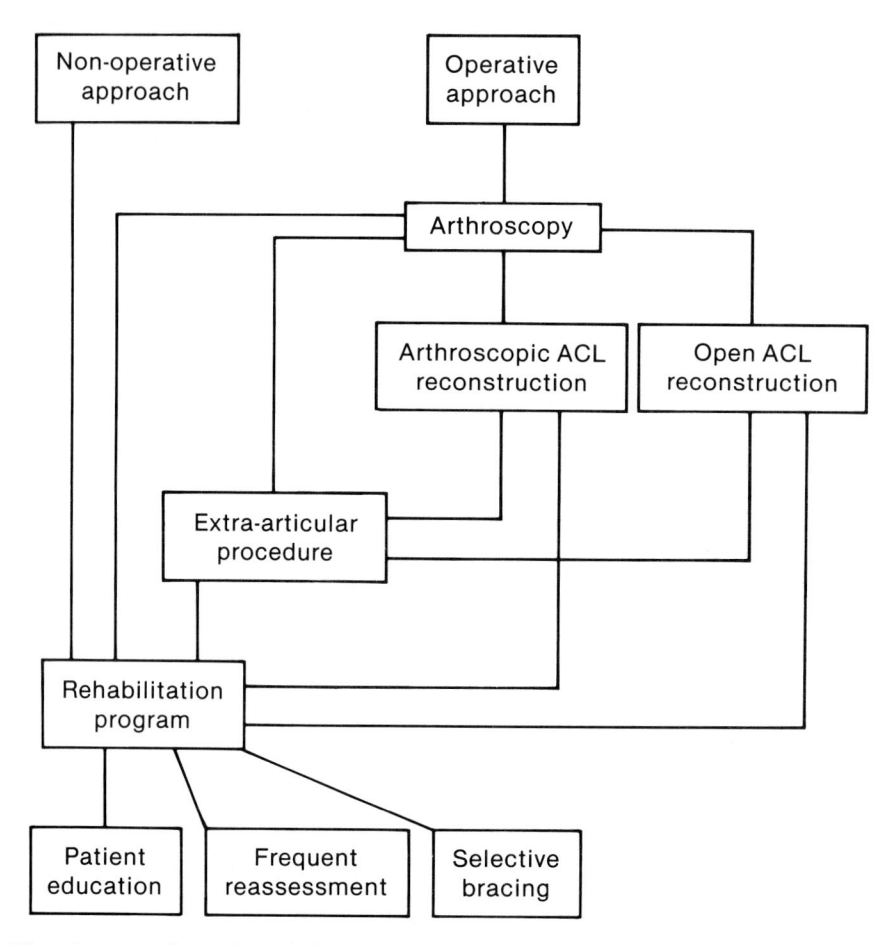

Fig. 9-1 *Overview of the management of anterior cruciate ligament injury.*

individual manifestation. Careful physical examination and diagnosis is the basis for appropriate patient education and supervised physical therapy. Certain patients will be best served by this management. These patients usually learn to compensate for the loss of their anterior cruciate ligament. The patient may experience no apparent or appreciated deficits and thus be able to function adequately in the activities of daily living.[23] The majority of anterior cruciate ligament injuries fall into this category and require no surgical reconstruction. In athletic populations, where the anterior cruciate ligament is the most commonly ruptured ligament in the knee, the nonoperative approach is not usually satisfying to the patient unless it is coupled with a significant change in activity level.

The second approach is basically an extension of the first. Because the anterior cruciate ligament seldom ruptures as an isolated injury, other injuries may occur at the same time or be present prior to the ligament rupture. These may include one or more meniscal tears, articular cartilage damage, chondromalacia, and degenerative arthritis. These changes may be present individually or in combination and need to be addressed in considering the alternatives. Other ligamentous and capsular instability may be associated with the nonfunctional or absent anterior cruciate ligament and requires careful delineation. After reviewing these injuries and their manifestations the surgeon may choose to perform limited arthroscopic surgery without an anterior cruciate ligament reconstruction.[5,8,9] Correcting meniscal tears (partial menisectomy or meniscal repair) and debriding cartilage defects can increase the chances for success with nonoperative management of the anterior cruciate ligament tear. Using this approach, an unpredictable instability has the potential to be reduced to a more predictable instability. If the instability always occurs with certain movements, the coordinated individual can adjust by using their good knee for certain functions. If another internal derangement is present, it may magnify the subluxation phenomena (amplifier effect). Arthroscopy is not necessary to diagnose the complete anterior cruciate ligament tear. Diagnosis is provided by careful preoperative physical examination of the involved knee. Occasionally anesthesia is necessary to clinically document the instability. The arthroscope is quite helpful in documenting the partially torn anterior cruciate ligament.[8]

The third option is to perform arthroscopic evaluation of the involved knee, addressing intra-articular cartilage or meniscal pathology. This may be followed by an arthroscopic or limited open repair, augmentation, or reconstruction of the anterior cruciate ligament. The techniques of arthroscopic anterior cruciate ligament repair, augmentation, and reconstruction have recently developed and are rapidly being refined to where an orthopedic surgeon proficient in arthroscopic surgery can do it quite precisely. This method incorporates the same precise placement required for open reconstruction of the ligament, and it has the advantages of smaller sized incisions and less disturbance of the extensor mechanism. The avoidance of the parapatellar arthrotomy incision and patellar dislocation results in less morbidity, fewer adhesions, and less long-term extensor mechanism pain. The patient experiences much less postoperative pain with this method. Postoperative range of motion and quadriceps strength return faster during the early rehabilitation period. This procedure has the potential of eventually being performed as an outpatient procedure. The long-term results of this approach are not yet available; however, early experience is encouraging.

Finally, the surgeon may choose to perform an arthroscopic evaluation with intra-articular surgery as indicated, followed by an open anterior cruciate ligament reconstruction. This is the more conventional and traditional operative approach. The exposure is more extensive using the open approach. Postoperative rehabilitation is hampered by increased pain and decreased range of motion in the early postoperative period. In addition, the aggravation of chondromalacia patella and patellar tendonitis in the long-term follow-up has been a factor associated with this surgical approach. The technique of careful preparation and placement of osseous tunnels along with careful preparation and placement of the graft can result in good long-term results by this method. Early motion is enhanced by a lateral parapatellar approach with medial dislocation of the patella as opposed to the more widely used medial parapatellar incision.

Numerous procedures for stabilization of the anterior cruciate deficient knee are present in the literature. These include intra-articular as well as extra-articular methods and combinations of both. Each method has its' advocates and proposed advantages. Once surgical stabilization is considered, the selection of the procedure depends on numerous factors, including: (1) acute versus chronic anterior cruciate ligament injury, (2) patient age and sex, (3) activity level, (4) degree of instability, (5) future athletic expectations, and (6) present level of disability. The overall results reported have been quite variable, relating to the experience of the surgeon, surgical technique, material used for the reconstruction, and overall patient compliance. Three basic types of materials are available for intra-articular reconstruction of the anterior cruciate ligament. These materials include autograft materials (patellar tendon, fascia lata, semitendinosis), allograft materials (freeze-dried patellar tendon, freeze-dried fascia lata, freeze-dried anterior cruciate ligament), and prosthetic ligaments. At this point, autograft materials have been used most commonly for intra-articular reconstruction.[24] Autograft materials have been used without extra-articular stabilization.[6] Allograft ligaments, ligament augmentation devices, and prosthetic ligaments are still in their investigational stages. The

Food and Drug Administration will require long clinical trials before release of further prosthetic ligaments and ligament augmentation devices. Until long-term follow-up has been reported, the widespread use of prosthetic materials will be delayed. As our familiarity with allograft materials, augmentation devices, and prosthetic ligaments improves, the surgical indications for each type of repair will become more evident. Further research and comparison of methods must be made before any widespread agreement emerges on the timing and methods of stabilization in the anterior cruciate deficient knee.

Extra-articular reconstruction

Many surgeons recommend an extra-articular augmentation in conjunction with an intra-articular reconstruction.[4] The rationale for this is twofold. First, during the initial stages of rehabilitation it may protect the intra-articular repair against the translational forces exerted anteriorly by the extensor mechanism on the tibia. Second, if extra-articular augmentation is placed isometrically, it may offer lasting capsular stability in the anterolateral region of the capsule. If used in conjunction with a prosthetic ligament, it offers the potential to minimize some of the peak stresses a prosthetic ligament could experience and to possibly prolong the ultimate life of the prosthetic material. Thus, used together, the intra-articular and extra-articular procedures may offer greater initial stability and may have a lower long-term failure rate than either one used alone. This is yet to be established in the literature.

An isolated extra-articular procedure has been proposed by Andrews et al. for mild to moderate, chronic anterolateral rotatory instability and in those patients having meniscal repairs without intra-articular stabilization.[12] Andrews et al. believe that this isolated extra-articular repair is also indicated in moderate to severe, acute anterolateral rotatory instability.[2] Patients who cannot afford the time of protecting the biological incorporation of the intra-articular graft may be candidates for this approach. Factors such as the time spent on crutches, the time away from work, and insurance coverage all enter into the decision. The extra-articular procedures alone require a more limited exposure, which is a desirable feature.

Extra-articular reconstructive procedures are an important consideration in the overall decision for anterior cruciate ligament reconstruction in non-athletic individuals. Isolated extra-articular repairs may be indicated for relatively inactive patients with mild anterolateral rotatory instability who will place low level demands on their repair. An example of this type of patient would be a person who experiences mild symptoms during activities of daily living with no high performance demands. Rosenberg has reported on a small group of patients in which an isolated iliotibial band tenodesis was performed.[26] He has reported that 80% of these patients believed that they were improved with this procedure. Paulos stresses the importance of placing the tenodesis at the isometric point on the femur to prevent stretching and ultimate loss of stability.[25] In addition, activity limitation and selection and good muscle conditioning of the lower extremities are important.

The use of extra-articular procedures in children with open growth plates is often a consideration if surgery is believed to be necessary before growth is complete. Osseous tunnels through open epiphyseal plates may cause early closure of the plates resulting in altered growth. Peripheral drill holes have a greater potential for growth disturbance than centrally placed drill holes in the region of the intercondylar notch. Larger drill holes have a greater propensity to close the plates than smaller drill holes. The surgeon must estimate the growth remaining in the epiphyseal plate based on bone age and make a decision concerning violation of the plate based on this information. If very little growth remains, it may be acceptable to drill through the plate. Some youngsters may best be cared for by waiting until growth is complete before any surgical intervention is performed. Milder functional instability can often be controlled with an extra-articular repair alone.

The choice of the extra-articular repair is an individual decision of the surgeon. Primary repair of an extra-articular capsular tear may be adequate in an acute injury if strong tissue reapproximation can be achieved. The iliotibial band tenodesis is designed to protect the joint from the anterior translational forces created by the pull of the quadriceps muscle during active extension. Krachow and Brooks located isometric points on the femur and tibia that allow full flexion and extension of the knee joint without significantly changing the length of the tenodesis (Fig. 9-2).[17] The femoral isometric point is located on the lateral femur just above the metaphyseal flare along its posterolateral aspect. The tibial point is located just anterior to Gerdy's tubercle. Moving the tibial point back to Gerdy's tubercle, the distance between the two points at 45 degrees of flexion is noted to lengthen by 1 cm during full flexion and

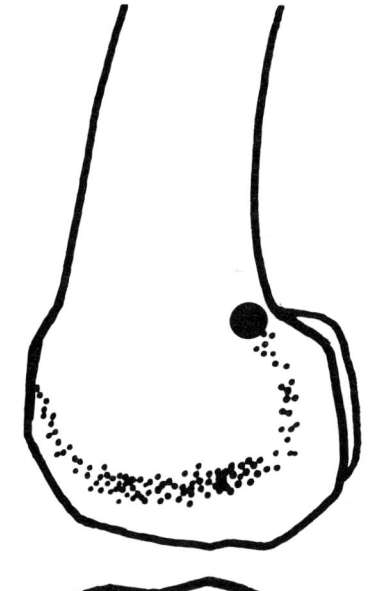

Fig. 9-2 *The isometric femoral and tibial points as described by Krachow and Brooks.*[17]

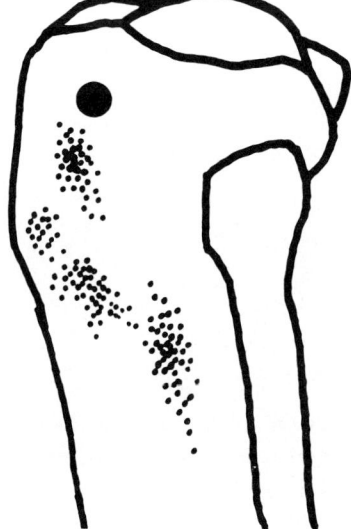

extension. By performing a tenodesis of the iliotibial band at 45 degrees of flexion leaving the attachment at Gerdy's tubercle intact, full flexion and extension is achieved.[14] While there is loosening in the effect of the tenodesis during flexion and extension of up to 1 cm, it does give additional stability in the range where the "pivot shift" phenomena is most disabling.

The iliotibial band with its dynamic muscle attachment can adjust to this change of length in the uninjured knee. The tenodesis

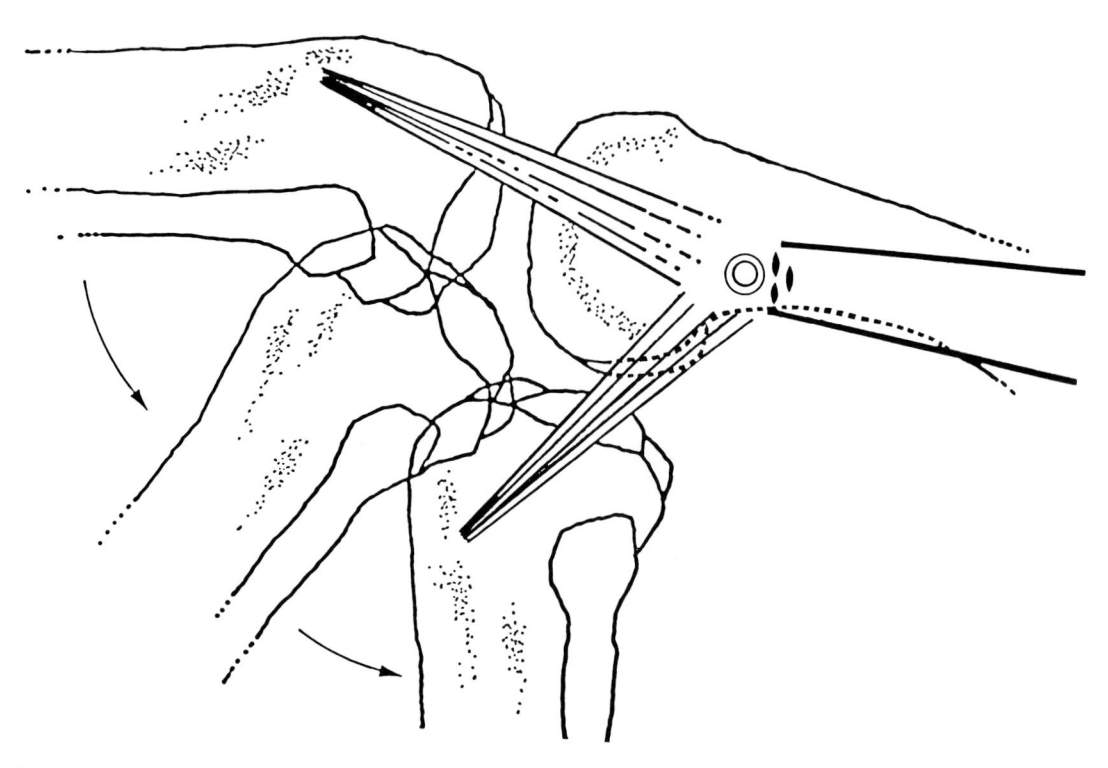

Fig. 9-3 *Tenodesis of the iliotibial band at the isometric femoral point uses the same screw used for securing the intra-articular reconstruction.*

effect alters the normal functioning of this important structure. It becomes a ligament that is extra-articular and not isometric through the range of motion. Close attention to detail allows one to approach isometry. The tenodesis is performed by securing the posterior portion of the iliotibial band to the lateral femur at the femoral isometric point using a 6.5 mm cancellous screw and spiked washer. This same fixation screw can also be used for securing the anterior cruciate graft as it emerges from the osseous tunnel in the femur. Before completely tightening the screw, multiple relaxing incisions are made in the iliotibial band proximal to the screw fixation in order to isolate the tenodesis and allow further tightening. These incisions also minimize the "dimpling effect" of the screw (Fig. 9-3). Using this approach, the anterior subluxation of the tibia is significantly reduced throughout the flexion and extension arc.

The Arnold-Kocher sling about the fibular collateral ligament to Gerdy's tubercle has also been reported as a successful extra-articular repair.[1] In this method of repair a strip of iliotibial band 1 cm wide and 8 cm in length is isolated. This fascial strip is passed beneath the fibular collateral ligament and doubled back on itself. It is sutured firmly at the fibular collateral ligament and back onto itself as it passes back toward Gerdy's tubercle. Superiority of any one of the many extra-articular repairs over another has not been established because no comparative studies have been performed. Multiple factors, including minimal exposure, low morbidity, and minimal added instability resulting from a failed extra-articular repair, make certain procedures more desirable than others.

Intra-articular reconstruction

Proponents of intra-articular reconstruction of the anterior cruciate ligament recommend this procedure for specific situations, including: (1) cruciate ligament injury in a highly athletic individual, (2) physically active individuals with functional instability and an unwillingness to alter their lifestyle, (3) frequent symptoms of instability with activities of daily living, (4) recurrent episodes of effusion, and (5) reported instability episodes after 6 months of intensive rehabilitation.[8,12] The patient's level of activity and willingness to alter his or her lifestyle is an overriding factor in choosing the appropriate method of management.

Acute anterior cruciate ligament deficiency

Acute reconstructions should only be undertaken after careful discussion of the available options with the patient and when the patient has an understanding of the time commitment for rehabilitation (Fig. 9-4). The advantages and disadvantages of acute versus chronic reconstruction or of no reconstruction at all is a subject that remains controversial. We believe that a surgical reconstruction of the acute anterior cruciate ligament rupture within 7 to 10 days is essential to obtain the best results. This is especially true in an athlete who wishes to return to a competitive level of athletics. The patient's anterior cruciate ligament should be repaired when possible and augmented with fascia lata, patellar tendon, or semitendinosis autograft or allograft, depending on the preference of patient and surgeon.[3] If the ligament is not repairable, then it can be replaced by a suitable autograft or allograft material. Autogenous patellar tendon-bone grafts are the most commonly used substitutes.[20,21] This biological graft has well-documented incorporation and revascularization after implantation. In addition, the bone-patel-

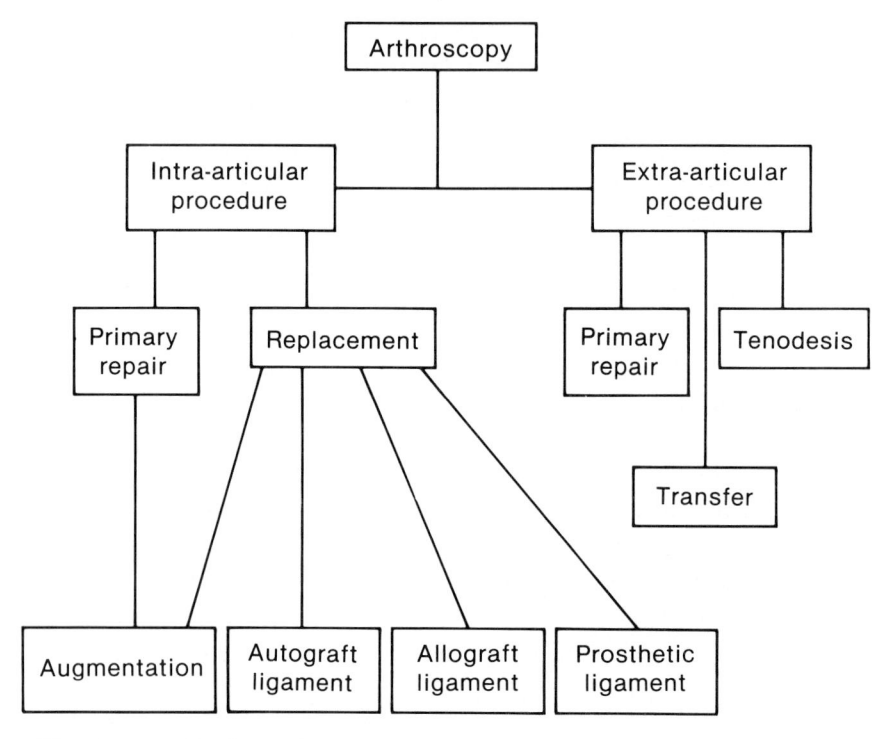

Fig. 9-4 *Decisions in acute anterior cruciate ligament reconstruction.*

lar tendon-bone complex allows for bony incorporation of the graft within the osseous tunnels.[11] Extra-articular augmentation may also be performed as a back-up and for early stability. Re-establishment of the control over excessive anterior translation of the tibia will presumably protect the knee from the degenerative changes that have been reported by Noyes and others as a result of recurrent subluxation episodes.[18,21]

Following an acute anterior cruciate ligament reconstruction, rehabilitation should be started as soon as the surgical technique allows. The acute repairs and reconstructions tend to have a greater problem with loss of extension and adhesions, which must be watched closely. Occasionally a closed manipulation or arthroscopic lysis of adhesions is necessary. If an acute reconstruction is deferred, the patient should begin a rehabilitation program immediately to minimize atrophy and the disuse changes that follow this injury. Future decisions concerning reconstruction of the anterior cruciate ligament are then based on the amount of chronic disability the patient experiences.

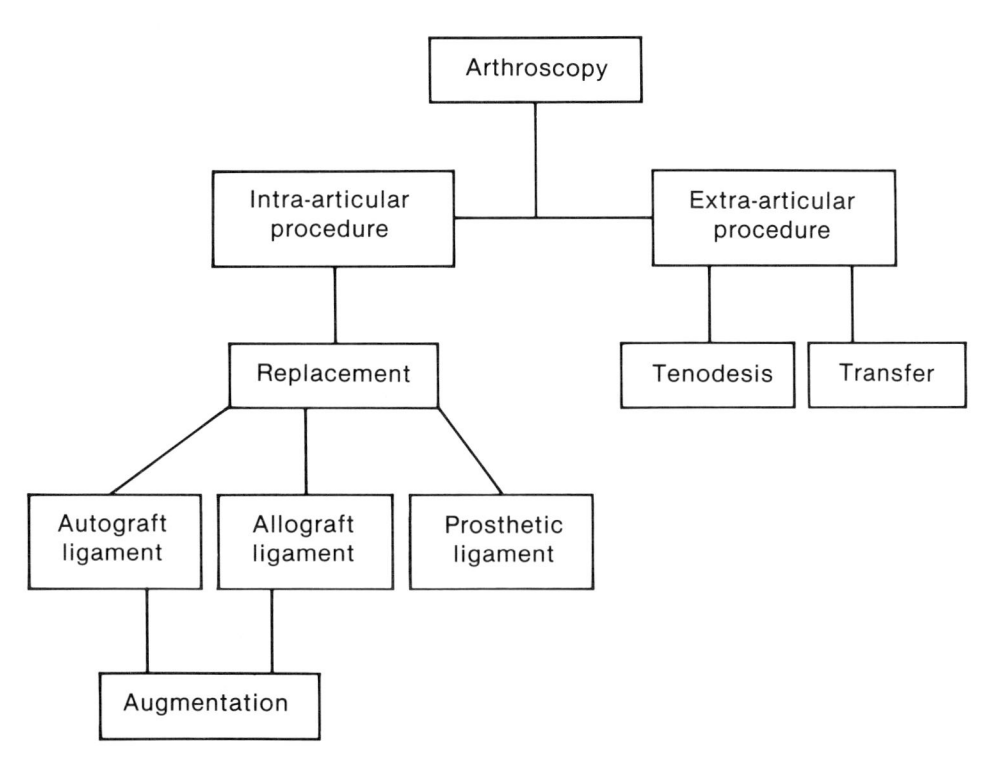

Fig. 9-5 *Decisions in chronic anterior cruciate ligament reconstruction.*

Chronic anterior cruciate ligament deficiency

Chronic anterior cruciate ligament deficient knees present some additional considerations to the acute repair (Fig. 9-5). The best surgical and nonsurgical management results reported have been in the acute anterior cruciate ruptures.[15] The acute group includes those anterior cruciate ligament ruptures that may have done well without physician management. Chronic surgical reconstructions are done on patients that have been selected as needing further treatment. This group includes patients with acute ruptures who either did not present for consideration of acute repair or reconstruction or who elected not to have an acute repair.[22] These are patients that did not do well following their acute ruptures over a period of time. They are the more symptomatic patients with a significant disability from their anterior cruciate ligament deficiency. They usually have varying degrees of associated capsular laxity. In addition, they may have intra-articular damage to the menisci and articular surfaces as a result of the original injury or recurrent subluxation episodes.[10] Other factors to consider include the preoperative presence of pain, deformity (pronounced genu varum), limitation of motion, and degenerative changes in the involved knee. The surgeon must be cautious with this type of patient not to promise too much, since the potential results are affected by the degree of degenerative arthritic changes present before surgical intervention. The progression of these changes has the potential to be decreased in many cases by performing a successful surgical reconstruction of the anterior cruciate ligament. Prior damage cannot be reversed, meaning that patellofemoral pain or compartmental pain may not be alleviated if they are a result of altered joint mechanics and/or degenerative cartilage changes.[16] A younger patient with these changes must be willing to significantly alter his or her lifestyle in order to protect the knee from further degenerative changes. In the older patient, considerations for future resurfacing arthroplasty may be necessary. It is much more difficult to reestablish a nearly normal functioning knee following a chronic reconstruction.[7] Each patient must be considered individually, and the reconstructive effort must be tailored to meet the individual's needs.

Athletically inclined individuals generally possess a relatively greater muscle mass and strength level than sedentary individuals. Their activity level and size places a high demand on any reconstruction. The patients are often in the younger age bracket, thus, any reconstruction will have a potentially longer lifespan. At this point in time, a biological graft that will revascularize and undergo collagen reorganization and that has the potential to respond to injury appears to be the desirable anterior cruciate replacement in this group. This includes both the autograft or allograft replacement materials in which a vascular supply develops.[21] Most prosthetic and/or ligament augmentation devices show fatigue and fail when placed under repetitive high level cyclic loadings over a long period of time and would thus be less desirable. In addition to the appropriate intra-articular reconstruction, the chronically unstable knee may benefit from an extra-articular augmentation. The purpose of the extra-articular augmentation would be to protect the biological graft during the initial period of revascularization and during incorporation of the graft into the osseous tunnels. The extra-articular procedure also has the potential of remaining a reinforcement after healing of the anterior cruciate ligament replacement is complete.

Less active patients who have chronic anterior cruciate ligament instability present a special problem in that they tend to be an older population. Their daily demands on the injured knee may actually be less because of their lower activity level. Few patients in this category actually require surgical reconstruction of the anterior cruciate deficient knee because of the lower level of disability the individual experiences and because of the fact that no repair is without risks and without some residual alteration in knee function. However, a small percentage of these patients do have disability related to activities of daily living. If a surgical reconstruction is performed in this group of patients, they are not likely to place the high peak loads on the implant that are encountered in athletic individuals. Carefully selected individuals may only require extra-articular stabilization. Biological ingrowth and revascularization, which are essential to the long-term success of an intra-articular repair in the younger population, may not be as critical in older patients. The usual prolonged rehabilitation program must be carried out if this approach is selected. These patients must understand this and be willing to complete the total program if they undergo a biological intra-articular reconstruction. In the future, older patients will probably be the first candidates for prosthetic ligament replacement because of the less extensive rehabilitation requirements following this procedure. Until this is available, the surgeon should be selective in performing an intra-articular reconstruction in the older patient. Severe degenerative joint changes will often preclude a lasting good result.[18]

The mechanics and condition of the opposite knee are also important in considering an anterior cruciate ligament reconstruction. Any limitations in the contralateral extremity may place increased demands on the reconstruction. The best results of anterior cruciate ligament reconstruction are obtained in patients with a normal contralateral knee. Activity modifications along with appropriate selection of sports activities must be discussed with the patient before undertaking any sort of reconstructive procedure. Ideally, the patient should be willing to continue with a maintenance strengthening and exercise program indefinitely to ensure lasting results. Avoidance of reinjury and recurrent effusions is an important part of the ongoing program. If the patient completely understands the scope of the problem, reinjury can usually be avoided.

The most difficult problems are encountered in patients with previous surgical reconstructions that have failed to stabilize the knee joint. In these situations, normal structures (patella tendon, iliotibial band, semi-tendinosis, etc.) may have been sacrificed for the previous reconstructions. The exact surgical procedures must be determined before further intervention, because new options need to be considered. Multiple failed procedures represent a strong indication for the prosthetic ligament, however, the ideal prosthetic ligament is not yet available. Allograft substitutions may play an important role in the future as their behavior in vivo becomes further defined. As long-term follow-up reports of allograft implants are released over the next few years, their role may become more apparent. The multiple operated knee must be carefully assessed and screened before any further surgical intervention to avoid increasing the potential disabilities.

Summary

Many variables have been identified both for the surgeon and the patient in considering ligament reconstruction for anterior cruciate ligament dysfunction. All of the surgical procedures devised to this point have the possibility of altering the joint biomechanics in ways that we may not predict preoperatively.[15] Supporting structures may stretch out with time postoperatively. Many procedures have the potential to result in a decreased range of motion by being too tight or by being nonisometric. In this case, they may actually capture the joint, preventing normal flexion and extension. The extensor mechanism has been a problem with pain at long-term follow-up. Abnormal cartilage wear has been reported, both in the patellofemoral joint and the tibiofemoral articulations. This wear may result from the original injury or from altered joint mechanics secondary to the injury and surgical repairs. The surgeon performing these procedures must be aware of these potential problems and be equipped to deal with them effectively. The overall picture of anterior cruciate ligament surgery is rapidly changing. The desire for the future is a graft or prosthesis that approaches an anatomical duplication of the original anterior cruciate ligament. Patellar tendon autologous grafts are considered at present to be state of the art, but they fall short of the normal anterior cruciate ligament structure and function. As new developments emerge and are successfully applied, the patient will be the ultimate beneficiary.

REFERENCES

1. Arnold, J.A., et al.: Natural history of anterior cruciate tears, Am. J. Sports Med. **7**: 305, 1979.
2. Andrews, J.R., and Sanders, R.: A "mini-reconstruction" technique in treating anterolateral rotatory instability (ALRI), Clin. Orthop. **172**:93, 1983.
3. Cabaud, H.E., Rodkey, W.G., and Feagin, J.A.: Experimental studies of acute anterior cruciate ligament injury and repair, Am. J. Sports Med. **7**:18, 1979.
4. Cabaud, H.E., Feagin, J.A., and Rodkey, W.G.: Acute anterior cruciate ligament injury and augmented repair, Am. J. Sports Med. **8**:395, 1980.
5. Chick, R.R., and Jackson, D.W.: Tears of the anterior cruciate ligament in young athletes, J. Bone Joint Surg. (Am.) **60**:970, 1978.
6. Clancy, W.G., Jr.: Anterior cruciate ligament functional instability, Clin. Orthop. **172**:102, 1983.
7. Clancy, W.G., Jr., et al.: Anterior cruciate ligament reconstruction using one-third of the patellar ligament, augmented by extraarticular tendon transfers, J. Bone Joint Surg. (Am.) **64**:352, 1982.
8. DeHaven, K.E.: Arthroscopy in the diagnosis and management of the anterior cruciate ligament deficient knee, Clin. Orthop. **172**:52, 1983.
9. DeHaven, K.E., and Collins, H.R.: Diagnosis of internal derangements of the knee, J. Bone Joint Surg. (Am.) **57**:802, 1975.
10. Fetto, J.F., and Marshall, J.L.: The natural history and diagnosis of anterior cruciate ligament insufficiency, Clin. Orthop. **147**:29, 1980.
11. Frank, C., et al.: Normal ligament properties and ligament healing, Clin. Orthop. **196**:15, 1985.
12. Friedman, M.J., et al.: Autogeneic anterior cruciate ligament (ACL) anterior reconstruction of the knee, Clin. Orthop. **196**:9, 1985.
13. Giove, T.P., et al.: Non-operative treatment of the torn anterior cruciate ligament, J. Bone Joint Surg. (Am.) **65**:184, 1983.
14. Ihle, C.L.: Personal communication, October, 1985.
15. James, S.L.: Biomechanics of knee ligament reconstruction, Clin. Orthop. **146**:90, 1980.
16. Johnson, R.J.: Five- to ten-year follow-up evaluation after reconstruction of the anterior cruciate ligament, Clin. Orthop. **183**:122, 1984.
17. Krachow, K.A., and Brooks, R.L.: Optimization of knee ligament position for lateral extraarticular reconstruction, Am. J. Sports Med. **11**:293, 1983.
18. Lynch, M.A., Henning, C.E., and Glick, K.R., Jr.: Knee joint surface changes, Clin. Orthop. **172**:148, 1983.
19. McDaniel, W.J., Jr., and Dameron, T.B., Jr.: The untreated anterior cruciate ligament rupture, Clin. Orthop. **172**:158, 1983.
20. Noyes, F.R., et al.: Biomechanical analysis of human ligament grafts used in knee-ligament repairs and reconstructions, J. Bone Joint Surg. (Am.) **66**:344, 1984.
21. Noyes, F.R., et al.: Intra-articular cruciate reconstruction, Clin. Orthop. **172**:71, 1983.
22. Noyes, F.R., et al.: The symptomatic anterior cruciate-deficient knee, Part I, J. Bone Joint Surg. (Am.) **65**:154, 1983.
23. Noyes, F.R., et al.: The symptomatic anterior cruciate-deficient knee, Part II, J. Bone Joint Surg. (Am.) **65**:163, 1983.
24. Paulos, L.E., et al.: Intra-articular cruciate reconstruction, Clin. Orthop. **172**:78, 1983.
25. Paulos, L.E.: Personal communication, October 1985.
26. Rosenberg, T.: Personal communication, October, 1985.

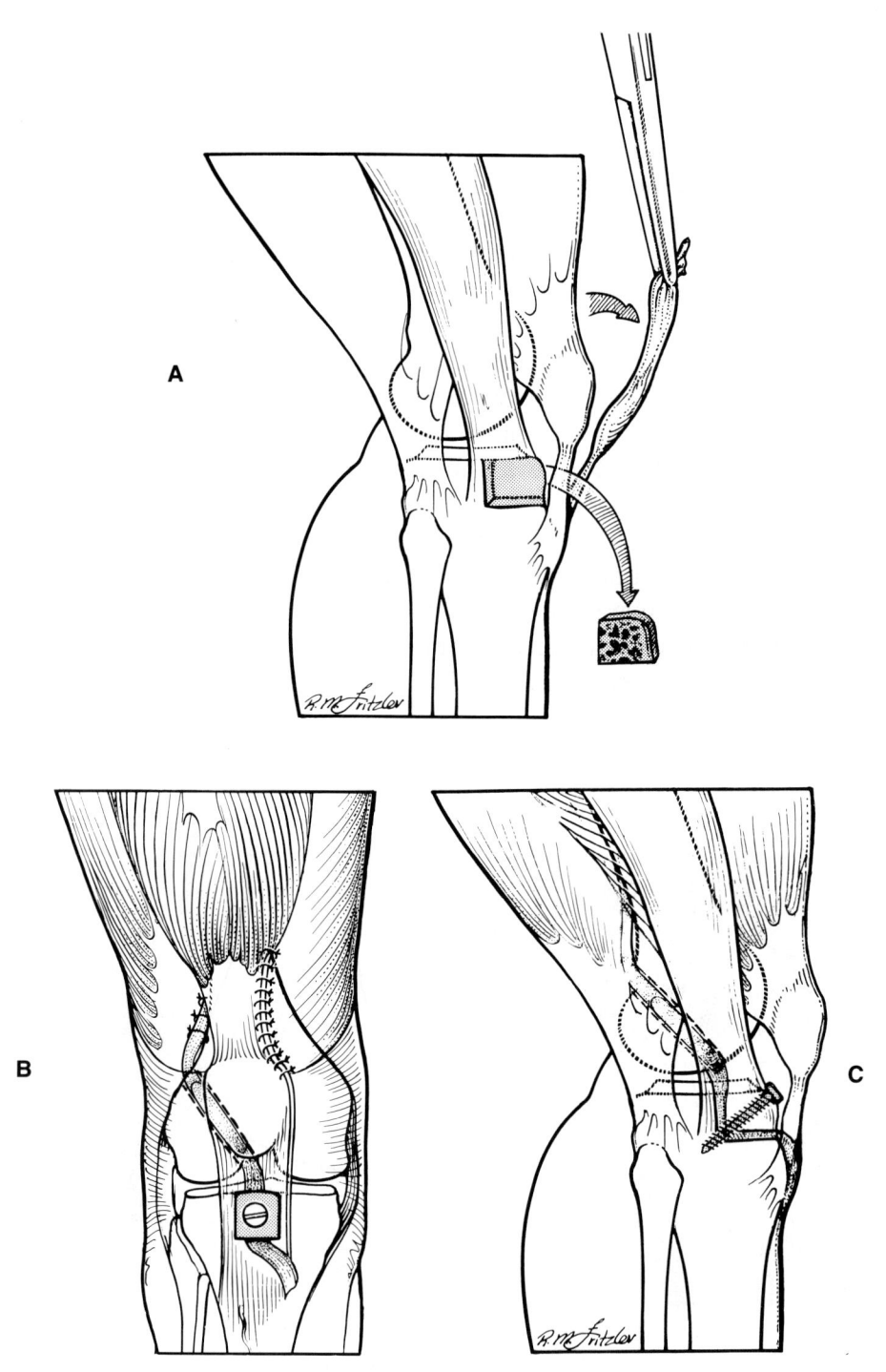

Fig. 10-2 *A,* An inferior tibial bone block is removed and replaced after the distal ligament had been placed in the resulting trough. *B* and *C,* The proximal aspect of the ligament is attached to the outer side of the lateral femoral condyle after being pulled through the intercondylar notch. The end of the graft is secured with screw fixation. (From Lam, S.J.S.: Reconstruction of the anterior cruciate ligament using the Jones procedure and its Guy Hospital modification, J. Bone Joint Surg. [Am.] **50:**1213, 1968.)

In a later follow-up study, Jones reported on modifications of his technique. Pin fixation of the bone block in the femoral condyle was introduced in place of pull-through suturing. Complications with these modifications included slipping of the bone block in two cases. Of the 46 cases in the follow-up report, a 90-degree drawer sign was present in 29 patients, and only 14 patients could get within 35 degrees of full extension.[25]

Further modifications were reported by Lam[28] at Guy's Hospital in 1968. The necessity for proper placement of the osseous tunnel in the intercondylar notch was noted. Lam described tunnel position in the intercondylar notch with the distance between the osseous tunnel and the tibial tuberosity remaining constant throughout the full arc of motion of knee movement. The weakest point in the new ligament was the junction between the patellar bone ends and the tendon; this point often extended out into the joint because of the short length of the graft. The modification involved taking the medial side of the extensor apparatus for additional length. An inferior tibial bone block was removed and subsequently replaced after the distal tendon had been laid in the resulting trough, and both ends of the graft were secured with a screw fixation (Fig. 10-2). The proximal aspect of the ligament was attached to the outer side of the lateral femoral condyle after being pulled through the intercondylar notch. Tension was applied to abolish the drawer sign intraoperatively. Six cases were reported with these modifications; five of the six had a good functional result; the only failure reported was in a 55-year-old patient.

Marshall et al[33] took the middle third of the patellar tendon, including the entire expanse overlaying the patella and the middle third of the quadriceps tendon, folded the middle portion taken from over the patella to strengthen it, and passed it through a tibial tunnel and over the top of the posterior lateral femoral condyle or through the lateral femoral condyle (Fig. 10-3). They described the marginal osteophyte deep in the intercondylar notch that should be removed with a gouge or osteotome so that the graft can pass without impingement (notchplasty) (Fig. 10-4). Of the 40 cases Marshall reported, rehabilitation was complicated in nine; two by painful staples requiring removal, two by recurrent synovitis, and five by patellar tendonitis. Twenty-four patients did not return to their previous activity level.

Wirth and Artmann[49] found in a study of 100 knees that when left attached to the tibial tubercle, the patellar graft was only long

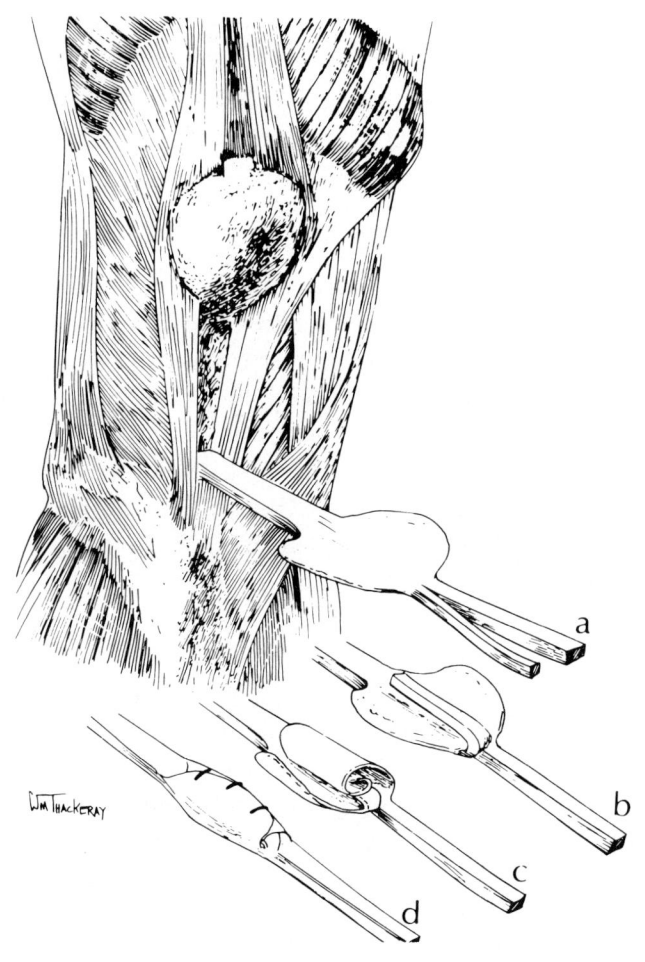

Fig. 10-3 *Harvesting and fashioning the patelloquadriceps substitution for the anterior cruciate ligament. (From Marshall, J.L., et al.: The anterior cruciate ligament: a technique of repair and reconstruction, Clin. Orthop. **143**:97, 1979.)*

enough to reach the insertion site on the lateral femoral condyle in 13% of patients.

Eriksson[15] also used the medial third of the patellar tendon and commented on the extreme importance of anchoring the ligament deep in the joint at its normal insertion.

Clancy et al.[11,12,13] further modified the patellar ligament anterior cruciate ligament reconstruction by recommending eccentrically placed tibial and femoral tunnels for more accurate ligament placement. A Kirschner's (K) wire is inserted starting just medial to the tibial tubercle and above the insertion of the sartorius muscle and exiting anteromedially to the anatomical center of the original ante-

Intra-articular surgical considerations

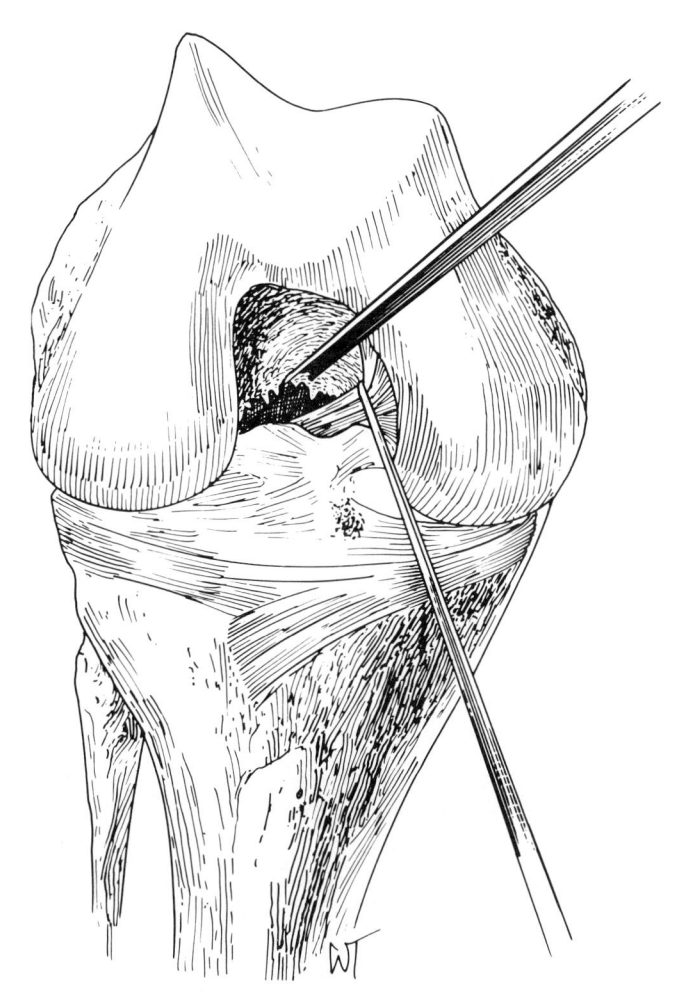

Fig. 10-4 *Removal of the medial osteophyte deep in the intercondylar notch. (From Marshall, J.L., et al.: The anterior cruciate ligament: a technique of repair and reconstruction, Clin. Orthop. **143**:97, 1979.)*

rior cruciate ligament. This K-wire is then used as a guide for a 9-mm cannulated drill. Placement of the K-wire at the anatomical center of the tibial anterior cruciate ligament attachment results in up to a 5-mm displacement of the patellar tendon (Fig. 10-5). With the knee then placed in a figure four position, the lateral femoral canal is created (Fig. 10-6). A second K-wire is placed posterior and superior to the anatomical center of the old anterior cruciate ligament so that when drilled the anterior and inferior circumference of the canal will coincide with the anatomical center, allowing proper pull on the graft, which was located anteriorly and inferiorly in the tunnel.

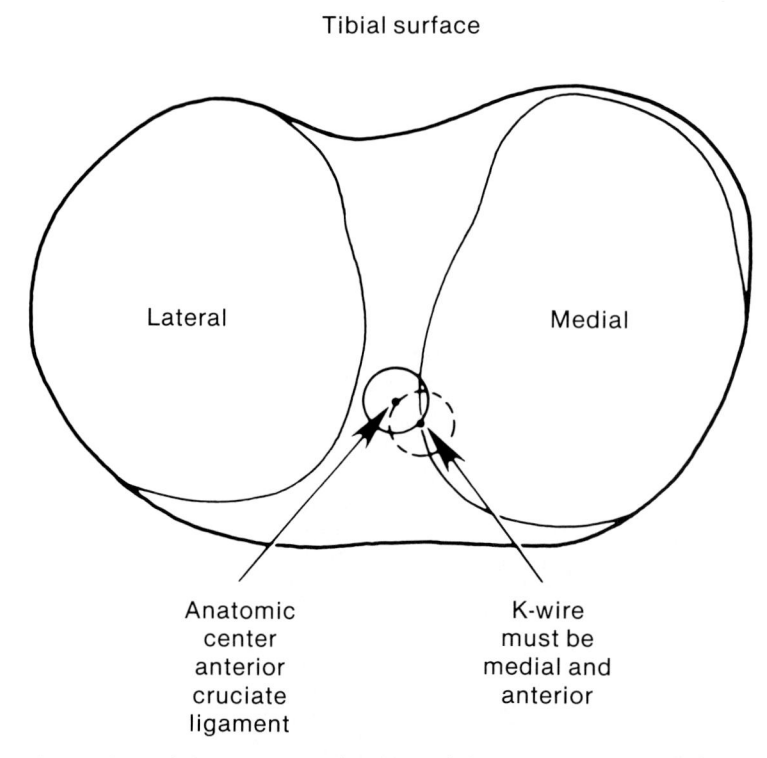

Fig. 10-5 *Relationship of the anatomical center of the anterior cruciate ligament and the placement of the K-wire and tunnel for fixation of a new anterior cruciate ligament patellar graft substitution. (From Clancy, W.G., et al.: Anterior cruciate reconstruction using one third of the patella ligament augmented by extra-articular tendon transfer, J. Bone Joint Surg. [Am.] 64:352, 1982.)*

If the K-wire were placed at the anatomical center, the resultant graft would lie up to 5-mm anteroinferiorly. Originally the medial third of the patella was taken as a graft with both tibial and patellar osseous ends. Later the middle third was used as a vascularized free graft instead (Fig. 10-7). The graft is rotated 180 degrees on its fat pad, which was left attached to the undersurface of the patella. The patellar bone is placed in the tibial canal, and the tibial bone is placed in the femoral canal. By releasing the tendon at both ends and rotating it 180 degrees the tendon can be slid as necessary to allow the positioning of the bony attachments in the osseous tunnels. Sutures from the patellar block are tied over an AO screw and washer placed at the edge of the tibial tunnel. The tibial bone sutures are tied over a button placed over the femoral canal site and

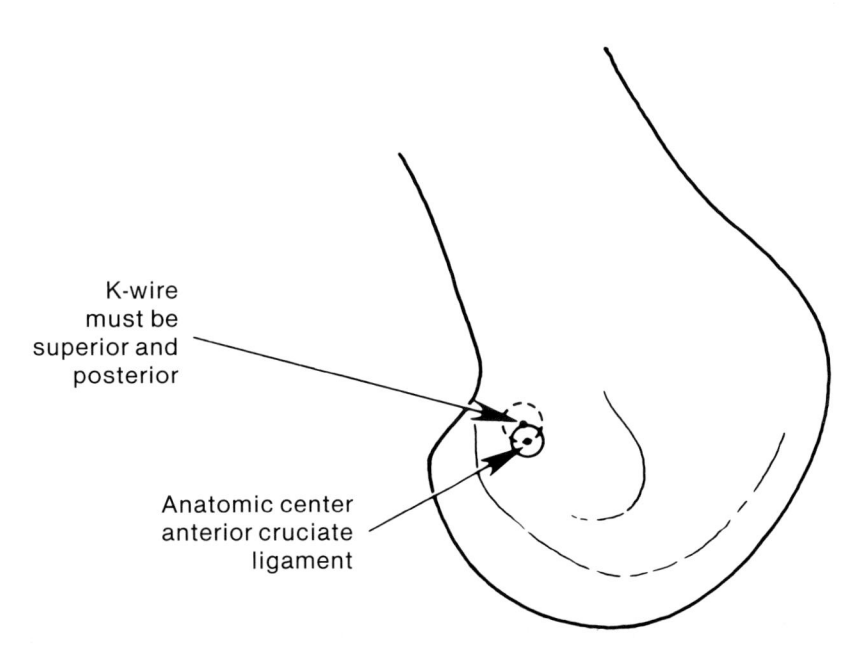

Fig. 10-6 *Relationship of the anatomical center of the anterior cruciate ligament and the placement of the K-wire and tunnel for graft placement. (From Clancy, W.G., et al.: Anterior cruciate reconstruction using one third of the patella ligament augmented by extra-articular tendon transfer, J. Bone Joint Surg. [Am.] 64:352, 1982.)*

tightened and then further secured to a staple placed proximal to the canal to take up any remaining slack. The procedure is then augmented laterally by a biceps tendon transfer and medially by a pes anserinus transfer. Fifty of the eighty patients reconstructed with this technique between 1976 and 1980 were reevaluated. Forty-four patients had resumed sports activities requiring acceleration, deceleration, and cutting. Eight patients had a trace pivot shift, and one had a mild pivot shift. Forty-one patients had no pivot shift phenomenon. Thirty patients had excellent results, seventeen had good, one had fair, and two had poor results based on subjective, objective, and functional criteria. The two failures were the result of chondromalacia and neuroma.[11] Five patients (10%) required operative manipulation to regain motion.

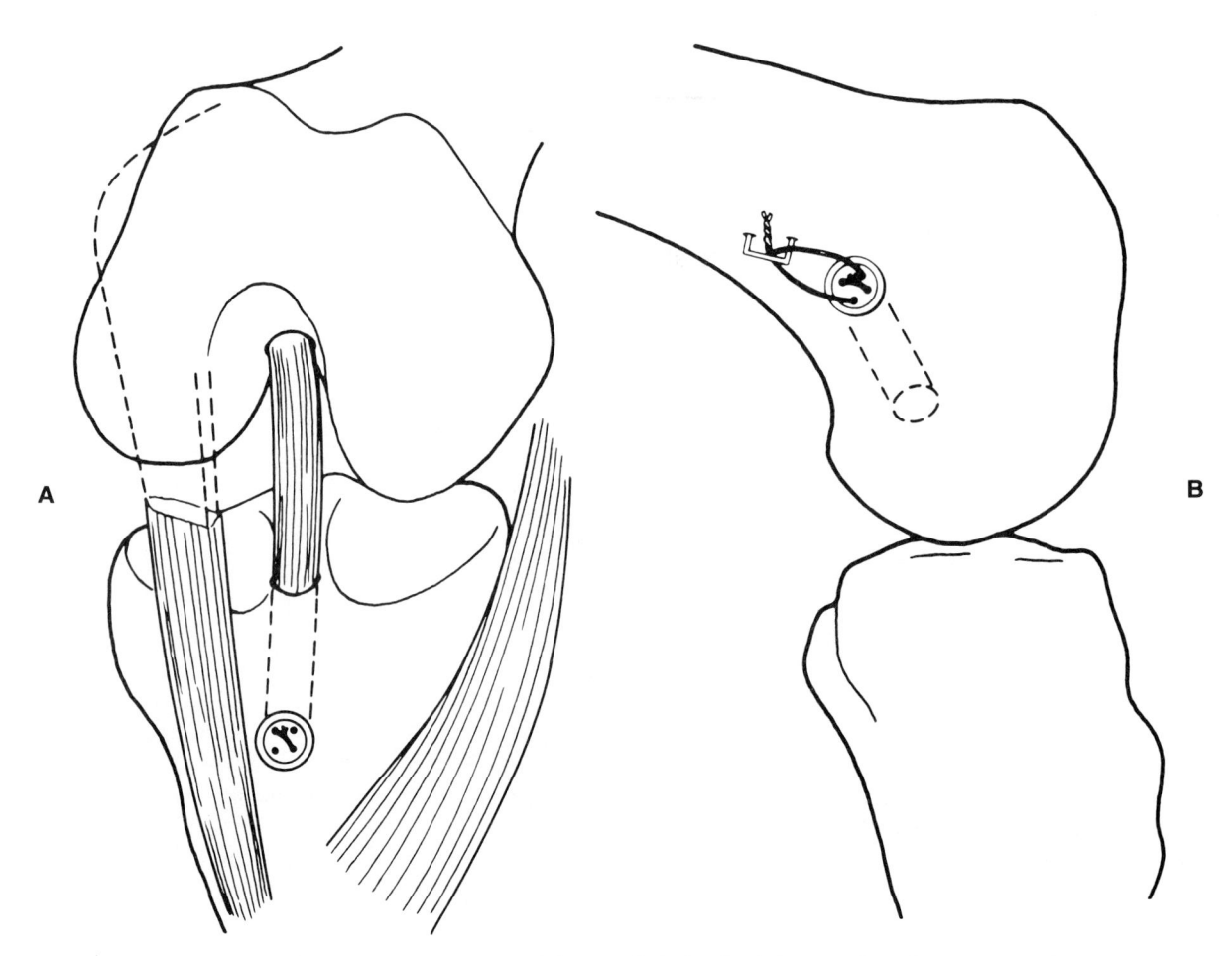

Fig. 10-7 **A** and **B**, Demonstration of the medial third of the patella taken as a graft with both tibial and patellar osseous ends. (From Clancy, W.G., et al.: Anterior cruciate reconstruction using one third of the patella ligament augmented by extra-articular tendon transfer, J. Bone Joint Surg. [Am.] **64**:352, 1982.)

Since 1980 over 300 vascularized patellar tendon grafts have been performed with the early results essentially unchanged from the earlier study.[13] Noyes et al.[36] have also recommended using a patellar tendon graft (usually the medial third) with its vascular and neural attachments on the hypothesis that the biological graft would undergo less necrosis and remodeling. The surgical procedure of the vascularized pedicle graft is demanding, and the eventual clinical results may not warrant the extra effort needed to preserve the blood supply of the graft.[40]

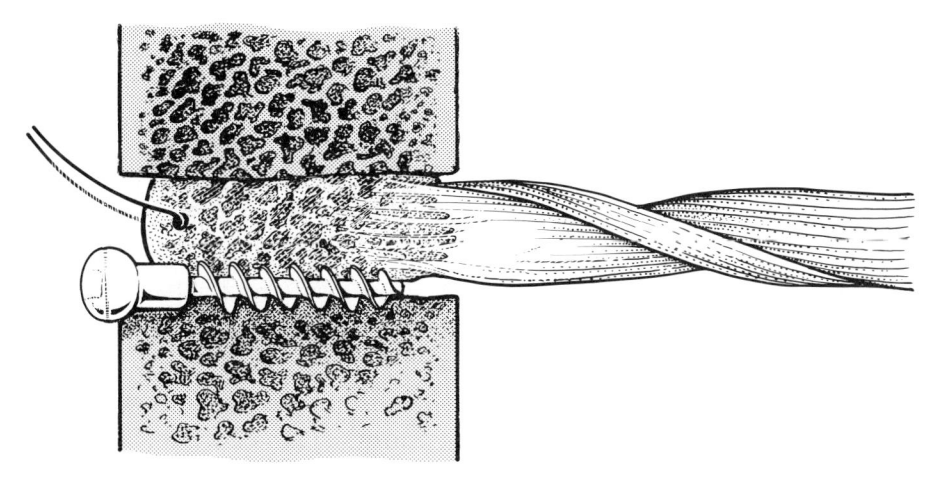

Fig. 10-8 *Fixation of bone block using cog-type screw fixation. (From Lambert, K.L.: Vascularized patella tendon graft with rigid internal fixation for anterior cruciate ligament insufficiency, Clin. Orthop.* **172**:*85, 1983.)*

Lambert[29] has modified the fixation technique by interposing an AO screw within the canals for fixation of the bone blocks, creating a cog type of fixation (Fig. 10-8). This improves immediate fixation to allow early motion.

The importance of placement of the femoral tunnel was stressed by Alin.[1] He showed on rearthrotomy of 11 middle third patellar tendon reconstructions of the anterior cruciate ligament that improper placement of the tendon led to laxity and subsequent inflammatory and degenerative changes. Macroscopic revascularization of the patellar tendon was demonstrated by ingrowth of vessels from the surrounding synovium. Arnoczky et al.[2] demonstrated with patellar tendon grafts in dogs the absence of perfusion of vessels from the osseous side to the patellar tendon graft. Failure of the osseous insertion of the graft to contribute to the revascularization process occurs initially after transplantation. The patellar tendon graft is essentially an avascular graft at insertion and requires the contribution of surrounding soft tissues of the knee to contribute to revascularization of the graft. Arnoczky suggested using the fat pad and synovial tissue to optimize graft revascularization. Throughout the period of intrinsic revascularization there was noted cellular proliferation that would eventually subside. At 1 year the transplanted graft had the histologic appearance of a normal ligament.

Intra-articular iliotibial band

One of the earliest reported anterior cruciate ligament reconstructions was described by Hey Groves in 1917.[21] In this case the iliotibial band was detached from its tibial insertion and pulled through a lateral femoral canal that was placed at the old insertion site of the anterior cruciate ligament and then brought through a tibial canal placed near the tibial insertion of the anterior cruciate ligament. In the same procedure he described reconstructing the posterior cruciate ligament with the semitendinosus. This was a single case report with a good result.

A modification of the Hey Groves technique was reported by O'Donoghue[38] in 1963. The iliotibial band graft was left attached distally, taken first through the tibial tunnel and then through the femoral tunnel. The remaining tissue was used to reconstruct the distal portion of the iliotibial band and the lateral collateral ligament. The distal portion of the iliotibial tract is an extremely dense, strong structure that makes a more effective ligament when passed across the joint space than does the longer thin proximal layer. The thinner portion was doubled over on itself to reinforce the lateral collateral ligament (Fig. 10-9). With the original Hey Groves procedure the thick portion of the iliotibial band is left intact and the thinner proximal portion is rolled up and passed through the tunnels. Of the 29 cases reported, 21 continued to have one grade or more anterior instability as compared to the opposite knee. There were four postoperative infections. Twenty-four patients returned to sporting activities. The patients selected for the operation were young, active, in good health, and exceedingly well motivated.

The bone-block iliotibial band transfer was first reported by Insall et al.[22] in 1981. The anterior distal part of the iliotibial tract with an attached bone block from Gerdy's tubercle was used as an intraarticular graft. It is important to use only the anterior two thirds of the iliotibial band, leaving the posterior one third to provide lateral stability. The bone-block and its attached band are brought into the intercondylar notch by the "over-the-top" technique. While applying as much traction as possible on the fascial graft, the bone-block is then fixed to a prepared slot in the anterior aspect of the tibia and held with an AO screw (Fig. 10-10). The procedure is recommended for insufficiency of the anterior cruciate ligament with anterior, anteromedial, or anterolateral laxity with unpredictable episodes of instability that do not improve after adequate rehabilitation. The procedure is contraindicated when there is posterior or

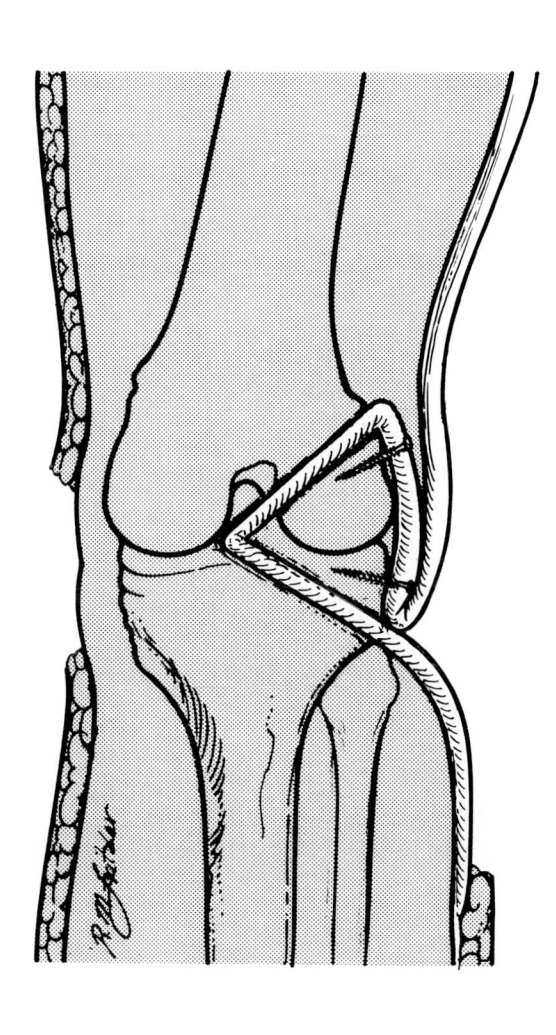

Fig. 10-9 *Final graft position with the strong, thick, distal portion of the iliotibial band passed through the knee. The thinner proximal tract is stapled along the lateral aspect of the knee to reinforce the lateral collateral ligament. (From O'Donoghue, D.H.: A method for replacement of the anterior cruciate ligament of the knee, J. Bone Joint Surg. [Am.] 45:905, 1963.*

single-plane lateral laxity. Twenty-four patients were reported, all with positive anterior drawer tests preoperatively. The pivot shift was tested in ten knees preoperatively; the Lachman test was performed on only four patients. Both tests were positive in all knees tested. Postoperatively, all knees had full extension; only one knee had flexion limited to 110 degrees. Occasional pain was noted from five patients, and one patient underwent later patellectomy. Other complications included one knee with skin necrosis, a subcutaneous hematoma in one knee, and two knees requiring manipulation under general anesthesia at 6 weeks to regain flexion of 125 and 130 degrees respectively. Some laxity was noted in most knees by the anterior drawer and Lachman tests at follow-up.

Scott and Schosheim[42] modified the bone-block iliotibial band

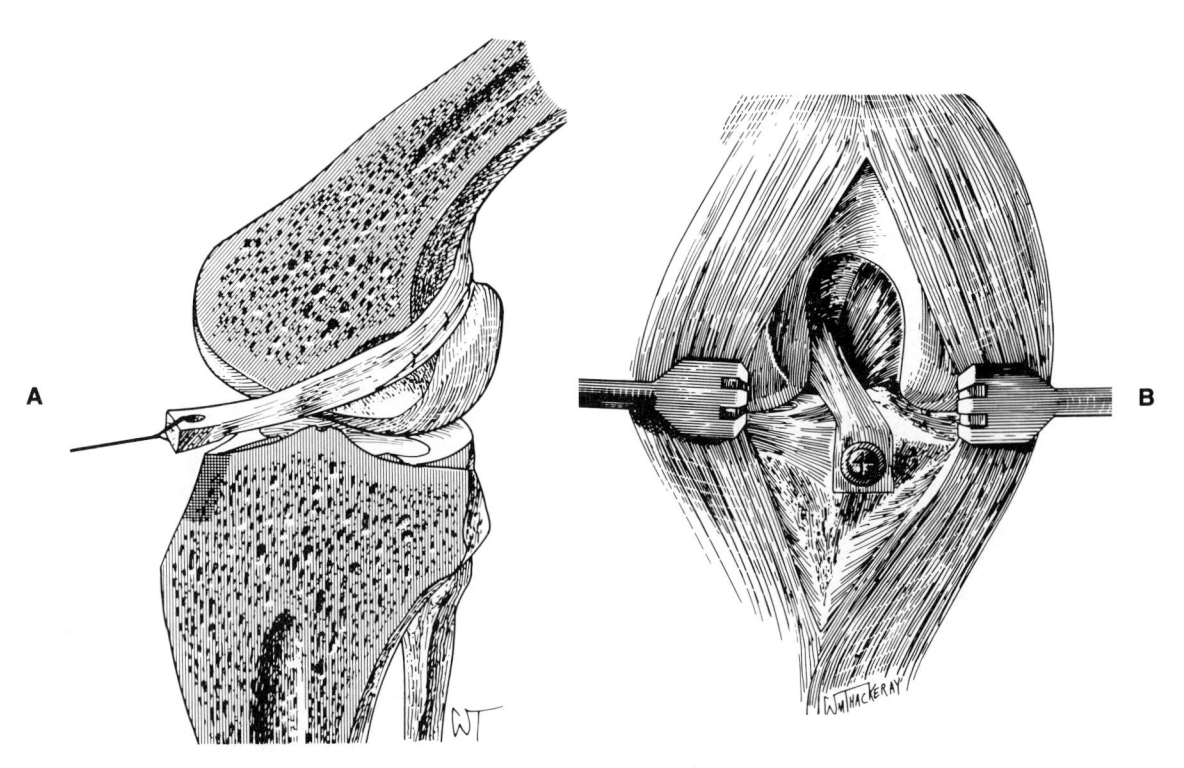

Fig. 10-10 *A,* The over-the-top placement of the iliotibial humeral graft. *B,* Position of the transfer following fixation of the bone block with a screw. (From Insall, J., et al.: Bone block transfer for anterior cruciate deficiency, J. Bone Joint Surg. [Am.] **63:**560, 1981.)

transfer by limiting the posterior dissection of the iliotibial band to 4 cm. This is unlike the original description, which took equal length anterior and posterior limbs of approximate 13 cm in length.

This alteration allows maintenance of the attachment of the iliotibial band to the lateral intermuscular septum and restricts mobility, giving a better static stability. A trough is created in the tibia deep enough so that the AO cancellous screw is below the plateau level. The tourniquet is released before insertion of the bone block to minimize proximal tension and to allow a taut fit.

In a follow-up study, Scott et al.[43] reported on the 2 to 7 year follow-up of their modified procedure. Ninty-four percent of the patients had negative pivot shift, 84% had a 1+ or less anterior drawer test, and 81% had a negative Lachman test. Of the 110 patients (111 knees) in this series, decreased extension as compared to the unoperated side was noted in 30 knees (0 to 5 degrees in 25 and 6 to 10 degrees in 5). Limited flexion was noted in 46 knees (less than 10 degrees in 35, 15 degrees in 6, and 20 degrees in 5). Little additional motion was gained after the first year. There were few complications. The bone-block crumbled intraoperatively in two patients and required alternate fixation and then casting for 6 weeks. Ten patients required further surgery; six patients required removal of the intra-articular screw, one required meniscectomy, and three required lysis of adhesions.

Revascularization was necessary for the proximally based transfer of the iliotibial band. During rearthrotomy for screw removal the grafts all appeared viable.[43]

Eighteen knees (16%) had acceptable results with a 2+ or more anterior drawer test and a positive Lachman test. It was believed that these were the result of combined instability patterns. The authors now augment the intra-articular transfer with an extra-articular technique (pes anserinus transfer medially, proximal advancement of the medial or lateral collateral ligament, artificial extra-articular enhancement, or a combination).[43]

Intra-articular semitendinosus

Augustine[3] was the first to suggest the use of the semitendinosus as a dynamic reconstruction of the anterior cruciate ligament. The semitendinosus tendon is left attached proximally, released from its insertion, and passed through the intracondylar groove and into the tibial tunnel. Some residual laxity was expected with this procedure. O'Donoghue[38] noted that if the semitendinosus was strong enough to act as the anterior crciate ligament, it should do so without having to be transferred.

Kennedy et al.[27] studied the behavior of the semitendinosus tendon in animals in an intra-articular environment both as a distally attached graft and as a free graft. At 26 weeks these grafts had half the tensile strength on Instrom testing as normal semitendinosus tendons. On nuclear scanning those tendons with increased blood flow as compared to normal semitendinosus tendons demonstrated microscopic fiber degeneration.

Using the semitendinosus tendon as a distally (tibial) based graft was recommended by Cho.[10] The semitendinosus tendon is released at its muscular tendinous junction, and the proximal muscle belly is sutured to the other medial hamstrings. Tunnels are prepared in both the tibia and the lateral femoral condyles as previously

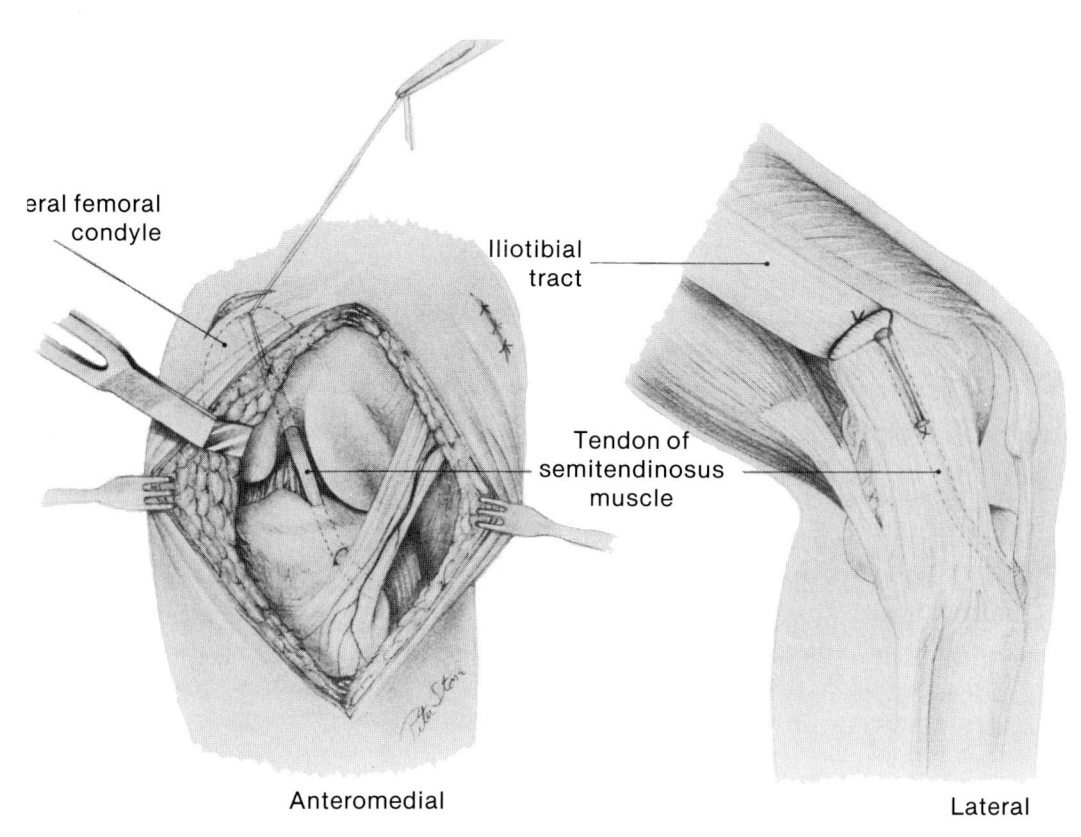

Fig. 10-11 *The semitendinosus muscle is passed through the knee by way of the tunnels in the fibula and lateral femoral condyle and sutured to the iliotibial level. (From Cho, K.O.: Reconstruction of the anterior cruciate ligament by semitendinous tenodesis, J. Bone Joint Surg. [Am.] 57:608, 1975.)*

described. The tendon is then passed through the tibial tunnel, across the joint, and into the femoral tunnel. The proximal end of the tendon usually will not reach the end of the canal so the attached sutures are tied over the iliotibial band, and bone-tendon union is expected to occur during the postoperative cast immobilization (Fig. 10-11). Only seven cases were reported by Cho with an average 21.5 month follow-up. Two cases had continued anterior laxity postoperatively, but both had genu recurvatum and generalized ligamentous laxity. One case required rearthrotomy for patellar subluxation that allowed direct observation of the semitendinosus tendon at approximately 8 months. The tendon was noted to be hypertrophied and covered with thickened, mildly inflamed synovium. Two patients had loss of motion but were able to return to work.

Lipscomb et al.[32] reported on 78 patients with torn anterior cruciate ligaments who were treated using the technique described by Cho. Special attention was given to placing the tendon as far posteriorly as possible in the lateral femoral condylar notch to follow as closely as possible the anatomical path of the original ligament. Reefing of the posterolateral capsule was performed routinely when anteromedial instability was present. Associated meniscectomy was performed in 71 patients, and reefing of the posteromedial capsule was performed in 35. Of the 71 reconstructions with associated medial meniscectomy, 60 reconstructions showed improved stability, and all 35 reefing procedures had good results. Fourteen percent (11 patients) had significant residual anterior and anteromedial rotatory instability.

The transformation of the transferred semitendinosus tendon into a functioning anterior cruciate ligament still has not been documented. The histologic studies done on a ruptured semitendinosus transfer of 16 months duration demonstrated fibrocartilaginous metaplasia and appeared to be viable as a whole. Collagen fibers were noted to be oriented in multiple directions like the anterior cruciate ligament, and the entire tendon was covered with synovium. However, the reconstruction that was augmented with extra-articular medial and lateral procedures failed.[41]

A modification of the Cho technique has been reported by Zarins.[50] A combined intra-articular/extra-articular reconstruction is performed using both the semitendinosus tendon and the iliotibial band and a lateral capsular reefing (Fig. 10-12).

> The semitendinosus is divided at the musculotendinous junction. The posteromedial capsule is reefed in a double-breasted manner. An oblique drill hole is made in the proximal tibia. A strip of iliotibial tract is fashioned and left attached to Gerdy's tubercle. The fibular collateral ligament is dissected free of the underlying lateral capsule. The lateral capsule is reefed deep to the lateral collateral ligament. Both transfers are passed along an identically parallel course: through an oblique drill hole in the anteromedial tibia, across the knee joint, over the top of the lateral intermuscular septum, and deep to the fibular collateral ligament. Both transfers are pulled tightly and sutured to one another.[50]

No follow-up has been reported with this procedure.

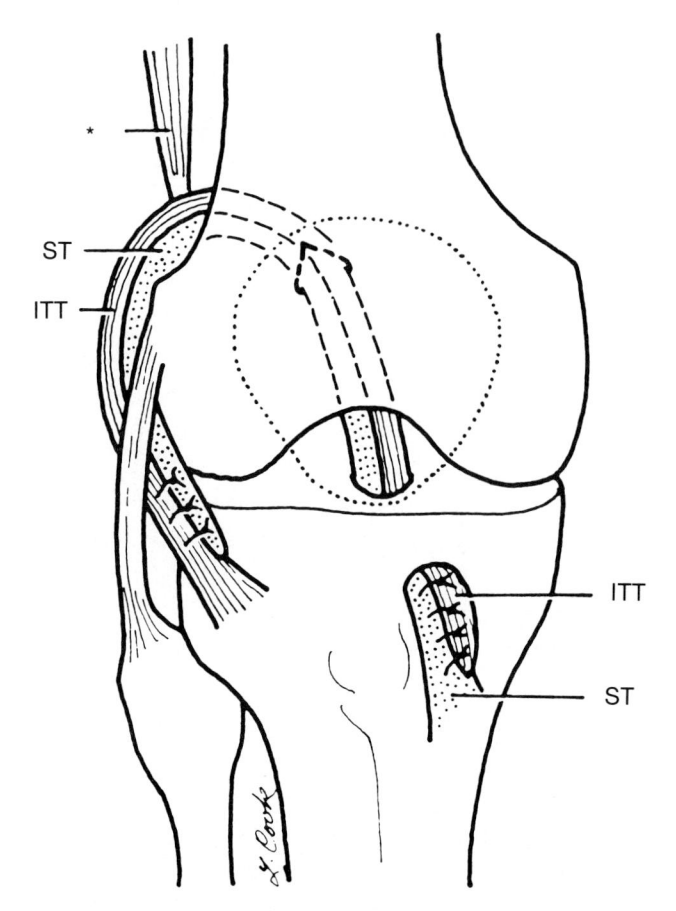

Fig. 10-12 *Semitendinosus tendon (ST) and iliotibial tract (ITT) transfers used as a combined anterior cruciate ligament reconstruction.*, Lateral intermuscular septum. (From Zarins, B.: Combined intra-articular and extra-articular reconstruction for anteriortibial subluxation, Orthop. Clin. North Am.* **16:**223, 1985.)

Intra-articular gracilis substitution

Use of the gracilis tendon as a free sliding substitution for the anterior cruciate ligament was first publicized in 1950 in *Zeitschuilt fur Orthopaidie und Ihre Grenzgebiete* by Lindemann.[30] duToit reported his results with the Lindemann procedure in 1967.[14] In this technique the free sliding gracilis tendon is substituted for the chronically torn anterior cruciate ligament by passing it through a posterolateral perforation in the posterior capsule of the knee joint and through the intracondylar notch. It is secured by tunnel fixation in the proximal tibia just anterior to the distal attachment of the previous anterior cruciate ligament[14] (Fig. 10-13).

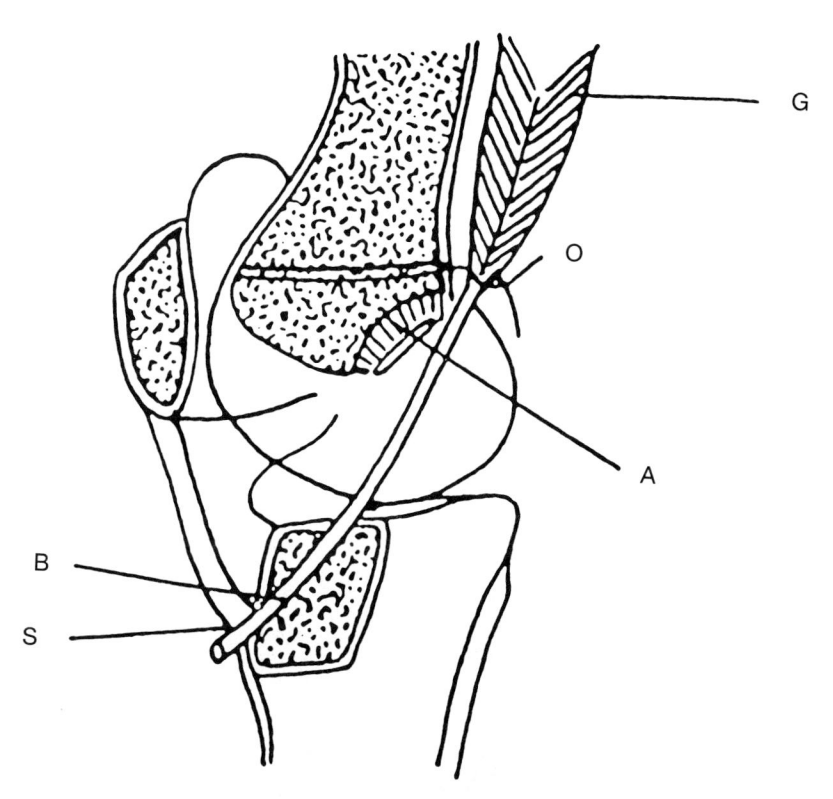

Fig. 10-13 *Anterior cruciate substitution using the gracilis muscle (G). The gracilis muscle is laced through a bony tunnel (B) and sutured to the infrapatellar tendon (S) as an anterior cruciate ligament. O, Capsule opening; A, anterior capsule. (From du Toit, G.T.: Kneejoint cruciate ligament substitution: the Lindemann procedure, S. Afr. J. Surg. 5(1):25, 1967.)*

The theoretical advantages of this procedure are twofold: (1) the living tendon with intact proprioceptors presumably gives greater awareness of tension than a free denervated piece of fascia, and (2) the free-sliding gracilis tendon does not stretch because the muscle tone preserves its tension.[14]

The knee is approached through an anteromedial arthrotomy. The incision is then extended proximally along the border of the sartorius muscle and distally to the pes anserinus. The gracilis is identified and freed. The distal end of the gracilis is divided and grasped with a clamp. The knee is flexed to 90 degrees, and the areolar tissue is bluntly dissected from the intermuscular septum and the posterior aspect of the femur, taking care to protect the popliteal vessels. A long, curved forceps is then pushed from the anterior direction through the intercondylar notch and through the lateral portion of the posteromedial capsule. The forceps are then spread to widen the hole and to grasp the distal end of the gracilis tendon and pull it through the openings. A tibial tunnel is fashioned just medial to the patellar tendon and exiting near the normal tibial attachment of the anterior cruciate ligament. A strong suture is placed through the gracilis to pull it through the tibial tunnel; this is done under moderate tension with the knee flexed to 50 degrees. The gracilis tendon should be firmly pulled distally but not to the degree likely to cause sloughing by tension ischemia. The tendon will usually emerge through the tunnel 2 to 3 cm and should be secured with multiple sutures.

duToit reported 12 cases using the gracilis transfer. Eleven patients were subjectively improved, one patient noted no improvement, and two patients lost a few degrees of flexion. There were no infections.[14]

Intra-articular meniscal anterior cruciate ligament reconstruction

The menisci have been suggested as materials for reconstruction of the anterior cruciate deficient knee based on the theory that the menisci are already avascular and that they rely on the synovial bathing of the knee joint for their nutrition.[31] The menisci are readily available without requiring a large surgical exposure. Many of their collagen bundles are longitudinally arranged,[8] and their strength appears to be comparable to that of the anterior cruciate ligament.[21]

Using an anteromedial arthrotomy, the medial meniscus is totally removed and the posterior aspect is trimmed to obtain a graft of uniform width. A 7- to 8-mm cannulated drill is used to create both the tibial and the posterior border of the lateral femoral condylar canal. A smaller hole is made at an angle to the first canal to create a cortical bridge. The menisci are then placed in the knee and pulled into both canals, using the cortical bridge to tie sutures over[47] (Fig. 10-14). A modification of this technique has been described, in which the anterior attachment of the medial meniscus is preserved[21] (Fig. 10-15).

Lindstrom reported 22 cases of anterior cruciate ligament reconstruction using this procedure. There were four failures (18%) with pronounced residual drawer symptoms.[31] Tillberg reported on 45 cases of anterior cruciate ligament reconstruction using the meniscus. Of the 45, six patients (13%) developed complications—four of the reconstructions elongated, one proximal attachment failed, and one patient developed infection. Fourteen patients (31%) had 3- to 10-mm anterior instability as compared to the opposite knee. Of the

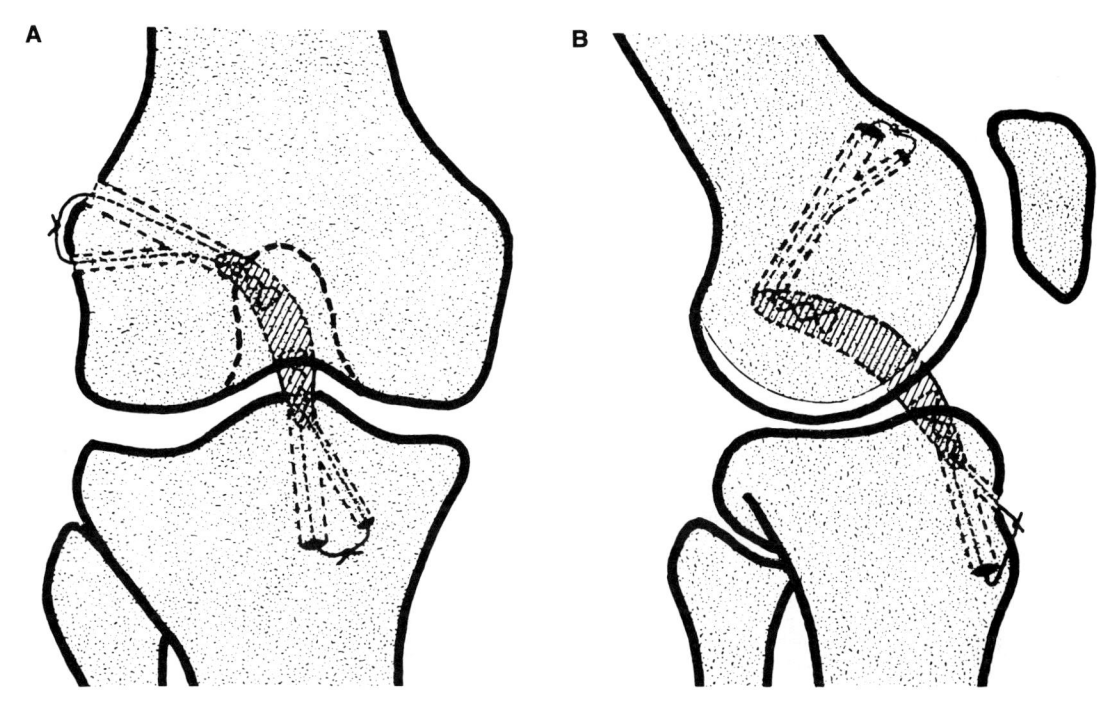

Fig. 10-14 *A* and *B*, Placement of the meniscus through bony tunnels to substitute for the anterior cruciate ligament. (From Tillberg, B.: Late repair of torn cruciate ligaments using the menisci, J. Bone Joint Surg. [Br.] **59:**15, 1977.)

45 cases, 22 patients reported some intermittent instability of the knee.[47]

Smillie reported good results in 17 of 20 cases using the meniscus for isolated anterior cruciate ligament tears. Despite his results Smillie did not advocate this technique.[46]

Walsh reported 13 anterior cruciate ligament reconstructions using the menisci and leaving the anterior attachment of the meniscus intact. All cases were unimproved, and seven were significantly worse following reconstruction. Five cases required re-exploration, during which the meniscal transplant was found to be degenerated and loose.[48]

Menisci substitutions were compared to patellar tendon substitutions by Ivey et al.[23] The only observed difference between the two methods was an average loss of 6 degrees of flexion with the patellar tendon substitutions. In each case the menisci were damaged, and the authors did not advocate the sacrifice of a normal menisci for reconstruction of the anterior cruciate ligament.

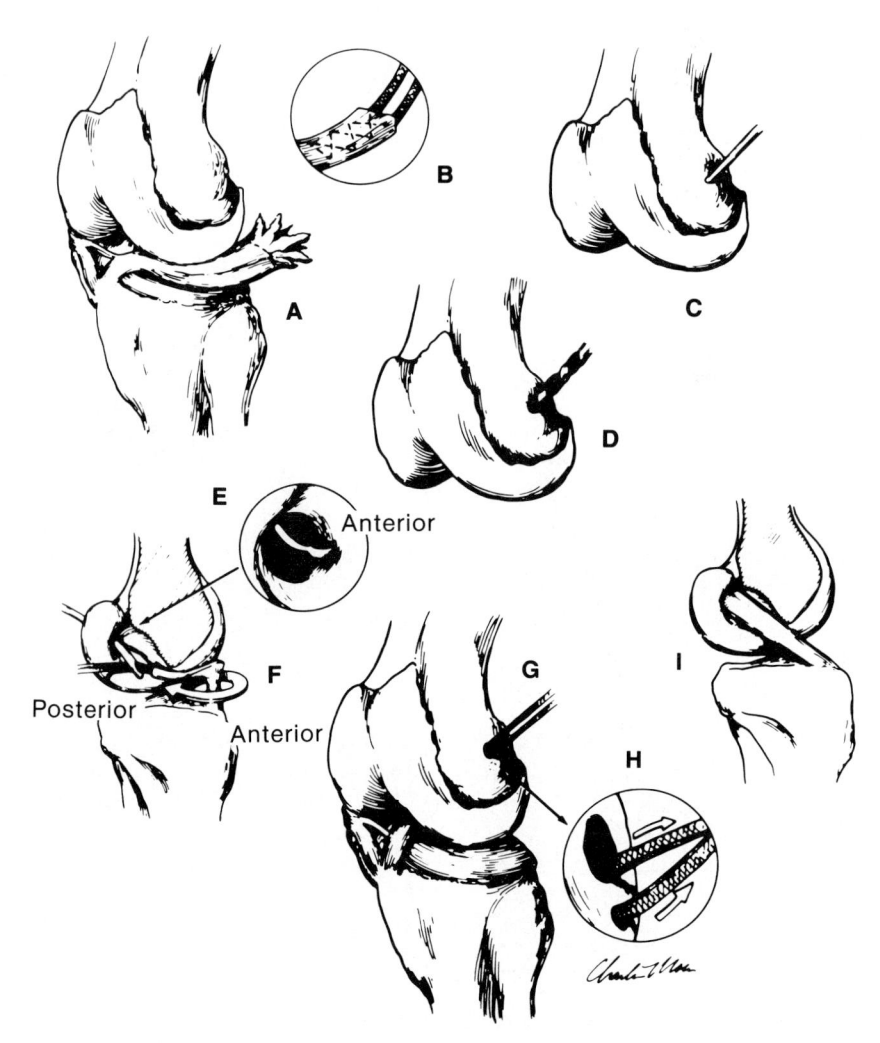

Fig. 10-15 *A through H, Modified technique of anterior cruciate ligament substitution using the medial meniscus with the anterior attachment preserved. (From Ivey, F.M., et al.: Intra-articular substitution of anterior cruciate insufficiency, Am. J. Sports Med. 8:405, 1980.)*

Summary

Reconstruction of the anterior cruciate ligament has progressed a great deal in the last 80 years. However, open arthrotomy techniques for anterior cruciate ligament reconstruction have had associated complications. The intra-articular procedures reported to date have had a number of complications, including loss of extension, loss of flexion, patellofemoral joint pain, patellar tendonitis, continued or recurrent laxity, chronic knee pain, and inability of the patient to return to previous activity level. The ideal reconstruction would require minimal exposure and no dislocation of the patella, would allow immediate range of motion and weight bearing, would not require sacrificing the secondary stabilizing structures of the knee for an autograft, and would allow the patient to return to previous sporting activities in the shortest time possible.

The use of an autograft has required the sacifice of other stabilizing structures about the knee. The sacrifice of secondary stabilizing structures is an already unstable anterior cruciate deficient knee may contribute to greater knee pathology.

Continued attempts at improving anterior cruciate ligament reconstruction has led to use of the arthroscopic technique. This technique allows minimal dissection of the soft tissue, which can eliminate a significant amount of the postoperative morbidity. In arthroscopic techniques the patella is not everted, and trauma to the patella and patellofemoral joint is minimized, reducing the incidence of postoperative patellofemoral joint pain and patellar tendonitis. The continued improvements in surgical equipment will allow easier and more reproducible graft placement.

New graft materials, such as allograft augmentation and prosthetic ligaments, will allow the surgeon to waive the use of any secondary stabilizing structures. The ideal anterior cruciate ligament graft has yet to be developed. The work currently underway with both allograft and prosthetic graft replacements is quite promising.

Osseous tunnels can be prepared on a reproducible basis either in the traditional, open surgical technique or arthroscopically through limited arthrotomy. Certain principles of osseous tunnel placement have been developed and have become common in most procedures. These principles include: (1) proper placement of drill guides for isometric placement of the osseous tunnel; (2) minimization of tunnel obliquity to decrease the bending moment placed on the graft at the tunnel entrance (proper obliquity of the tunnels makes passing the graft through the tunnels easier); (3) chamfering of the sharp edges of the tunnel entrance to further decrease the potential bending fatigue the graft experiences (if the bending fatigue is significant, utlimate failure of the graft may occur); (4) making the tunnel large enough to allow the graft to pass through without damage (the bone plugs need to fit tightly to promote bony ingrowth and not a surrounding fibrous layer); (5) using slow drilling techniques to minimize the amount of heat necrosis and further promote bony ingrowth.

REFERENCES

1. Alin, A.: Survival of part of patella tendon transposed for reconstruction of anterior cruciate ligament, Acta. Chir. Scand. **139:** 443-447, 1973.
2. Arnoczky, S.P., et al.: Anterior cruciate ligament replacement using patella tendon, J. Bone Joint Surg. (Am.) **64**(2):217-224, 1982.
3. Augustine, R.W.: The unstable knee, Am. J. Surg. **92:**380-388, 1956.
4. Battle, W.H.: A case after open section of the knee joint for irreducible traumatic dislocation, Clin. Soc. London Trans. **33:**232, 1900.
5. Bosworth, D.M., and Bosworth, B.M.: Use of fascia lata to stabilize the knee in cases of ruptured crucial ligaments, J. Bone & Joint Surg. **18:**178-179, 1936.
6. Butler, D., Noyes, F., Grood, E., et al.: Mechanical properties of transplants for the anterior cruciate ligament, Orth. Trans. **3:** 180-181, 1979.
7. Campbell, W.C.: Repair of the ligaments of the knee, Surg. Gynec. & Obst. **62:**964-968, 1936.
8. Campbell, W.C.: Reconstruction of the ligaments of the knee, Am. J. Surg. **43:**473-480, 1939.
9. Chick, R.R., and Jackson, D.W.: Tears of the anterior cruciate ligament in young athletes, J. Bone Joint Surg. (Am.) **60**(7):970-973, 1978.
10. Cho, K.O.: Reconstruction of the anterior cruciate ligament by semitendinous tenodesis, J. Bone Joint Surg. (Am.) **57**(5):608-612, 1975.
11. Clancy, W.C., et al.: Anterior cruciate reconstruction using one third of the patella ligament augmented by extraarticular tendon transfer, J. Bone Joint Surg. (Am.) **64**(3):352-359, 1982.
12. Clancy, W.C.: Anterior cruciate ligament functional instability, Clin. Orthop. **172:** 102-106, 1983.
13. Clancy, W.C.: Intraarticular reconstruction of the anterior cruciate ligament, Orthop. Clin. North Am. **16**(2):181-189, 1985.
14. duToit, G.T.: Knee joint cruciate ligament substitution: the Lindemann procedure, S. Afr. J. Surg. **5**(1):25-30, 1967.
15. Eriksson, E.: Reconstruction of the anterior cruciate ligament, Orthop. Clin. North Am. **7**(1):167-179, 1976.
16. Eriksson, E.: Ivar Palmer: a great name in the history of cruciate ligament surgery, Clin. Orthop. **172:**3-10, 1983.
17. Feagin, J.A., and Curl, W.W.: Isolated tear of the anterior cruciate ligament, Am. J. Sports Med. **4:**95-100, 1976.
18. Fetto, J.F., and Marshall, J.L.: The natural history and diagnosis of anterior cruciate insufficiency, Clin. Orthop. **147:**29-38, 1980.
19. Galen, C.: On the usefulness of the parts of the body, (Translated by May, M.T.), Ithaca, 1968, Cornell University Press, pp. 22, 90, 197, and 550.
20. Goetjes, H.: Uber verletzungen der ligamenta cruciata des kniegelenks, Dtsch. Z. Chir. **123:**221, 1913.
21. Hey Groves, E.W.: Operation for the repair of the crucial ligaments, Lancet **2:**674-675, 1917.
22. Insall, J., Joseph, D.M., Aglietti, P., et al.: Bone block transfer for anterior cruciate deficiency, J. Bone Joint Surg. (Am.) **63**(4): 560-569, 1981.
23. Ivey, F.M., et al.: Intra-articular substitution of anterior cruciate insufficiency, Am. J. Sports Med. **8:**405, 1980.
24. Jones, K.G.: Reconstruction of the anterior cruciate ligament, J. Bone Joint Surg. (Am.) **45**(5):925-932, 1963.
25. Jones, K.G.: Reconstruction of the anterior cruciate ligament using the central one third of the patella ligament (a follow-up report), J. Bone Joint Surg. (Am.) **52**(7): 1302-1308, 1970.
26. Kennedy, J.C.: Natural history and management of acute and chronic problems. Part Four, presented at AAOS instruction course: The Athletic Knee in 1981 and Arthroscopy, Palm Beach, Florida, 1981.
27. Kennedy, J.C., Roth, J.C., Mendenhall, U.V., et al.: Presidential address: intra-articular replacement of the anterior cruciate ligament deficient knee, Am. J. Sports Med. **8:**1-8, 1980.

28. Lam, S.J.S.: Reconstruction of the anterior cruciate ligament using the Jones procedure and its Guy Hospital modification, J. Bone Joint Surg. (Am.) **50**(6):1213-1224, 1968.
29. Lambert, K.L.: Vascularized patella tendon graft with rigid internal fixation for anterior cruciate ligament insufficiency, Clin. Orthop. **172**:85-89, 1983.
30. Lindemann, K.: Über den plastischen ersatz kreutzbänder durch gestielte schnenueupflanzung, Ztschr. Orthop. **79**(2):316, 1950.
31. Lindstrom, N.: Cruciate ligament plastics with meniscus, Acta. Ortho. Scand. **29**:150-153, 1959.
32. Lipscomb, A.B., Johnston, R.K., Snyder, R.B., et al.: Secondary reconstruction of the anterior cruciate ligament in athletes by using semitendinous tendon, Am. J. Sports Med. **7**(2):81-84, 1979.
33. Marshall, J.L., et al.: The anterior cruciate ligament: a technique of repair and reconstruction, Clin. Orthop. **143**:97-106, 1979.
34. Mayo Robsin, A.W.: Ruptured crucial ligaments and their repair by operation, Am. Surg. **37**:716, 1903.
35. McDaniel, W.J., and Dameron, T.B.: Untreated ruptures of the anterior cruciate ligament, J. Bone Joint Surg. (Am.) **62**:696-705, 1980.
36. Noyes, F.R., Butler, D.L., Paulos, L.E., et al.: Intra-articular cruciate reconstruction, Clin. Orthop. **172**:71-77, 1983.
37. O'Donoghue, D.H.: Surgical treatment of fresh injuries to the ligaments of the knee, J. Bone Joint Surg. (Am.) **32**:738, 1950.
38. O'Donoghue, D.H.: A method for replacement of the anterior cruciate ligament of the knee, J. Bone Joint Surg. (Am.) **45**(5):905-924, 1963.
39. Palmer, I.: On injuries to the ligaments of the knee joint, Acta. Chir. Scand. (Suppl.) **53**:1-282, 1938.
40. Paulos, L.E., Butler, D.L., Noyes, F.R., et al.: Intra-articular cruciate reconstruction, Clin. Orthop. **172**:78-84, 1983.
41. Puddu, G., and Ippolito, E.: Reconstruction of the anterior cruciate ligament using the semitendinous tendon: histological study of a case, Am. J. Sports Med. **11**:14-16, 1983.
42. Scott, W.N., and Schosheim, P.M.: Intra-articular transfer of the iliotibial muscle tendon unit, Clin. Orthop. **172**:97-101, 1983.
43. Scott, W.N., Ferriter, P., and Marino, M.: Intra-articular transfer of the iliotibial tract, J. Bone Joint Surg. (Am.) **67**(4):532-538, 1985.
44. Snook, G.A.: A short history of the anterior cruciate ligament and the treatment of tears, Clin. Orthop. **172**:11-13, 1983.
45. Stark, J.: Two cases of rupture of the crucial ligaments of the knee joint, Edinb. Med. Surg. **74**:267, 1850.
46. Smillie, I.S.: Injuries to the knee joint, ed. 3, Baltimore, 1962, Williams & Wilkins.
47. Tillberg, B.: Late repair of torn cruciate ligaments using the menisci, J. Bone Joint Surg. (Br.) **59**(1):15-19, 1977.
48. Walsh, J.J.: Meniscal reconstruction of the anterior cruciate ligament, Clin. Orthop. **89**:171-177, 1972.
49. Wirth, J.C., and Artmann, M.: Ist die Lange der Pattelarsehue fur die vor dere Kruzbandplastik aursreichend, Arch. Orthop. Unfall. Chir. **79**:149-152, 1974.
50. Zarins, B.: Combined intra-articular and extra-articular reconstruction for anterior tibial subluxation, Orthop. Clin. North Am. **16**(2):223-225, 1985.

11

The role of extra-articular anterior cruciate ligament stabilization

JAMES R. ANDREWS

WILLIAM G. CARSON, Jr.

Treatment of the patient with a torn anterior cruciate ligament is one of the most controversial problems confronting the orthopedic surgeon. Once the decision has been made to surgically stabilize the knee, even more controversy exists over the type of surgical repair to be used. Surgical procedures designed to stabilize the knee include combinations of intra-articular and extra-articular procedures* and extra-articular procedures alone.†

It is obvious from the many different procedures described to stabilize anterior cruciate laxity that the search continues for the ideal surgical procedure. This ideal procedure should provide adequate tissue for a strong repair, allow early range of motion, control both anterior and posterior excursion of the knee, and provide rotatory stability. In addition, it should provide long-term stability to the knee with minimal stretching of the repaired tissues over time.

Anatomical instability differs in many ways from functional instability. A surgical procedure performed to correct instability of the knee resulting from a torn anterior cruciate ligament should eliminate functional instability and provide anatomical stability to the knee. In this chapter we review the role of extra-articular procedures designed to control anterolateral rotatory instability in the case of anterior cruciate ligament laxity. A common goal of these procedures is the elimination of the pivot-shift phenomenon and the resulting functional instability.

---

*References 1, 11-13, 16, 38, 39, 58, 59, 73, and 74.
†References 1-6, 14, 17, 18, 20, 21, 26, 34, 41, 45, 52, 56, 68 and 69.

Classification of knee ligament instability

Extra-articular procedures are used to stabilize rotatory instability about the knee, particularly anterolateral rotatory instability. The three types of rotatory instabilities that are commonly recognized are anterolateral, anteromedial, and posterolateral. Classification is based on the premise that the posterior cruciate ligament is intact and that the tibia rotates around this intact ligament. The direction of the tibial movement describes the instability. Thus in anterolateral rotatory instability the tibia moves in an anterolateral direction on the femur (Fig. 11-1). A torn anterior cruciate ligament alone can cause this instability; however, lesions of the lateral capsular ligament and of the iliotibial band may also be present.

In anteromedial rotatory instability the tibia moves in an anteromedial direction on the femur (Fig. 11-2). Lesions in the medial capsule, tibial collateral ligament, and posterior oblique ligament produce a milder form of this type of instability, even with an intact anterior cruciate ligament. When the anterior cruciate ligament is torn, the resulting laxity is more severe.

The least common form of rotatory instability, posterolateral rotatory instability, indicates a posterolateral rotation of the tibia on

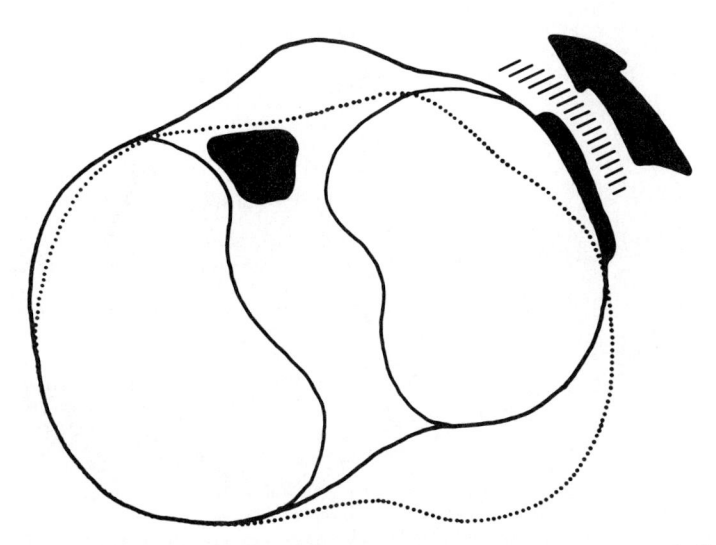

Fig. 11-1 *Anterolateral rotatory instability. Arrow indicates direction of tibial movement. Shaded area represents the iliotibial band. (From T. Boers, Nederlands Tijdschrift voor Fysiotherapie, 95:5, 1985. By permission.)*

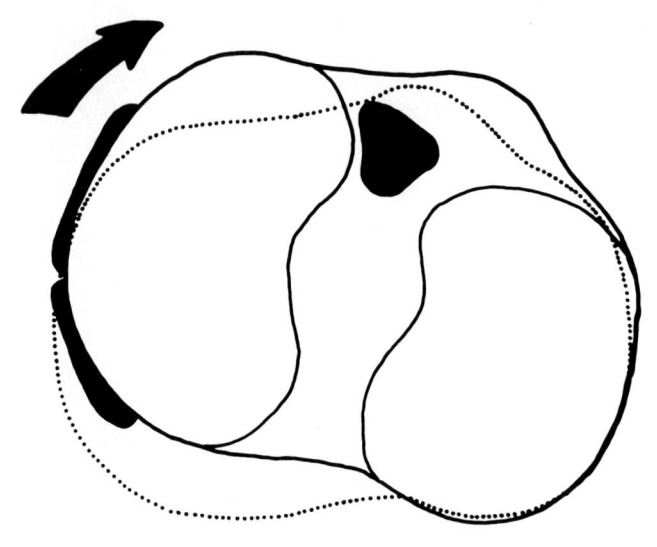

Fig. 11-2 *Anteromedial rotatory instability. Arrow indicates the direction of tibial movement. (From T. Boers, Nederlands Tijdschrift voor Fysiotherapie, 93:5, 1985. By permission.)*

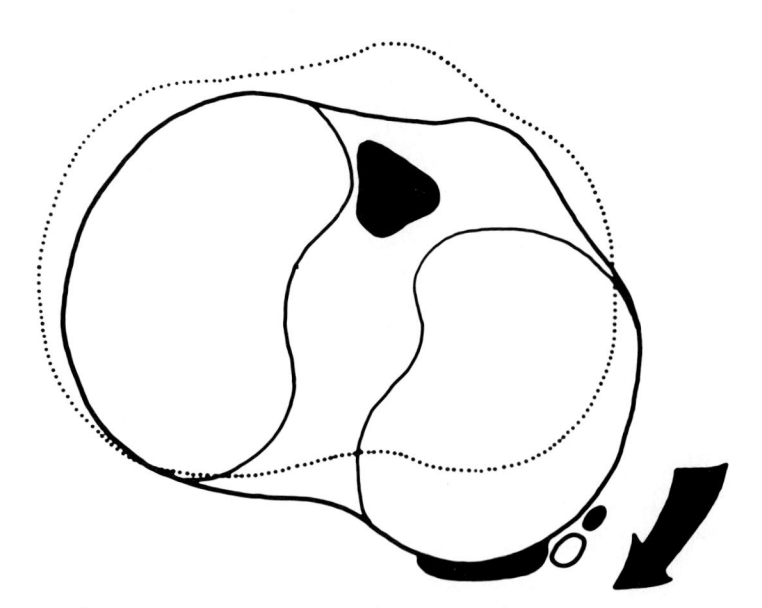

Fig. 11-3 *Posterolateral rotatory instability. Arrow indicates direction of tibial movement. (From T. Boers, Nederlands Tijdschrift voor Fysiotherapie, 95:5, 1985. By permission.)*

the femur (Fig. 11-3). A lesion in the arcuate ligament, the fibular collateral ligament, the popliteus tendon, or the lateral capsular ligament typically produces this type of instability.

Rotatory instabilities may exist in combined forms. The combination that occurs most often is anteromedial and anterolateral rotatory instabilities.

Indications for surgery and patient selection

Several extra-articular procedures have been successful in controlling anterolateral rotatory instability. Deciding which surgical procedure to use may be a difficult decision. However, an even more difficult decision may be encountered when trying to identify which patient with an anterior cruciate ligament injury will benefit from surgery and which patient will respond to conservative treatment.[44] Although some authors report satisfactory results with nonoperative treatment for the torn anterior cruciate ligament,[25] others report progressive deterioration of their patients' knees resulting in significant functional disability.[53-55] In 103 patients treated nonoperatively for an anterior cruciate ligament injury, Noyes et al.[53] demonstrated that 82% could actually return to sports. However, 35% subsequently reinjured the knee within 6 months, and 51% reinjured the knee within 1 year of the original injury. This group of patients was also noted to have significant problems with functional disability, meniscal damage, and arthritic changes.

Noyes et al.[54] also reported on 81 patients who were treated nonoperatively with rehabilitation, activity modification, counseling, and functional bracing. In this group of patients with an isolated anterior cruciate ligament injury, 36% were improved by this treatment program, 32% believed that their knee progressively deteriorated, and 32% remained unchanged.

Thus the dilemma remains with regard to which patients with an isolated anterior cruciate ligament injury will have a functionally stable knee with rehabilitation and activity modifications and which patients will progressively deteriorate with a nonoperative approach. The variables involved are many. The surgeon must consider the patient's age, the sport the patient is involved in, the actual position of the player in that particular sport, and the patient's own expectations and motivation.

The risk of reinjury varies with the specific sport. Football, basketball, soccer, and gymnastics remain high-risk sports, and racquetball, tennis, softball, jogging, and snow skiing are somewhat less demanding.[27] Even within a particular sport, variations exist in the requirements placed on the anterior cruciate ligament. A muscular, short-statured offensive lineman may well be able to compete with a torn anterior cruciate ligament. However, a defensive back or running back may require stabilization of the ligament since greater demands are placed on his knee as a result of the rapid pivoting, twisting, and changes of momentum required by his position.

Therefore there are three decisions the orthopedic surgeon must make when treating the patient with an anterior cruciate ligament lesion: (1) Can the patient modify activity levels and rehabilitate the knee by nonoperative treatment? (2) Will the patient benefit by a surgical procedure? (3) Which surgical procedure is appropriate when surgery is indicated?

The pivot-shift phenomenon

An understanding of the surgical procedures designed to control anterolateral rotatory instability (ALRI) must be based on the ability to identify the pivot-shift phenomenon.[10]

As mentioned previously, anterolateral rotatory instability is defined as the abnormal anterior subluxation of the lateral tibial plateau in relation to the lateral femoral condyle as the knee approaches full extension.[19,35,38,40,48] This rotatory instability occurs around an intact posterior cruciate ligament.[33] Anterolateral rotatory instability is secondary to partial or complete loss of the anterior cruciate ligament and may be made more severe by attenuation of the lateral supporting structures of the knee. Norwood et al.[51] demonstrated that in 36 knees with acute anterolateral rotatory instability, a tear of the anterior cruciate ligament was found, as well as a tear of the middle one third of the lateral capsular ligament. Norwood and Hughston[50] demonstrated a torn anterior cruciate ligament and a tear of the middle one third of the lateral capsular ligament in 18 patients who were evaluated with acute combined anterolateral and anteromedial rotatory instability. If damage occurs to the anterior cruciate ligament and to the lateral structures, the most severe pivot-shift phenomenon results. Thus the lateral tibial plateau subluxes anteriorly as the knee approaches full extension. As the knee is brought from extension into flexion, the anterolateral portion of the tibial plateau, which was subluxed with the knee in extension, is suddenly reduced to its normal position. In a normally functioning knee the anterior cruciate ligament is the guide to the screw-home mechanism, progressively tightening as the knee is brought from a flexed to an extended position. The anterior cruciate ligament guides the knee into a few degrees of external rotation as it approaches terminal extension, thus locking the knee in a stable position for weight bearing. When the anterior cruciate ligament is lost, this guide is lost, and the anterolateral portion of the tibia is allowed to rotate internally and sublux anteriorly.

The iliotibial tract plays an important role in producing the lateral pivot-shift phenomenon.[72] As the anterolateral portion of the tibial plateau is subluxed in the extended position, the iliotibial band is anterior to the transverse center of rotation. As the knee is brought from an extended into a flexed position, the iliotibial tract glides posterior to this transverse center of rotation. At approximately 30 degrees of flexion the iliotibial tract fibers inserting into the tibia abruptly reduce the anterolateral portion of the tibial plateau in relation to the lateral femoral condyle.[9] The result is the pivot-shift phenomenon.

A variety of tests may be used to demonstrate the pivot-shift phenomenon. Some tests start with the knee in flexion and demonstrate anterolateral subluxation of the lateral tibial plateau with the knee in full extension.[33,45] Other tests begin with the knee in extension and demonstrate reduction of the subluxed lateral plateau when the knee is brought from an extended to a flexed position.[23,24,36,52,65] These tests are performed with the patient in the supine position. Thus the examiner is able to detect the subluxation of the tibia as it reduces on the femur. However, when the patient is in a weight-bearing position, this subluxed portion of the tibia is perceived by the patient as posterior subluxation of the lateral femoral condyle on the tibia.[42] The patient experiences this sensation when the tibia is fixed and when the femoral condyle is rotated posteriorly; the patient may describe hyperextension of the knee. Therefore, if a patient states that the knee is hyperextending, many times it is a lateral pivot-shift phenomenon that is occurring.

A patient may still demonstrate anterolateral rotatory instability and not demonstrate a lateral pivot-shift phenomenon in very mild and subtle instabilities. The instability can be demonstrated, however, by performing the anterior drawer test with the patient's foot in the neutral position while applying equal anterior pressure to both the medial and lateral aspects of the tibia. If the anterolateral plateau comes further forward than the medial aspect, an anterolateral rotatory instability may exist.[33,38] A positive Lachman test[70] is the most sensitive examination for establishing the integrity of the anterior cruciate ligament.

Principles of extra-articular procedures to control anterolateral rotatory instability

The goal of an extra-articular procedure performed to correct anterolateral rotatory instability is to prevent the anterior subluxation of the lateral tibial plateau in relation to the lateral femoral condyle. Most of the procedures described in this section use some portion of the iliotibial tract to keep the tibia posterior to the transverse center of rotation of the knee. Placement of the extra-articular portions of the iliotibial tract is crucial in realizing this goal.[42] The iliotibial tract can either be left distally or proximally attached or it can be used to create a simple tenodesis effect. When the iliotibial tract is released distally or proximally, it is routed beneath the fibular collateral ligament so that it is posterior to the transverse center of rotation at all times. The iliotibial tract acts as a reinforcement against anterior subluxation of the lateral tibial plateau. In this position it parallels the course of the anterior cruciate ligament and may be thought of as an extra-articular anterior cruciate ligament—one that is better positioned to resist rotatory movements. The ideal position of a reconstruction to control anterior and posterior excursion of the joint is in the center of the joint; however, in this position the intra-articular placement creates a lever arm about the center of rotation that is too short to be truly effective in controlling rotatory movements.[36,38,42] Because of the peripheral location of the extra-articular procedures, the lever arm is nearly twice as effective in resisting rotatory torques. (This is analogous to turning a steering wheel at the center of the hub versus at the peripheral rim.) Thus, because of this interplay between anterior and posterior forces and rotatory components, intra-articular and extra-articular repairs are at many times used in conjunction.* Most of the lateral extra-articular procedures function as a static reinforcement to anterior subluxation of the lateral tibial plateau; however, some lateral extra-articular procedures are theorized to function in a dynamic fashion.† The biceps tendon can be transferred anteriorly and distally to provide an additional dynamic support to a lateral extra-articular repair.‡

*References 1, 11, 13, 16, 22, 38, 39, 58, 59, and 74.
†References 17, 18, 26, 41, 56, and 68.
‡References 11, 13, 14, 16, 18, 37, 47, 49, 66, and 69.

Surgical procedures to control anterolateral rotatory instability

Losee procedure

In 1978 Losee et al. reported the results of 50 patients who underwent the "sling and reef" procedure.[45] Similar to the original MacIntosh procedure,[46] the Losee procedure also used a section of the iliotibial tract left attached distally to provide a reinforcement to prevent anterior subluxation of the lateral tibial plateau. In addition, this procedure provided for a reefing of the posterolateral corner of the knee through the arcuate complex and the lateral half of the gastrocnemius muscle. Of 50 patients with a 1 to 6 year-follow-up, good results were obtained in 82%. All patients were satisfied with the procedure and 70% returned to their pre-injury status.

In the Losee procedure a section of iliotibial tract that is approximately 18-cm long and 1.5-cm wide is released proximally and left attached distally to Gerdy's tubercle (Fig. 11-4). This strip of iliotibial tract is brought from an anterior position to a posterior position through a bony tunnel in the lateral femoral condyle. The anterior entrance point for the bony canal is determined by placing the strip of iliotibial tract at various points on the lateral femoral condyle just anterior to the fibular collateral ligament insertion in a attempt to find the location that will prevent the strip's pulling loose when the knee is flexed 90 degrees. The exit location of the bony canal is over the posterior aspect of the lateral femoral condyle through the insertion of the lateral head of the gastrocnemius in the posterior capsule. If the tunnel is properly placed, pulling on the transferred portion of the fascial strip should reduce anterior subluxation of the lateral tibial plateau. The iliotibial tract may be sutured to the entrance and exit holes of the bony tunnel for additional fixation of sutures. The iliotibial tract is then woven through the tendon of the origin of the lateral head of the gastrocnemius muscle at a point approximately 1-cm distal and 0.5-cm medial to the posterior exit of the bony tunnel. It is then passed horizontally and laterally to encircle approximately 1 cm of the gastrocnemius tendon at its origin. A second reefing stitch may be placed through the gastrocnemius tendon. This stitch starts 1.5-cm medial and 0.5-cm distal to the point of the exit of the previous stitch. The strip is then directed distally and laterally and passes through the arcuate ligament. It is then passed beneath the fibular collateral ligament distal to the joint line superior to Gerdy's tubercle. As the iliotibial tract is woven through the lateral gastrocnemius tendon, posterior capsule, and arcuate liga-

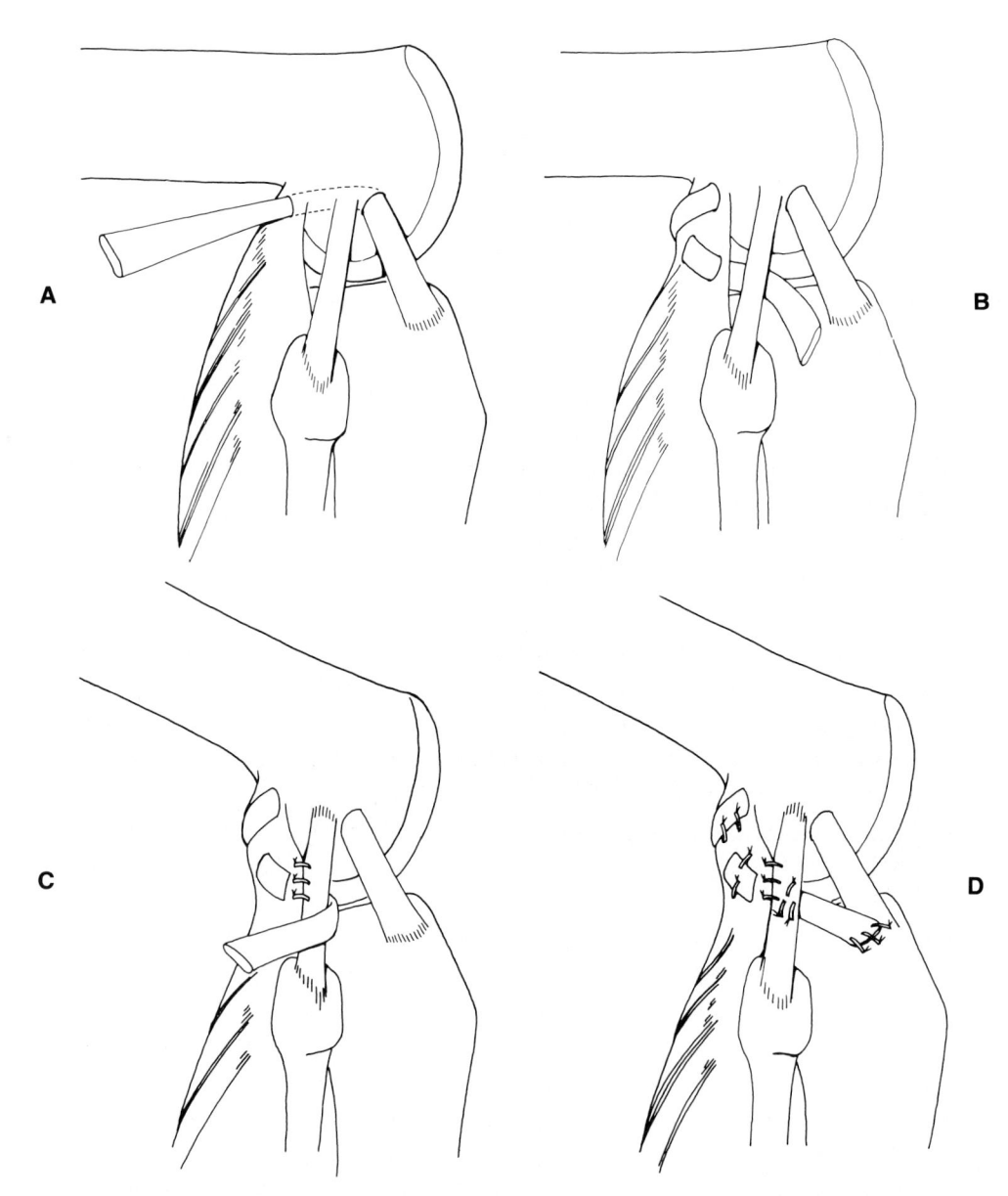

Fig. 11-4 Losee procedure. **A,** A strip of iliotibial band is released proximally and passed through a tunnel in the lateral femoral condyle. The strip exits through the origin of the lateral head of the gastrocnemius. **B,** The strip is woven through the gastrocnemius tendon and passed beneath the fibular collateral ligament. **C,** After the strip is sutured to the fibular collateral ligament, it is brought anteriorly, passed through to its origin at Gerdy's tubercle, and tightened. **D,** Sutures are placed along the strip's course, anchoring it to adjacent capsule and ligament tissues.

ment and as it is pulled anteriorly, the entire lateral gastrocnemius complex is pulled anteriorly as well and thus tightens the posterolateral corner of the knee. The posterior capsule and lateral gastrocnemius muscle are then sutured to the fibular collateral ligament and additional sutures may be placed along the course of the iliotibial tract to anchor it to adjacent tissues. It has been suggested that the defect in the iliotibial tract be closed if the cut edges of the fascia lata can be reapproximated without excessive tension.[45] The leg is then placed in a long leg cast for approximately 6 weeks with the knee in approximately 30 to 45 degrees of flexion and with the tibia externally rotated.

Lateral tenodesis procedure

Like the Losee procedure described previously, the lateral tenodesis procedure described by James[36,38] uses a strip of the iliotibial tract left attached distally and provides a static reinforcement to prevent anterior subluxation of the lateral tibial plateau in relation to the lateral femoral condyle. This procedure also provides a tightening of the posterolateral corner of the knee similar to that described by Losee, et al.[45] This procedure is used for the more severe forms of chronic anterolateral rotatory instability and is usually combined with an intra-articular reconstruction of the anterior cruciate ligament.

A 20-cm long and 2- to 2.5-cm wide strip of iliotibial tract is released proximally and left attached distally to Gerdy's tubercle. A bony tunnel is made in the lateral femoral condyle, beginning just proximal and anterior to the insertion of the fibular collateral ligament. The tunnel is directed posteriorly and slightly medially and exits just above the lateral femoral condyle through the insertion of the lateral gastrocnemius tendon. A soft-tissue tunnel is created through the arcuate ligament, through the gastrocnemius tendon, and beneath the fibular collateral ligament (Fig. 11-5). After the bony and soft-tissue tunnels are developed, the iliotibial tract is passed under the fibular collateral ligament and through the previously created soft-tissue tunnel in the arcuate ligament and gastrocnemius tendon. It is then brought back anteriorly and once again passed through this same passage, forming a loop around the fibular collateral ligament, arcuate ligament, and gastrocnemius tendon. This loop effect provides a tightening of the posterolateral corner of the knee and draws the gastrocnemius tendon and arcuate ligament anteriorly toward the fibular collateral ligament. The strip is

178 The anterior cruciate deficient knee

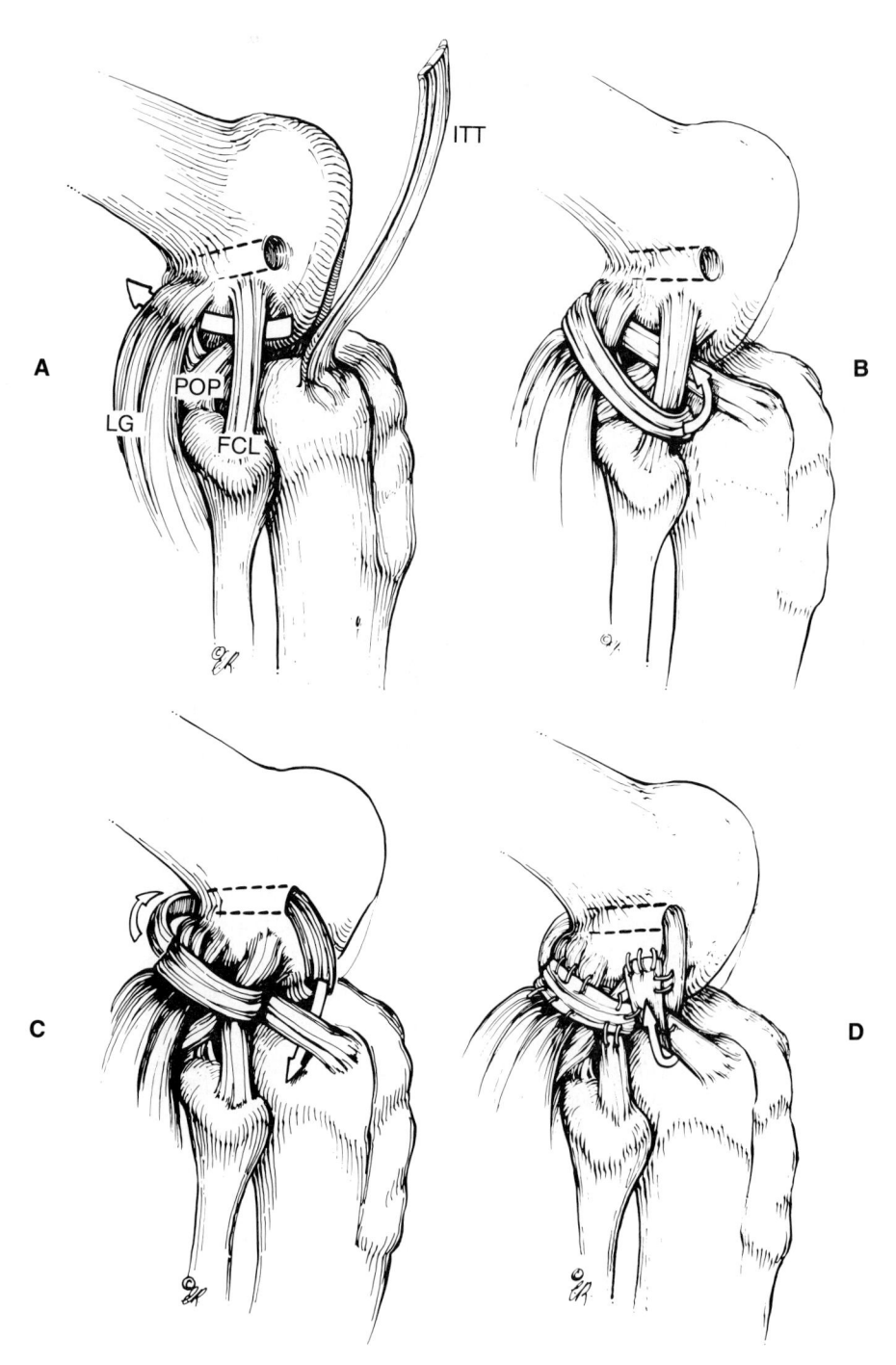

Fig. 11-5 *For legend see opposite page.*

then passed through the previously created bony tunnel from a posterior to anterior position and then distally beneath the iliotibial tract that is still attached to Gerdy's tubercle. The free strip of iliotibial tract may then be brought proximally and sutured under tension to the insertion of the fibular collateral ligament. The defect of the iliotibial tract is then closed, occasionally requiring a lateral retinacular release directly adjacent to the lateral border of the patella. The leg is then placed in a long leg cast in approximately 30 degrees of flexion.

Using a 200 point rating system (100 objective and 100 subjective points), 25 patients undergoing this lateral procedure were reviewed with the average length of follow-up being 19 months.[38,39] The procedure was performed for severe chronic anterolateral rotatory instability and was combined in all cases with either a semitendinosus or patellar tendon intra-articular reconstruction. Of these cases, 87% were improved, the anterior drawer test was eliminated or decreased in 87%, and the lateral pivot shift was eliminated in 100%.

Modified MacIntosh procedure[60,71]

Another procedure that uses a portion of the iliotibial band as a reinforcement for anterior subluxation of the lateral tibial plateau is that described by Arnold et al.[5,6] In this procedure a strip of iliotibial band that is approximately 15- to 18-cm long and 2-cm wide is obtained from the strongest section of the iliotibial tract (usually located over the posterior border of the tract approximately 1- to

Fig. 11-5 *Lateral tenodesis procedure, as described by James.[38] **A**, A 20-cm strip of iliotibal tract (ITT) is released proximally and left attached at Gerdy's tubercle. A bone tunnel is made through the lateral femoral condyle. A soft-tissue tunnel is made under the fibular collateral ligament (FCL) and through the arcuate ligament and gastrocnemius tendon, **B**, The strip of ITT is passed under the fibular collateral ligament and through the soft-tissue tunnel in the arcuate ligament and the gastrocnemius tendon. **C**, The strip is brought back and passed through the same passage, forming a loop around the fibular collateral ligament, arcuate ligament, and gastrocnemius tendon. The strip is then passed through the bone tunnel and distally under the oblique limb. **D**, The end is brought back proximally to be sutured under tension to the insertion of the fibular collateral ligament. The iliotibial tract defect is closed. (LG, lateral gastrocnemius; POP popliteus tendon.) (From James, S.L.: Knee ligament reconstruction. In Evarts, C.M., editor: Surgery of the musculoskeletal system, vol. 3, New York, 1983, Churchill Livingstone Inc., p. 7:69. By permission.)*

2-cm anterior to the intermuscular septum). This strip of iliotibial tract is freed proximally and left attached distally to Gerdy's tubercle. The strip is then passed under the more proximal portion of the fibular collateral ligament near its insertion in an anterior to posterior direction; it is then looped back on itself and secured with a staple to an area of denuded bone just distal to Gerdy's tubercle (Fig. 11-6). The iliotibial tract is then sutured to the fibular collateral ligament for additional stability. The defect in the iliotibial tract is left unclosed and appears to cause no significant postoperative problems.[5,6,38] The patient is placed in a knee brace with the knee flexed 55 degrees. The knee is progressively extended over a 6-week period. In 1979 Arnold et al. reported on the results of 132 patients who underwent this procedure with a 6 to 32 month follow-up. Using a 100 point rating scale, the average score obtained by this

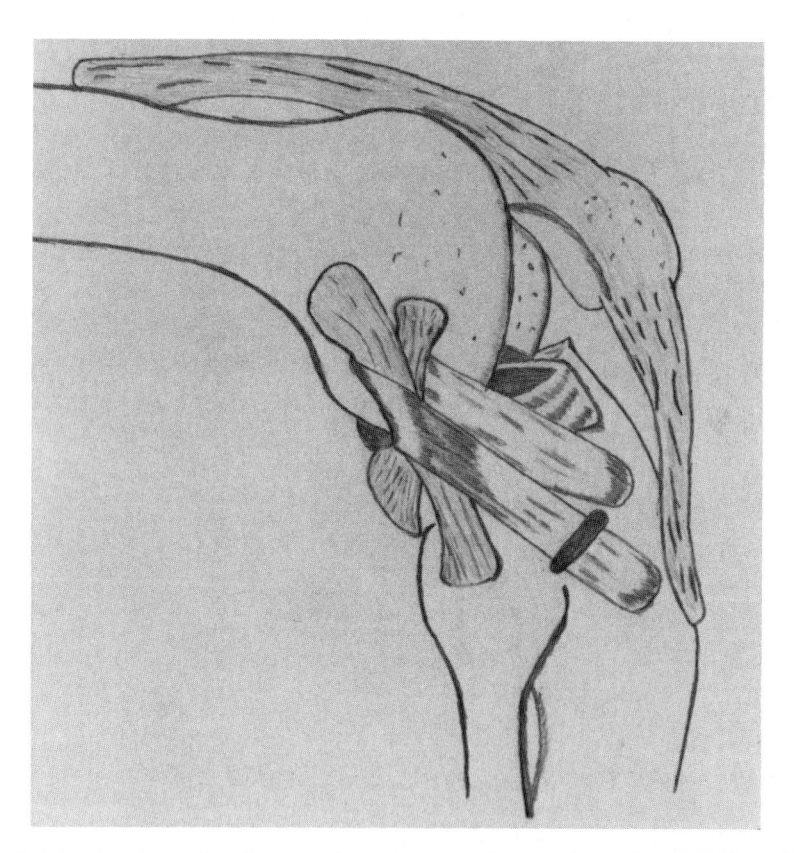

Fig. 11-6 *A lateral extra-articular tenodesis to control anterolateral instability. (From Arnold, J.A.: A lateral extra-articular tenodesis for ACL deficiency of the knee, Orthop. Clin. North Am. **16**(2):219, 1985. Reprinted with permission from W.B. Saunders Co.)*

patient population was 89 points, and all patients had elimination of the lateral pivot-shift phenomenon postoperatively.[6]

Combined intra-articular and extra-articular reconstruction

Zarins and Rowe have described a combined intra-articular and extra-articular approach to the management of anterolateral rotatory instability.[73,74] The principle behind this technique is a simultaneous

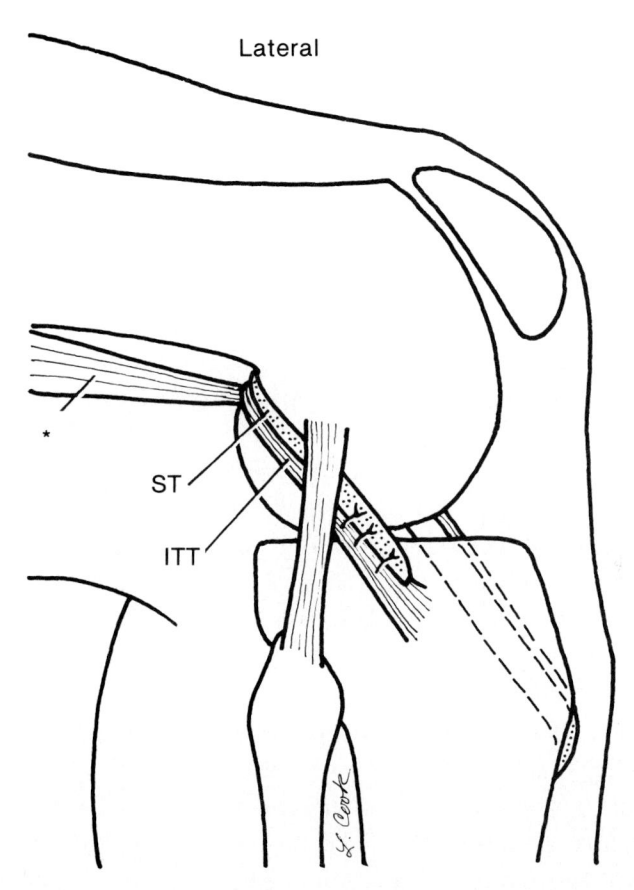

Fig. 11-7   Combined intra-articular and extra-articular reconstruction, as described by Zarins and Rowe.[74] The distally based semitendinosus (ST) graft is brought through the joint, over the top of the lateral femoral condyle, and deep to the fibular collateral ligament; it is sutured to Gerdy's tubercle. A strip of iliotibial tract (ITT) is passed in the opposite direction, beneath the fibular collateral ligament, over the top of the lateral femoral condyle, through the joint, and into the tibial drill hole (Courtesy Bertram Zarins, M.D.). (From Carson, W.G.: Extra-articular reconstruction of the anterior cruciate ligament: lateral procedures, Orthop. Clin. North Am. 16(2):201, 1985. By permission of W.B. Saunders Co.)

over-the-top transfer of the semitendinosus tendon and a strip of the iliotibial tract plus posteromedial and lateral capsular reefings.

A strip of iliotibial tract measuring approximately 24 cm in length and 2.5 cm in width is left attached to Gerdy's tubercle and is released proximally. In addition, a distally-based section of semitendinous tendon is released proximally. The semitendinosus tendon is brought through a drill hole in the tibia intra-articularly, through the posterior capsule adjacent to the lateral femoral condyle, and over the top of the lateral femoral condyle above the insertion of the lateral intermuscular septum. The semitendinosus tendon is then brought down across the posterolateral capsule and beneath the fibular collateral ligament. The iliotibial tract is then routed in the opposite direction beneath the fibular collateral ligament, through the posterior capsule, above the intermuscular septum, and intra-articularly to exit through the tibial drill hole (Fig. 11-7). The semitendinosus tendon and iliotibial tract are then sutured to each other, and both tendons are sutured to the posterolateral capsule for additional support. The transferred tendons are not sutured to the fibular collateral ligament. The iliotibial tract is closed to the level of the superior pole of the patella but is left open distal to this. A long leg cast is applied with the knee in approximately 60 degrees of flexion.

There were 287 of these combined intra-articular and extraarticular procedures performed between 1977 and 1983. Examination of the first 100 consecutive patients, all with a follow-up greater than 3 years, demonstrated a negative pivot shift in 90% and a negative or trace positive Lachman test in 80%.

Iliotibial band tenodesis

A lateral extra-articular procedure to control anterolateral rotatory instability was described by Andrews[1-4,67]; it is a tenodesis of the iliotibial tract similar to the procedure described by Hughston.[51,61] This procedure consists of a tenodesis of the iliotibial tract to the lateral femoral condyle. Two isometric bundles are created along the fibers of the posterior part of the tract.

An arthroscopic examination is performed to detect any intra-articular pathology. Following the arthroscopic procedure the limb is re-prepared and draped. With the knee flexed approximately 90 degrees, a 10-cm, longitudinal, hockey stick incision is made over the lateral aspect of the knee. The iliotibial band and tract are identified, and the iliotibial tract is divided longitudinally over an area of approximately 10 cm. This splitting incision is placed approximately 4 cm anterior to the most posterior border of the iliotibial tract. The anterior edge of the iliotibial tract and the vastus lateralis are retracted with a Chandler retractor placed over the anterior surface of the distal femur. Fatty tissues are cleared away from the lateral portion of the distal femur, thus exposing the linea aspera and the distal insertion of the lateral intermuscular septum. After the lateral femoral condyle region is cleaned of all soft tissue, the area is "fish-scaled" with an osteotome to provide a bleeding, bony base; this promotes a proliferative healing response of the iliotibial tract to the bone.

At this point a medial skin incision is made, beginning at the level of the adductor tubercle and directed along the longitudinal axis of the tibia (the knee is still flexed 90 degrees). This incision is usually 2 to 3 cm in length. The inferior border of the vastus medialis obliquus muscle is exposed and retracted superiorly after the fascia

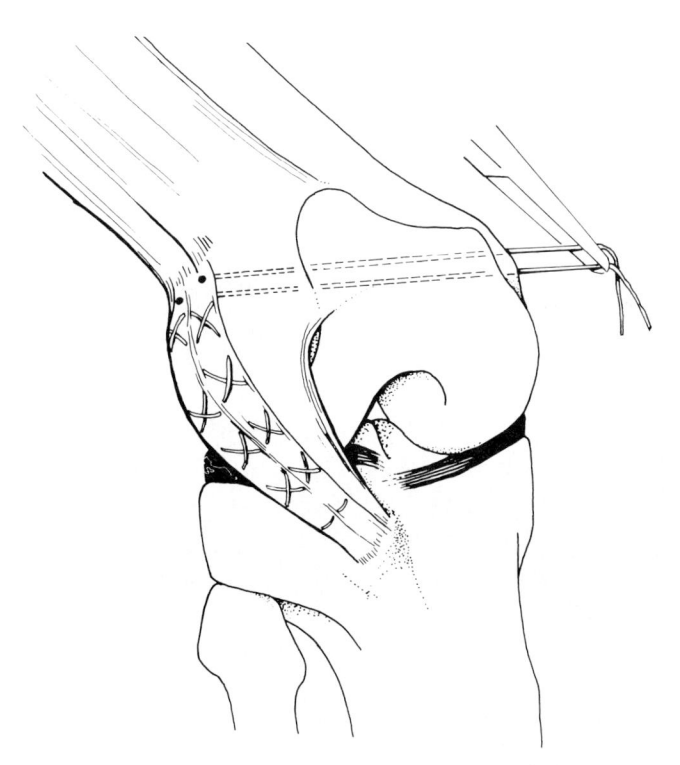

Fig. 11-8 *Andrews' iliotibial band tenodesis. The iliotibial tract is attached to the distal femur by two parallel rows of Bunnell sutures that are tied to each other on the medial side of the femur. This creates a "ligament" that extends from the linea aspera to Gerdy's tubercle.*

has been divided. The medial metaphysis of the femur is then exposed, this will be the future site of suture attachment. Two Beath needles are used to drill holes in a medial direction through the femur. The sutures will be passed through these holes and later tied over a 1-cm bone bridge medially. The first hole is drilled at the distal insertion of the lateral intermuscular septum on the linea aspera as close to the posterior femoral cortex as possible. The second hole is drilled approximately 1-cm anterior and 0.5-cm distal to the first hole.

A ligament is made from the iliotibial tract by creating two bundles from the lower third of the tract using #5 Tycron sutures. The lower bundle is created first by crisscrossing these sutures at a 45 degree angle, 1.5 cm wide, along the posterior border of the iliotibial tract for approximately 4 to 5 cm. A second crisscross suture is then placed in line with the anterior hole. The suture ends are then placed through the eyes of the Beath needles and pulled through the femur to exit medially (Figs. 11-8 to 11-10). Tension is

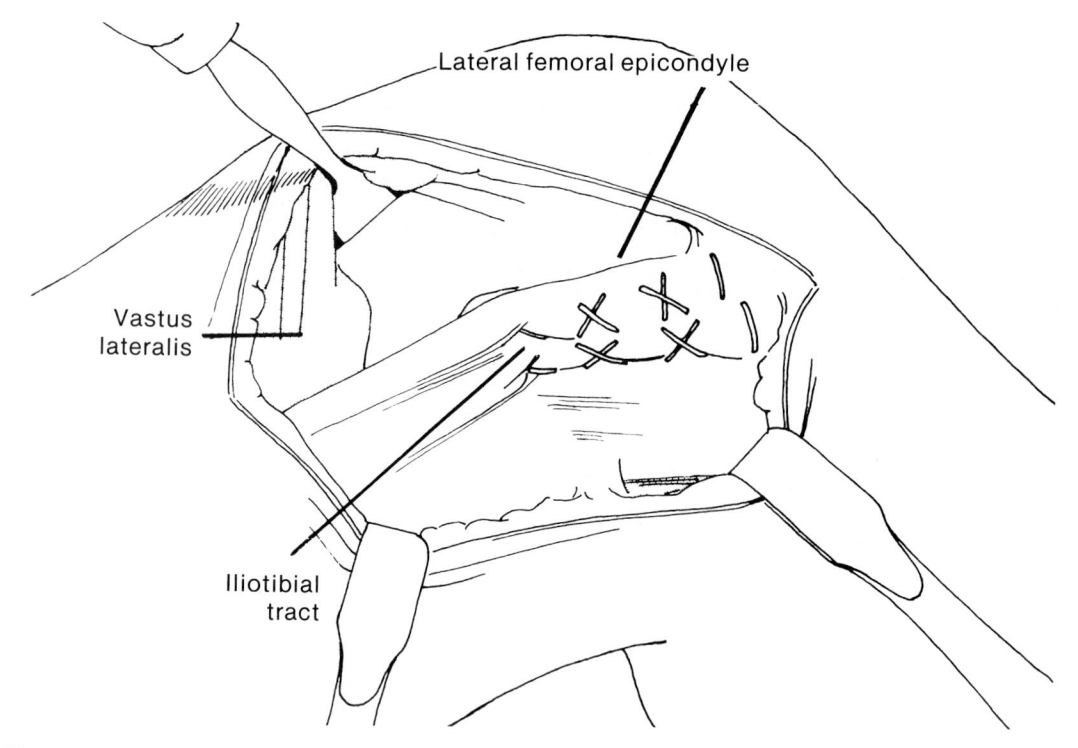

Fig. 11-9 *Fixation of the iliotibial tract to the distal femur. (From Andrews, J.R., Sanders, R.A., and Morin, B.: Surgical treatment of anterolateral rotatory instability: a follow-up study, Am. J. Sports Med.* **13**:*112-119, 1985.)*

then applied to the sutures, and the anterior and posterior bundles are observed during range of motion of the knee. If correct placement has been achieved, the anterior bundle will be relatively tight in flexion and the posterior bundle will be relatively tight in extension. If the iliotibial band tenodesis is not isometric, either the drill holes are repositioned or a second attempt at suturing may be required. If it is possible to sublux the tibia or if the lateral pivot-shift test is positive, the repair is too loose. Conversely, if the iliotibial tract cannot be pulled against the lateral femur or if the range of motion is not full, the repair is too tight. Once the proper placement is verified, the sutures are tied medially with the knee in approximately 45 degrees of flexion and with the tibia externally rotated.

The extremity is immobilized for approximately 4 weeks in a cylinder cast in 30 to 45 degrees of flexion; once the cast is removed range of motion is begun. At the present time a series of patients with acute injuries that were started on immediate protected motion is being studied. Patients begin with motion from 40 to 70 degrees

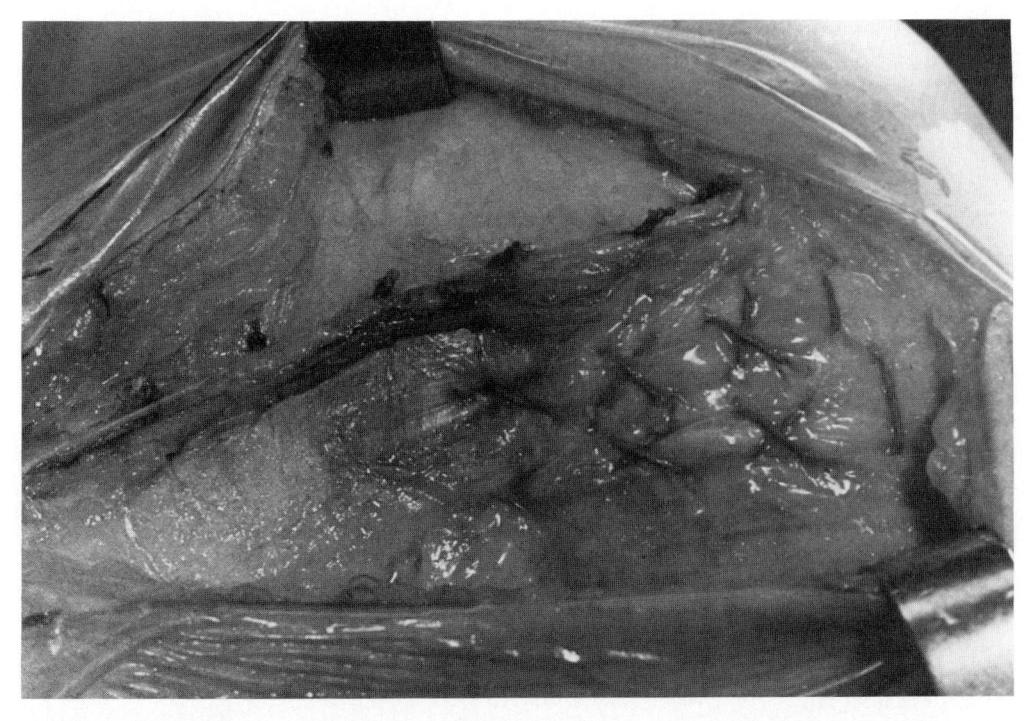

Fig. 11-10 *Photograph of the completed reconstruction showing the final and important step of closing the iliotibial tract incision. (From Andrews, J.R., Sanders, R.A., and Morin, B.: Surgical treatment of anterolateral rotatory instability: a follow-up study, Am. J. Sports Med. 13:112-119, 1985.)*

and increase to 15 to 90 degrees of motion at 3 weeks. The last 15 degrees of terminal extension are protected for a full 6-week period in a hinged knee immobilizer. Chronic cases are still immobilized in a 45 degree bent cylinder cast for a full 6 weeks.

Iliotibial band tenodesis has been used in acute and chronic anterolateral rotatory instability since 1977. In a review of 62 knees corrected with this procedure, 31 for acute and 31 for chronic anterolateral rotatory instability, objective satisfactory results were obtained in 94% and subjective improvement was noted in 92% (follow-up was greater than 2 years).[4] Of these patients, 93% returned to athletic activity requiring rapid change of momentum or pivoting activities. This procedure offers the advantage of a simple longitudinal incision that preserves the vascularity of the iliotibial tract and the linear arrangement of its fibers, thereby preserving its strength. In addition, the absence of any dissection between the iliotibial tract and the tibia preserves the fibrous connections of the iliotibial tract to the lateral capsule and lateral condyle and yields additional support to the lateral aspect of the knee.

This procedure has been effective when performed as described. We have had no experience with modifications of this technique, such as the use of staples or a screw and washer to hold the iliotibial band to the lateral aspect of the distal femur. By simply stapling or screwing the iliotibial band to the femur, a very important aspect of this surgical procedure is neglected, the creation of two bundles or bands by the Bunnell suture. By using #5 Tycron for these sutures, one actually augments the tract by creating a bandlike structure and provides a proliferative response making it a stronger structure. The suture material also acts as a device to actually increase the inherent tensile strength of the iliotibial tract. This newly created ligamentous structure is then anchored to the femur and tied on the medial side of the femur over the femoral condyle area. To simply staple or screw the iliotibial band would not add the additional support that is required, and the tract might pull away from the femur as a result of a concentration of stress. As mentioned previously, this should be an isometric repair. If, upon testing the knee in flexion and extension, the newly created ligamentous band is not isometric, either the sutures can be replaced or the drill holes can be repositioned.

Anteromedial rotatory instability

Injury to the posterior oblique ligament, medial capsule, tibial collateral ligament, and, in the more severe forms, the anterior cruciate ligament can give rise to anteromedial rotatory instability (AMRI).[29,31,62-64] Treatment of acute anteromedial rotatory instability requires the surgical repair of the various torn structures. In addition, reattachment of the anterior cruciate ligament, to either the femur or the tibia, may be attempted and combined with an acute intra-articular augmentation or an extra-articular procedure as described earlier.

The goal of surgery for chronic anteromedial rotatory instability is to stabilize the knee to prevent excessive valgus opening and antermedial rotation of the tibia. The simplest surgical procedure that will achieve an improved level of function is obviously the most desirable. For a knee with mild anteromedial rotatory instability and no significant valgus instability a dynamic restraint in the form of a pes anserinus transfer has been successful.[62,63] However, if the anteromedial rotation of the tibia is combined with significant valgus deformity, a reinforcement or reefing of the posterior oblique ligament is often required.[29,34,43,64] If, in addition to the anteromedial rotation of the tibia and the valgus instability, there exists significant anterior excursion of the tibia, then an intra-articular reconstruction would be warranted as well.[11,13,15,16,24] With these more severe forms additional reinforcement to the posterior oblique ligament may be provided by a semimembranosus advancement,[43,64] and if a marked valgus instability exists, then a sartorial advancement[64] or medial capsular advancement[57] can provide additional stability.

Posterolateral rotatory instability

Injuries to the arcuate ligament, popliteus tendon, lateral half of the posterior capsule, and lateral capsular ligament can result in posterolateral rotatory instability (PLRI). Injuries to the lateral gastrocnemius muscle, biceps femoris, iliotibial tract, fibular collateral ligament, and anterior cruciate ligament may also be associated. Often the posterior cruciate ligament has some stretching, but essentially it remains intact for this rotatory instability to occur. The treatment of acute posterolateral rotatory instability is the surgical repair of the torn extra-articular structures.[7,8,15] Should the anterior cruciate ligament be avulsed from the femur or the tibia, it is surgically reattached. Controversy does exist, however, regarding the repair of a mid-substance anterior cruciate ligament tear in combination with posterolateral rotatory instability.

The goal of surgery for this chronic instability is to restore the integrity of the structure of the posterolateral corner of the knee and to provide sufficient moment arm for resisting external tibial rotation. One of the most effective procedures in providing stability and support for the posterolateral corner of the knee is an "en masse" anterior and distal advancement of the arcuate complex and its osseous attachment.[30,32,38]

Summary

The common goals of all extra-articular procedures to control anterolateral rotatory instability of the knee are to create a restraining mechanism for control of the abnormal anterior subluxation of the lateral tibial plateau and thus to eliminate the lateral pivot-shift phenomenon and functional instability. These goals are most readily achieved by positioning some portion of the iliotibial tract posterior to the transverse center of rotation of the knee to provide a reinforcement for the lateral tibial plateau as the knee approaches terminal extension.

All of the procedures discussed in this chapter have been used successfully. There are many technical details inherent in each of these surgical procedures, and the reader is referred to the original articles for a more explicit description of these points. For the individual surgeon to participate in and view the actual surgical procedure that he or she intends to perform would be the ideal situation.[28] Various workshops where surgical procedures of the knee are actually performed and studied are currently available and of great value to the surgeon.

Of equal importance to the technical demands of these procedures is selection of the appropriate procedure for each patient. The selection must be based on many factors. The most important factor is the identification of the patient with a high level of athletic activity who is unwilling to modify his or her activity level to compensate for a deficient anterior cruciate ligament. This "at risk" patient will place different demands on the knee from those of the recreational athlete. Obviously, each patient requires an individualized treatment plan based on the following factors: (1) the severity of damage to the knee; (2) specific athletic activity; (3) frequency of sports participation; (4) expectations and motivation; (5) willingness to modify activity level; and (6) willingness to accept an intensive rehabilitation program.

Equally important to the technical details and patient selection in achieving a successful outcome are the various postoperative rehabilitation protocols. Each protocol is specifically designed for a certain surgical procedure, and there is no simple rehabilitation program that may be applied to all acute or chronic knee ligament procedures. Whereas "early" range of motion may be desirable and appropriate for certain extra-articular procedures, it may be detrimental to others, such as an iliotibial tract tenodesis that depends on the adherence of the iliotibial tract to the lateral femoral condyle for a successful result. Thus the physician should be familiar with the appropriate rehabilitation protocol for each of the different procedures.

In conclusion, successful treatment of anterior cruciate ligament lesions requires that the physician: (1) be aware of the various technical intricacies of each surgical procedure; (2) make the appropriate decision regarding the indications for surgery; and (3) choose the appropriate rehabilitation protocol.

REFERENCES

1. Andrews, J.R.: Management of acute anterolateral rotatory instability of the knee, Strategies in Orthopaedic Surgery (Upjohn), vol. 1(3), 1981.
2. Andrews, J.R., and Sanders, R.: A "mini-reconstruction" technique in treating anterolateral rotatory instability (ALRI), Clin. Orthop. **172**:93-96, 1983.
3. Andrews, J.R., and Axe, M.J.: The classification of knee ligament instability, Orthop. Clin. North Am. **16**(1):69-82, 1985.
4. Andrews, J.R., Sanders, R.A., and Morin, B.: Surgical treatment of anterolateral rotatory instability: a follow-up study, Am. J. Sports Med. **13**:112-119, 1985.
5. Arnold, J.A.: A lateral extra-articular tenodesis for anterior cruciate ligament deficiency of the knee, Orthop. Clin. North Am. **16**(2):213-222, 1985.
6. Arnold, J.A., Coker, T.P., Heaton, L.M., et al.: Natural history of anterior cruciate tears, Am. J. Sports Med. **7**:305, 1979.
7. Baker, C.L., Norwood, L.A., and Hughston, J.C.: Acute posterolateral rotatory instability of the knee, J. Bone Joint Surg. (Am.) **65**:614-618, 1983.
8. Baker, C.L., Norwood, L.A., and Hughston, J.C.: Acute combined posterior cruciate and posterolateral instability of the knee, Am. J. Sports Med. **12**:204-208, 1984.
9. Cabaud, H.E., and Slocum, D.B.: The diagnosis of chronic anterolateral rotatory instability of the knee, Am. J. Sports Med. **5**:99-105, 1977.

10. Carson, W.G.: Extra-articular reconstruction of the anterior cruciate ligament: lateral procedures, Orthop. Clin. North Am. **16**(2):191-211, 1985.
11. Clancy, W.G.: Anterior cruciate ligament functional instability: a static intra-articular and dynamic extra-articular procedure, Clin. Orthop. **172**:102-106, 1983.
12. Clancy, W.G.: Intra-articular reconstruction of the anterior cruciate ligament, Orthop. Clin. North Am. **16**(2):181-189, 1985.
13. Clancy, W.G., Nelson, D.A., Reider, B., et al.: Anterior cruciate ligament reconstruction using one-third of the patellar ligament, augmented by extra-articular tendon transfers, J. Bone Joint Surg. (Am.) **64**:352-359, 1982.
14. DeHaven, K.E.: Acute ligament injuries and dislocations. In Evarts, C.M., editor: Surgery of the musculoskeletal system, New York, 1983, Churchill Livingstone Inc., pp. 5-30.
15. DeLee, J.C., Riley, M.B., and Rollwood, C.A.: Acute posterolateral rotatory instability of the knee, Am. J. Sports Med. **11**:199-203, 1983.
16. Drez, D.: Modified Eriksson procedure for chronic anterior cruciate instability, Orthopedics **1**(1):30-36, 1978.
17. Ellison, A.E.: Distal iliotibial-band transfer for anterolateral rotatory instability of the knee, J. Bone Joint Surg. (Am.) **61**:330-337, 1979.
18. Ellison, A.E.: The pathogenesis and treatment of anterolateral rotatory instability, Clin. Orthop. **147**:51-55, 1980.
19. Fetto, J.F., and Marshall, J.L.: Injury to the anterior cruciate ligament producing the pivot-shift sign: an experimental study on cadaver specimens, J. Bone Joint Surg. (Am.) **61**:710-714, 1979.
20. Fleming, R.E., Blatz, D.J., and McCarroll, J.R.: Lateral reconstruction for anterolateral rotatory instability of the knee, Am. J. Sports Med. **11**:303-307, 1983.
21. Fox, J.M., Blazina, M.E., Del Pizzo, W., et al.: Extra-articular stabilization of the knee joint for anterior instability, Clin. Orthop. **147**:56-61, 1980.
22. Fried, J.A., Bergfeld, J.A., Weiker, G.G., et al.: Two to five years evaluation of anterior cruciate reconstruction using patellar tendon and Ellison iliotibial band transfer, Orthop. Trans. **7**(3):485, 1983.
23. Galway, H.R., and MacIntosh, D.L.: The lateral pivot shift: a symptom and sign of anterior cruciate ligament insufficiency, Clin. Orthop. **147**:45-50, 1980.
24. Galway, R.D., Beaupré, A., and MacIntosh, D.L.: Pivot shift: a clinical sign of symptomatic anterior cruciate insufficiency, Proc. Can. Orthop. Assoc. J. Bone Joint Surg. (Br.) **54**:763, 1972.
25. Giove, T.P., Miller, S.J., Kent, B.E., et al.: Non-operative treatment of the torn anterior cruciate ligament, J. Bone Joint Surg. (Am.) **65**:184-192, 1983.
26. Hanks, G.A., Joyner, D.M., and Kalenak, A.: Anterolateral rotatory instability of the knee: an analysis of the Ellison procedure, Am. J. Sports Med. **9**:225-232, 1981.
27. Holden, D.L., and Jackson, D.W.: Treatment selection in acute anterior cruciate ligament tears, Orthop. Clin. North Am. **16**(1):99-109, 1985.
28. Hughston, J.C.: Complications of anterior cruciate ligament surgery, Orthop. Clin. North Am. **16**(2):237-240, 1985.
29. Hughston, J.C., and Eilers, A.F.: The role of the posterior oblique ligament in repairs of acute medial (collateral) ligament tears of the knee, J. Bone Joint Surg. (Am.) **55**:923-940, 1973.
30. Hughston, J.C., and Norwood, L.A.: The posterolateral drawer test and external rotational recurvatum test for posterolateral rotatory instability of the knee, Clin. Orthop. **147**:82-87, 1980.
31. Hughston, J.C., and Barrett, G.R.: Acute anteromedial rotatory instability: long-term results of surgical repair, J. Bone Joint Surg. (Am.) **65**:145-153, 1983.
32. Hughston, J.C., and Jacobson, K.E.: Chronic posterolateral rotatory instability of the knee, J. Bone Joint Surg. (Am.) **67**:351-359, 1985.

33. Hughston, J.C., Andrews, J.R., Cross, M.J., et al.: Classification of knee ligament instabilities. Part II. The lateral compartment. J. Bone Joint Surg. (Am.) **58**:173-179, 1976.
34. Ireland, J., and Trickey, E.L.: MacIntosh tenodesis for anterolateral instability of the knee, J. Bone Joint Surg. (Br.) **62**:340-345, 1980.
35. Jakob, R.P., Hassle, H., and Steubli, H.: Observations on rotatory instability of the lateral compartment of the knee, Acta Orthop. Scand. (Suppl.) **52**(191):1-32, 1981.
36. James, S.L.: The knee. In D'Ambrosia, R.D., editor: Musculoskeletal disorders: regional examination and differential diagnosis, Philadelphia, 1977, J.B. Lippincott Co., pp. 440-486.
37. James, S.L.: Biomechanics of knee ligament reconstruction, Clin. Orthop. **146**:90-101, 1980.
38. James, S.L.: Knee ligament reconstruction. In Evarts, C.M., editor: Surgery of the musculoskeletal system, New York, 1983, Churchill Livingstone Inc., pp. 31-104.
39. Jensen, J.E., Slocum, D.B., Larson, R.I., et al.: Reconstruction procedures for anterior cruciate ligament insufficiency: a computer analysis of clinical results, Am. J. Sports Med. **11**:240-248, 1983.
40. Johnson, L.L.: Lateral capsular ligament complex: anatomical and surgical considerations, Am. J. Sports Med. **7**:156, 1979.
41. Kennedy, J.C., Stewart, R., and Walker, D.M.: Anterolateral rotatory instability of the knee joint, J. Bone Joint Surg. (Am.) **60**:1031-1039, 1978.
42. Krackow, K.A., and Brooks, R.L.: Optimization of knee ligament position for lateral extra-articular reconstruction, Am. J. Sports Med. **11**:293-302, 1983.
43. Larson, R.L.: Chronic medial instability. In Evarts, C.M., editor: Surgery of the musculoskeletal system, New York, 1983, Churchill Livingstone Inc., pp. 34-56.
44. Larson, R.L.: The knee—the physiological joint, J. Bone Joint Surg. (Am.) **65**:143-144, 1983.
45. Losee, R.E., Johnson, T.R., and Southwick, W.O.: Anterior subluxation of the lateral tibial plateau: a diagnostic test and operative repair, J. Bone Joint Surg. (Am.) **60**:1015-1030, 1978.
46. MacIntosh, D.L., and Darby, T.A.: Lateral substitution reconstruction. Proc. Can. Orthop. Assoc. J. Bone Joint Surg. (Br.) **58**:142, 1976.
47. Marshall, J.L., Girgis, F.G., and Zelko, R.R.: The biceps femoris tendon and its functional significance, J. Bone Joint Surg. (Am.) **54**:1444-1450, 1972.
48. McLeod, W.D., Moschi, A., Andrews, J.R., et al.: Tibial plateau topography, Am. J. Sports Med. **5**:13-18, 1977.
49. Narechania, R.G., Clancy, W.G., and Branham, R.: Biomechanical aspects of biceps tendon transfer. Presented at the Annual Meeting of the American Society of Biomechanics, Ann Arbor, Michigan, October 26, 1978.
50. Norwood, L.A., and Hughston, J.C.: Combined anterolateral-anteromedial rotatory instability of the knee, Clin. Orthop. **147**:62-67, 1980.
51. Norwood, L.A., Andrews, J.R., Meisterling, R.C., et al.: Acute anterolateral rotatory instability of the knee, J. Bone Joint Surg. (Am.) **61**:704-709, 1979.
52. Noyes, F.R., Bassett, R.W., Grood, E.S., et al.: Arthroscopy in acute traumatic hemarthrosis of the knee: incidence of anterior cruciate tears and other injuries, J. Bone Joint Surg. (Am.) **62**:687-695, 1980.
53. Noyes, F.R., Mooar, P.A., Matthews, D.S., et al.: The symptomatic anterior cruciate-deficient knee. Part I. The long-term functional disability in athletically active individuals, J. Bone Joint Surg. (Am.) **65**:154-162, 1983.
54. Noyes, F.R., Matthews, D.S., Mooar, P.A., et al.: The symptomatic anterior cruciate-deficient knee. Part II. The results of rehabilitation, activity modification, and counseling on functional disability, J. Bone Joint Surg. (Am.) **65**:163-174, 1983.
55. Noyes, F.R., McGinniss, G.H, and Grood, E.S.: The variable functional disability of the anterior cruciate ligament-deficient knee, Orthop. Clin. North Am. **16**(1):47-67, 1985.
56. Odensten, M., Lysholm, J., and Gillquist, J.: Long term follow-up of a distal iliotibial transfer (DIT) for anterolateral instability of the knee, Orthop. Trans. **7**(3):484, 1983.

57. O'Donoghue, D.H.: Reconstruction for medial instability of the knee: technique and results in sixty cases, J. Bone Joint Surg. (Am.) **55**:941-955, 1973.
58. Paulos, L.E., Butler, D.L., Noyes, F.R., et al.: Intra-articular cruciate reconstruction. II. Replacement with vascularized patellar tendon, Clin. Orthop. **172**:78-84, 1983.
59. Ritter, M.A., Leaming, E.S., and McCarroll, J.R.: Preliminary report on the Jones, Ellison, Slocum (JES) repair for symptomatic anterior cruciate deficient knees, Am. J. Sports Med. **11**:89-94, 1983.
60. Sisk, T.D., and Canale, S.T.: Traumatic affections of joints. In Edmonson, A.S., and Crenshaw, A.H., editors: Campbell's operative orthopaedics, St. Louis, 1980, The C.V. Mosby, p. 967.
61. Sisk, T.D., and Canale, S.T.: Traumatic affections of joints. In Edmonson, A.S., and Crenshaw, A.H., editors: Campbell's operative orthopaedics, St. Louis, 1980, The C.V. Mosby Co., p. 972.
62. Slocum, D.B., and Larson, R.L.: Pes anserinus transplantation: a simple surgical procedure for control of rotatory instability of the knee, J. Bone Joint Surg. (Am.) **50**:226-242, 1968.
63. Slocum, D.B., Larson, R.L., and James, S.L.: Pes anserinus transplant: impressions after a decade of experience, Am. J. Sports Med. **2**:123-136, 1974.
64. Slocum, D.B., Larson, R.L., and James, S.L.: Late reconstruction of the ligamentous injuries of the medial compartment of the knee, Clin. Orthop. **100**:23-56, 1974.
65. Slocum, D.B., James, S.L., Larson, R.L., et al.: Clinical test for anterolateral rotatory instability of the knee, Clin. Orthop. **118**:63-69, 1976.
66. Sullivan, J.G., DeHaven, K.E., and Lovelock, J.E.: Primary anterior cruciate ligament repair with extra-articular augmentation. Presented at the American Academy of Orthopaedic Surgeons Annual Meeting, Anaheim, California, March 11, 1983.
67. Sydnor, R.W., and Andrews, J.R.: Combined arthroscopy and "mini-reconstruction" techniques in the acutely torn anterior cruciate ligament, Orthop. Clin. North Am. **16**(2):171-179, 1985.
68. Teitge, R.A., and Indelicato, P.A.: Distal iliotibial band transfer for anterolateral rotatory instability: progress report, Orthop. Trans. **2**:24, 1978.
69. Torg, J.S., and Cooley, L.: Anterior cruciate ligament substitution utilizing fibular head osteotomy with lateral collateral ligament and biceps tendon advancement techniques, Orthop. Trans. **7**(3):485, 1983.
70. Torg, J.S., Conrad, W., and Kalen, V.: Clinical diagnosis of anterior cruciate ligament instability in the athlete, Am. J. Sports Med. **4**:84-93, 1976.
71. Tregonning, R.J.A.: MacIntosh fascia lata substitution for chronic anterior cruciate insufficiency: an early report on 45 procedures, J. Bone Joint Surg. (Br.) **64**:134, 1982.
72. Wood, M.R., and Dandy, D.J.: The cause and mechanics of the pivot shift phenomenon, J. Bone Joint Surg. (Br.) **61**:519, 1979.
73. Zarins, B.: Combined intra-articular and extra-articular reconstructions for anterior tibial subluxation, Orthop. Clin. North Am. **16**(2):223-226, 1985.
74. Zarins, B., and Rowe, C.R.: Anterior cruciate ligament reconstruction using semitendinosus tendon and iliotibial tract, Orthop. Trans. **4**(3):291, 1980.

12

Anterior cruciate ligament autografts

WILLIAM G. CLANCY, Jr.

J. MICHAEL RAY

Anterior cruciate ligament injuries should no longer be considered the enigma they were in the 1970s. Certainly, we do not have all the answers, but certain facts have been firmly established.

First, anterior cruciate ligament insufficiency can lead to any or all of the following: meniscal tears, stretching out of the secondary restraints, functional instability, and late traumatic arthritis.

Second, Marshall,[23] McDevitt,[26] Cabaud,[6,7] and Arnoczky[5] have documented that early traumatic arthritis will usually develop in animals if the anterior cruciate ligament is sectioned. Jacobsen,[18] Fried,[14] ourselves,[9] and others have documented that significant destructive articular injury was evident in a large percentage of those patients undergoing surgical reconstruction for chronic anterior cruciate ligament instability. The average age for these patients was 25 years and the average time interval from injury to surgery was approximately 3 years. It has been documented by many authors that meniscal tears were present in the vast majority of patients with functional anterior cruciate ligament insufficiency, and the literature is quite clear as to the long-term consequences of meniscectomy in an otherwise stable knee.[3,13,19,20]

Third, there have been published a variety of intra-articular procedures that can provide excellent static and functional stability in 75% to 95% of the patients followed from 2 to 8 years. Successful repair of peripheral intra-body meniscal tears combined with intra-articular stabilization has been documented.[10]

Diagnosis and treatment recommendation

Description of the Lachman test, in which an anterior drawer test is performed at 20 to 30 degrees of flexion, by Torg[33] has been the single most important recent contribution to clinical examination of the possibly anterior cruciate injured knee. This test has proved to be over 95% accurate in diagnosing both acute and chronic anterior cruciate ligament deficiencies. The pivot-shift test as described by Gallway and MacIntosh[15] has enabled us to reproduce the patients sensation of giving way and allows the examiner to establish correlation between static laxity and functional instability.

The pivot-shift test has been used by most surgeons in the evaluation of the acutely injured knee to predict the probability of the patient going on to develop functional instability. In an 8-year prospective study we found that the classical pivot shift was not a good predicator for conservative management when graded absent, trace, or mild.[11] It has come to our attention in the last few years that use of a modification of the pivot-shift test may be a better method in predicting which acute anterior cruciate ligament deficient knees will maintain long-term functional stability with nonoperative treatment.

In the classic description of the pivot-shift test, the patient's tibia is held in full extension and in internal rotation and an anterior and valgus force is applied and followed by knee flexion (Fig. 12-1). It has been our observation that in the majority of patients, the pivot-shift phenomenon can be increased significantly over the classic maneuver if the examiner holds the patient's tibia in external rotation before applying the anterior and valgus force (Fig. 12-2). It is our belief that internal rotation tightens the iliotibial band and thus decreases the full extent that the tibia can translate.

However, with the tibia in external rotation the tibia can now translate anteriorly to its full extent. Indeed, careful questioning of patients with chronic functional instability revealed that well over 90% of the episodes of instability occur when cutting or turning to the direction opposite to the injured knee (Fig. 12-3). This mechanism of instability produces external rotation and valgus of the affected knee, producing a pivot-shift and painful giving way. The examiner must make sure that there is no concomittant posterolateral laxity present. If there is some posterolateral laxity present, external rotation of the tibia in extension and maintenance of this rotation during flexion may eliminate or minimize the pivot-shift test since the tibia may be held in a posterolateral subluxed position as a result of the external rotation of the tibia. Indeed, if the pivot-shift test performed with the tibia in external rotation is graded less than when the tibia is held in internal rotation, associated posterolateral instability must be considered present.

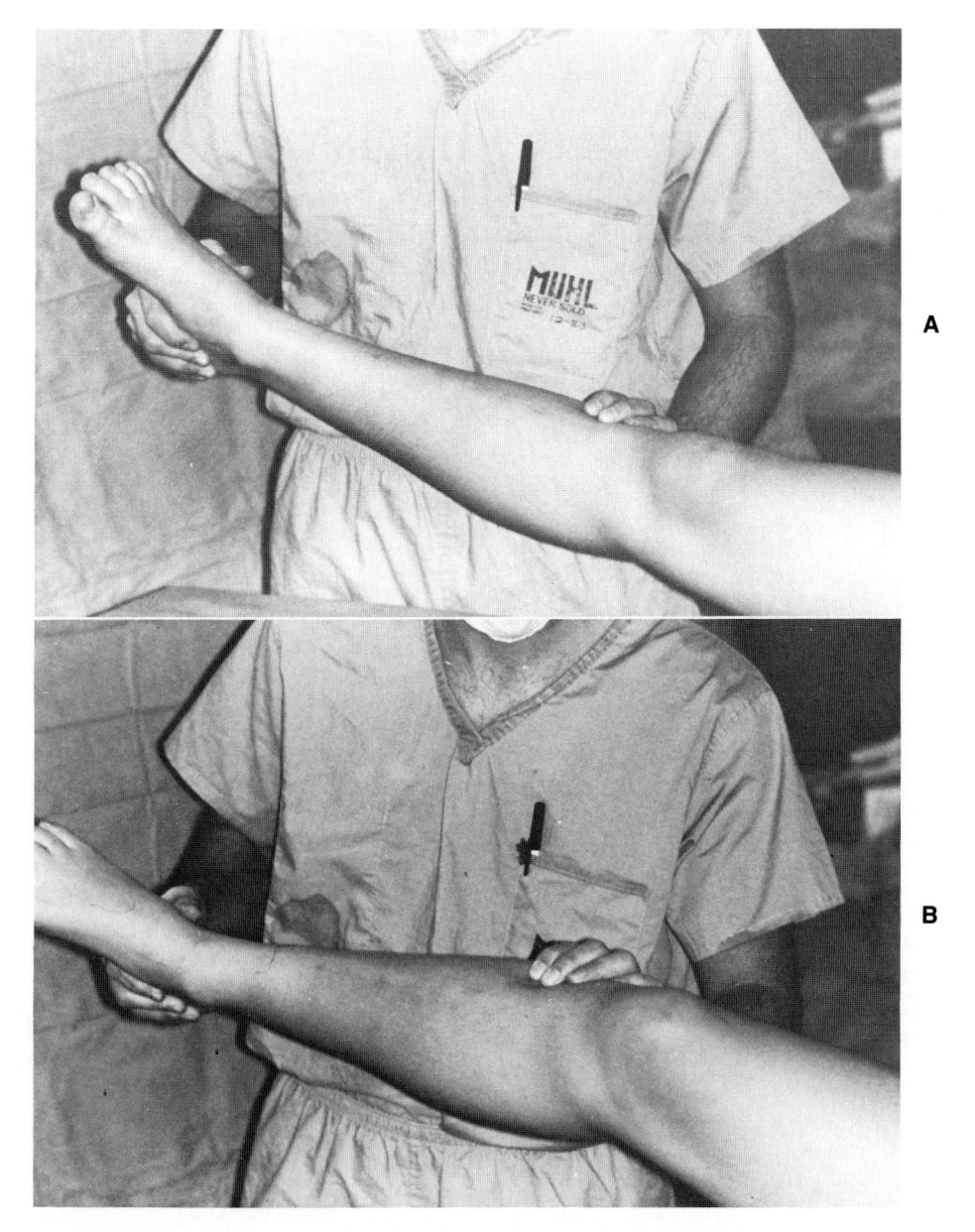

Fig. 12-1 *A,* In the classic pivot-shift test the examiner holds the tibia in internal rotation, and *B,* maintains this internal rotation through flexion.

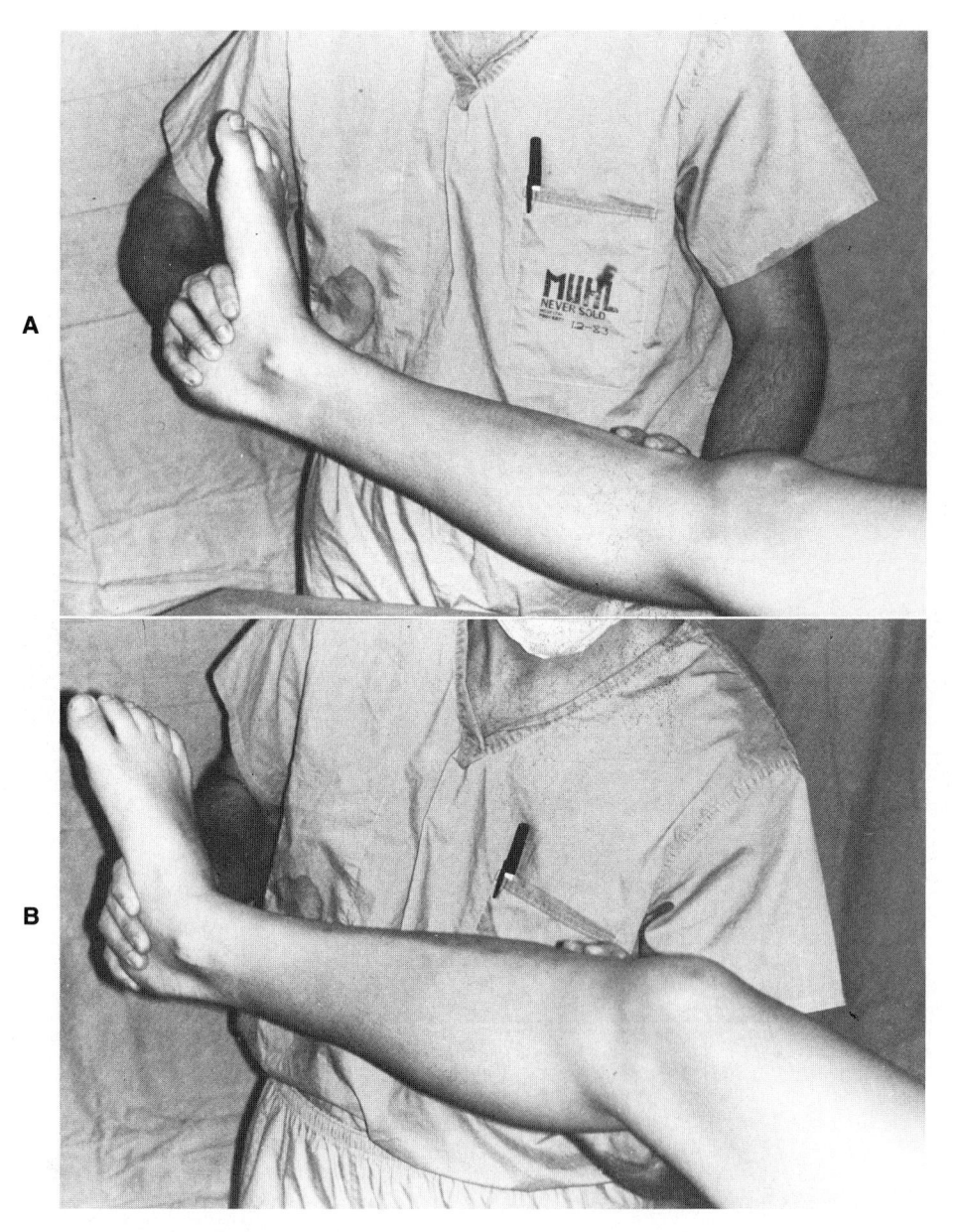

Fig. 12-2 *The modified pivot-shift test. **A**, In this test the examiner holds the tibia in external rotation, and **B**, maintains this external rotation through flexion.*

Anterior cruciate ligament autografts 197

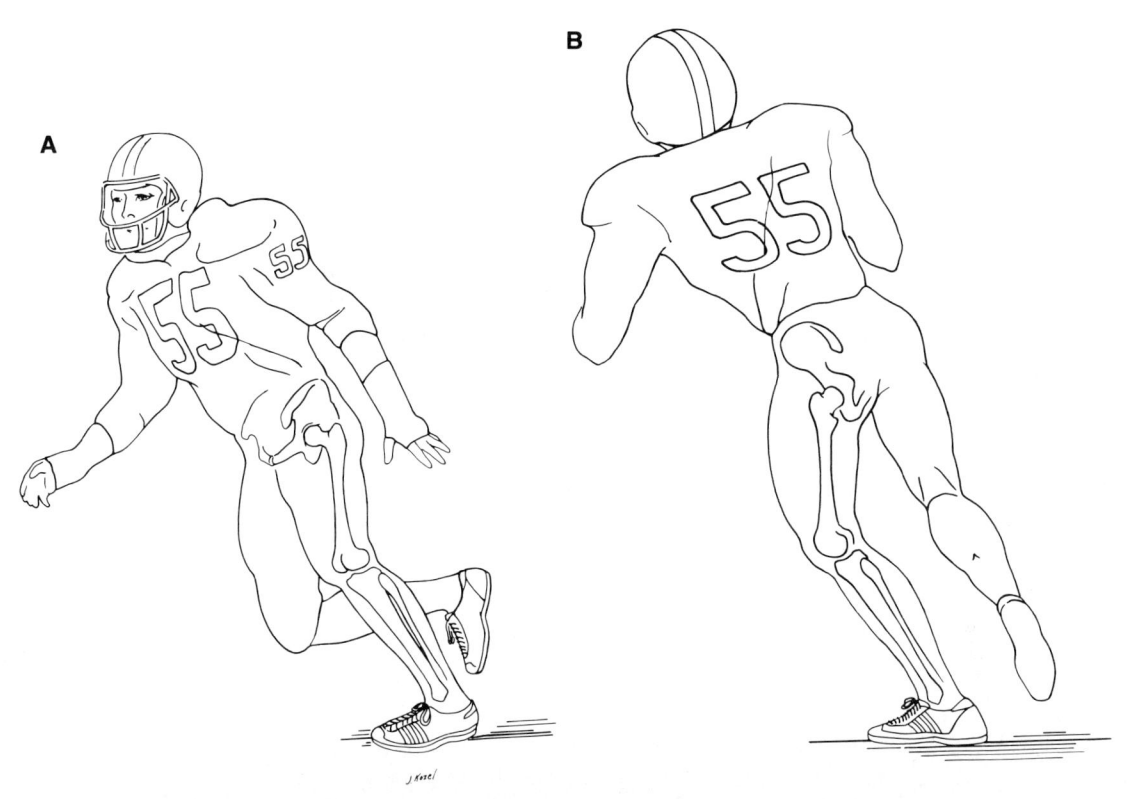

Fig. 12-3 *A, A football player about to cut to his right. B, With the abrupt change of direction, there occurs an external rotation of the tibia and a valgus force at the knee, reduplicating the modified pivot-shift test.*

Acute third degree anterior cruciate ligament tear

It is our present recommendation in evaluation of the acute anterior cruciate ligament injury that the pivot-shift test be performed with the tibia held first in internal rotation and then in external rotation. If the pivot shift is graded absent, trace, or mild in both positions, then conservative treatment is our usual mode of therapy.

Before using the modified pivot-shift test, a long-term perspective study of nonoperative and operative treatment of acute anterior cruciate ligament injuries was undertaken. The average 4-year follow-up revealed that 41% of the patients were graded as fair or as failures. Those patients with the most unstable knees, those with a pivot-shift test graded moderate or severe, underwent acute repair and patellar tendon augumentation. In this group, there was a 95% good to excellent result, no failures, and a 5% fair result.[10]

As a result of this study, our protocol in acute anterior cruciate ligament deficit is as follows:
1. If there is a repairable meniscal lesion, we recommend ligament repair, patellar tendon augmentation, and meniscal repair.
2. If the modified pivot-shift test is graded moderate or severe, we recommend ligament repair and patellar tendon augmentation.
3. If the modified pivot-shift test is graded absent, trace, or mild and if there is no meniscal pathology, nonoperative treatment is our usual recommendation, but we defer to the patient's decision, which he or she makes before receiving anesthesia. Surprisingly, 70% of the patients now desire surgical stabilization even if the examination revealed a pivot-shift test that was graded absent, trace, or mild.

Chronic anterior cruciate ligament functional instability

If the patient complains that his functional instability interferes with the desired lifestyle, if the modified pivot-shift test reproduces the instability, and if the patient is still symptomatic after a good rehabilitation program, an intra-articular anterior cruciate ligament reconstruction with a patellar tendon graft is our recommendation.

Biomechanical considerations of technique

The goal of any anterior cruciate ligament surgery should be not only to restore the knee joint to a functional, stable joint but to restore biomechanical stability. Although it is probably impossible to restore the normal biomechanics, particularly in those patients who have had a meniscectomy or stretched out secondary restraints, our goal should be restoration of functional stability and achievement of as much additional biomechanical stability as possible.

To date there is no universally accepted instrumentation devices that allow for accurate evaluation of biomechanical stability in all degrees of freedom. Therefore logic dictates that only an intra-articular procedure can achieve the desired result.

An intra-articular substitute should: (1) be biological; (2) be of sufficient tensile strength after transplantation; (3) maintain vascularity or revascularize readily; (4) be isometric; (5) not degenerate with time; and (6) yield consistently high clinical results. Other desirable qualities are: (1) allowing for early motion; (2) enabling the patient to return to work and sports in a relatively short period of time; (3) not requiring extensive surgical exposure; and (4) having minimal surgical complications.

Biomechanical strength of potential substitutes

The work of Noyes clearly documents that the patellar tendon with its bony insertions is by far the strongest and the most logical choice for intra-articular substitution for the anterior cruciate ligament.[27,28]

Our published research on anterior cruciate ligament substitutions in the monkey document that at 9 months the graft regained 80% of its pretransfer strength and that 50% of its initial strength had regenerated by 6 months.[12] If these data could be extrapolated to humans, then a successful patellar tendon graft as compared to a normal anterior cruciate ligament would be approximately 33% at 8 weeks, 55% at 3 months, 55% at 6 months, and 90% at 9 and 12 months. Unfortunately, this is purely speculative.

Vascular studies of patellar tendon grafts

Our study[12] and studies by Alm[1,2] clearly demonstrate that a patellar tendon graft rapidly revascularizes, that revascularization is almost complete at 8 weeks, and that the revascularization is mediated most predominantly through the endosteal vessels in the tibial and femoral tunnels. Vascularization studies by Arnoczky et al.[4] demonstrated that with their reconstructive procedure it took 16 to 20 weeks for the graft to revascularize and that revascularization was mainly by way of the fat pad and anterior and posterior synovium. It is important to note that in the study by Arnoczky et al., no femoral or tibial tunnels were created, and thus there could be no contribution to revascularization by endosteal vessels. A more recent study by our group has reconfirmed the overwhelming contribution by the endosteal vessels to graft revascularization.

Paulos and Noyes[30] developed the concept of trying to maintain vascularity to the patellar tendon graft. Their hope was that maintaining vascularity would result in a significantly smaller decrease in the graft's early tensile strength. Paulos and Noyes developed a medially based vascular pedicle. Since this is a technically difficult procedure and since there was the possibility that this procedure

Our studies indicated that if a bony tunnel was to be created in the tibia, the Kirschner wire (K-wire) should be placed slightly medial and anterior to the anatomical center of the cylindrical portion of the anterior cruciate ligament. Similarly, K-wire placement on the lateral femoral condyle had to be posterior and superior to the anatomical center of the insertion site of the anterior cruciate ligament. More recently, Graf has designed a commercially available strain gauge (Acufex Microsurgical Inc.) that will allow measurement of the approximate strain or change in graft length that the potential substitute will encounter (see Chapters 4 and 7). A K-wire hole is placed where the appropriate tunnel circumference will lie on the femur, and a suture is threaded through it and fixed on one end with a staple or button. The suture is run through the tibial tunnel, and the strain gauge is placed at the tibial tunnel exit site. The knee is placed through a range of motion, and any change in length is recorded directly from the strain gauge. Recently, Grood has stated that their studies revealed that there will be interstitial failure within the ligament or substitute if 5% to 10% strain occurs. We have selected a 2 to 3 mm strain as our limit of acceptability since Girgis and Marshall[16] revealed that the normal resting length of the anterior cruciate ligament is approximately 38 mm and that the range was 30 to 48 mm. Our average strain for the past 3 years has been approximately 1 to 1½ mm.

If we are performing an acute anterior cruciate ligament repair and a patellar tendon graft augmentation, the knee is first arthroscoped. A meniscal repair is performed either arthroscopically or by arthrotomy when there is a repairable tear of the lateral and/or medial meniscus.

A medial arthrotomy incision is used to expose the knee joint and the vastus medialis is freed proximally from its insertion to the intramuscular septum so that the patella can be subluxed. A notchplasty is performed when appropriate. The tibial tunnel is reamed, the patella is subluxed, and the knee is placed in a figure four position and flexed to approximately 110 degrees. This maneuver of varus, internal rotation, and flexion allows for adequate visualization of the posterior superior portion of the lateral femoral condyle so that the K-wire can be placed in the desired eccentric position from inside out. The K-wire can be over-drilled either from the inside out or from the outside in. Care must be taken to avoid reamer contact with the posterior cruciate ligament.

After the tunnels have been drilled in the acutely injured knee, a primary repair of the anterior cruciate ligament is performed, even if it is a midportion mop-end tear. Whip sutures are placed in either end of both portions of the tear, and the sutures are brought out through the appropriate tunnel. Our tensile testing studies have documented that the whip stitch technique is at least three times stronger than the loop suture technique described by Marshall.[23] The whip suture technique can better restore the height and width of the torn ends than any other suture technique tested.

In both acute and chronic cases, the central 10 mm of the patellar tendon along with its patellar and tibial bony attachments, which measure 10 mm in width, 4 mm in depth, and 25 mm in length, is harvested without any fat pad attachment. Three no. 5 nonabsorbable sutures are placed into each of the bony blocks, and the graft is pulled through the tunnels. An AO malleolar screw with a metal washer is placed just below the tibial tunnel, and the sutures are tied around it. The femoral sutures are placed through a button. The knee is flexed to 90 degrees with the patella reduced, and with a posterior drawer the first knot is laid down. The knee is then flexed to 30 degrees while maintaining a posterior drawer. The first knot is retightened and then multiple knots are tied. The knee is placed through a full range of motion, and a Lachman and pivot-shift test are performed. The suture ends on the femoral side are then looped around a staple placed 4 cm proximal to the femoral button and retightened.

Arthroscopic reconstruction of chronic anterior cruciate ligament instability

For the past several years, patients with chronic anterior cruciate ligament instability have had notchplasty, meniscal repairs, and drilling of the tibial and femoral tunnels performed through the arthroscope. It has been quite obvious that after arthroscopically assisted anterior cruciate ligament reconstruction patients have far less postoperative pain, can perform straight-leg raising several hours after surgery, do not develop severe muscle atrophy, and rapidly regain flexion and extension. To date, the clinical results are quite similar to those of open arthrotomy.

After the knee is thoroughly examined through the arthroscope, appropriate meniscal tears are repaired arthroscopically when indicated. If there is a peripheral lateral meniscus tear, a small longitudinal incision is made just superior to the biceps tendon and just posterior to the head of the fibula. The soft tissue is dissected down to the lateral capsule and lateral gastrocnemius tendon. A double-barreled curved cannula is placed into the lateral compartment through the anterior medial patellar portal and two needles with a 2-0 absorbable suture are passed through the cannula, through the meniscus, and out through the lateral capsule. The skin incision is manipulated so that all the needles can exit and be tied down over the lateral capsule without injury to the common peroneal nerve.

Any repairable medial meniscus tear is repaired in much the same fashion. A small longitudinal skin incision parallel to the pes tendons is made over the posterior medial corner of the knee; care is taken to avoid the saphenous nerve. All needles are directed out through this incision, and the sutures are tied over the capsule with the knee in full extension.

The intercondylar notch is inspected through the arthroscope, which is placed in the inferior medial patella portal. If there is marked narrowing of the notch, a notchplasty is performed using a ¼ inch osteotome or motorized burr. The osteotome is introduced through the medial parapatellar tendon portal. The remnant of the old anterior cruciate ligament is excised, particularly if it has fallen back and has scarred to the posterior cruciate ligament synovium. A medium-sized curette is then introduced into medial parapatellar tendon portal, and the lateral femoral condyle is completely cleaned. We have found that the curette is quicker and more efficient than the motorized devices.

The tibial tunnel is then created. A longitudinal skin incision is made starting at the lower portion of the medial parapatellar and carried down to the superior portion of the pes tendons. The Rosenberg/Acufex tibial drill guide is then introduced through the medial parapatellar portal while under direct vision of the arthroscope, which is placed in the inferior medial patellar portal. Placement of the drill guide should be such that the K-wires will exit slightly anterior and medial to the anatomical center of the anterior cruciate ligament insertion on the tibia. After the K-wire enters the joint, it is over reamed by a 9 mm cannulated reamer.

A motorized burr or small curette is then introduced and placed against the posterior superior aspect of the lateral femoral condyle approximately at the junction of where the posterior aspect of the femoral condyle joins the roof of the femur. A small hole is made, and this location should be posterior and superior to the anatomical insertion of the anterior cruciate ligament. This burr hole allows the surgeon to use a drill guide or K-wire without having either shift off the lateral condyle as a result of the acute angle of introduction. We seldom use a drill guide since most are designed to create a femoral tunnel that is too perpendicular to the shaft of the femur. A tunnel that is too perpendicular can create significant shear forces on the graft with motion. Since the tunnel should be directed more vertically and more parallel to the femoral shaft, a K-wire is passed through the skin of the anteromedial joint line and into the joint, after the knee is placed in a figure four position and flexed to 110 degrees. Once the K-wire is placed in the starter hole in the lateral femoral condyle, it is then drilled out through the lateral femoral shaft.

A lateral skin incision is made, the fascia overlying the vastus lateralis is incised, and the entire vastus lateralis is retracted superiorly, giving access to the distal insertion of the intramuscular septum. The K-wire is then reamed retrograde under arthroscopic control.

If the surgeon desires to use the Acufex strain gauge, then a second K-wire is placed 4.5 mm anterior and inferior to the first K-wire. The second K-wire is removed, and a suture and suture passer are passed through this K-wire hole into the knee joint and pulled out through the previously drilled tibial tunnel. A no. 5 Ethibon suture is tied to a button, and the suture is passed through the femoral and tibial tunnels. The strain gauge is applied to the tibial suture, the knee is placed through a range of motion, and the strain recorded by the gauge is monitored. If satisfactory tunnel placements are achieved, then the middle 10 mm of the patellar tendon with its bony attachments is developed as a free graft. The remaining portion of the technique is as previously described.

Rehabilitation

At surgery, a plastic stirrup is applied to hold the knee in 5 degrees of extension. A custom fitted polyethylene nonhinged half-shell flexed to only −5 degrees of full extension is applied at the third post-operative day. For 6 weeks the shell is removed three times a day for 30 minutes to allow the patient to perform active and passive range of motion exercises. The patient actively extends from 90 to 45 degrees of flexion and then passively extends 45 degrees to full extension. If a meniscal repair if performed, then no motion is allowed for 5 weeks. Patients are allowed 50% weight bearing as soon as they begin walking with crutches and are progressed to 70% by 2 weeks. Full weight bearing without crutches is allowed at 6 weeks, and hamstring isotonic exercises are begun at this time. Quadriceps progressive resistance exercises are begun at 3 to 4 months. Electrical stimulation of the hamstrings is begun 3 days after surgery and quadriceps stimulation is begun at 4 weeks with the knee flexed to 45 degrees. In those cases that can be very closely monitored, flutter kicking in the swimming pool has been started at 2 to 3 weeks after surgery.

Other biological substitutes for intra-articular anterior cruciate ligament stabilization

Lipscomb has reported overall good results in 84% of patients with use of semitendinous and gracilis tendon as intra-articular substitutes.[21] His technique of tunnel placement is quite similar to that which we described earlier. Lipscomb has further reported long-term follow-up studies of hamstring strength measurements at 1 year and documented that there was no deficit present when compared to the opposite leg.[22] Chiroff has described the histology of semitendinous substitution in dogs, documented the progressive incorporation of the tendon into bone in the femoral tunnel, and noted the revascularization and recollagenization within the intra-articular portion of the graft.[8]

Zarins has recently found an 89% good to excellent result in his long-term follow-up of combining the fascia lata and semitendinous as an intra-articular substitute.[35] He uses a 25 mm wide strip of the fascia lata that is tubed, brought over the top of the lateral femoral condyle, and brought out through the tibial tunnel. He places the semitendinous tendon through the tibial tunnel, over the top of the lateral femoral condyle, and down to Gerde's tubercle. However, Zarins has subsequently modified his technique in order to attain a more isometric graft. He now creates a bony trough in the lateral femoral condyle instead of placing the graft over the top of the lateral femoral condyle.

Pitfalls of intra-articular substitution

Tibial tunnel placement must be posterior enough so that the anterior femoral notch does not cut the graft at extension. The posterior aspect of the tibial tunnel should lie just in front of the anterior medial tibial spine.

The femoral tunnel will most often be placed too anterior if the surgeon tries to place a K-wire from the inside out and if the knee is placed over the table and flexed to only 90 degrees. The normal anterior tibial step-off forces K-wire placement to be more superior and anterior in order to get firm purchase on the lateral femoral condyle. However, if the K-wire is placed more horizontally, it will tend to slide off the condyle posteriorly. Therefore, if a small starter hole is made with a burr or small curette, the K-wire can be drilled correctly from inside out, and it will exit just superior to the intramuscular septum insertion on the lateral femur.

When drilling the tunnels, the surgeon must not allow the reamer to get too hot or the walls of the tunnel may undergo burn necrosis and the possibility of graft nonunion may arise.

Passage of the bony grafts can be made easier if a hole is made in a metal ruler the size of the reamer used to create the bony tunnels and if this is used to measure the diameter of the bony blocks.

It should be remembered that smaller diameter tunnels are required in those patients with small femoral condyles, otherwise graft placement will be too anterior because the tunnel is inappropriately too large. The bone blocks should be fashioned accordingly.

Summary

Although there is some interest in primary arthroscopic repair of the anterior cruciate ligament, it is important to note several facts. First, there has never been a published report of successful primary repair alone in any animal model. Second, the reports in the literature of open, primary repair alone have yielded less than acceptable static results by our present criteria, particularly in view of the superior results of primary repair and graft augmentation. Third, reports by Cabaud,[6,7] ourselves,[11] and others document clearly that primary repair and graft augmentation consistently yield superior results in both the animal model and in humans. Fourth, seldom is the anterior cruciate ligament completely avulsed from either of its femoral or tibial attachments. Since anatomical repositioning is mandatory to achieve an excellent result, it would seem to be nearly impossible to achieve this with arthroscopic stapling in all but the rare cases.

Although patellar tendon reconstruction or augmentation of acute tears best fulfills the requirements for a successful biological substitute, other biological substitutes have been used quite successfully in augmenting the acute tear and in reconstructing the chronic anterior cruciate ligament unstable knee.[9,21,35]

20. Johnson, R.J., Kettelkamp, D.B., Clar, W., et al.: Factors affecting late results after meniscectomy, J. Bone Joint Surg. (Am.) **56:**719-729, 1974.
21. Lipscomb, A.B., Johnston, R.K., Snyder, R.B., et al.: Secondary reconstruction of anterior cruciate ligament in athletes by using the semitendinosus tendon: preliminary report of 78 cases, Am. J. Sports Med. **7:**81-84, 1979.
22. Liscomb, A.B., Johnston, R.K., Snyder, R.B., et al.: Evaluation of hamstring strength following use of semitendinosus and gracilis tendons to reconstruct the anterior cruciate ligament, Am. J. Sports Med. **10:**340-342, 1982.
23. Marshall, J.L., and Olsson, S.E.: Instability of the knee: a long-term experimental study in dogs, J. Bone Joint Surg. (Am.) **53:**1561-1570, 1971.
24. Marshall, J.L., Warren, R.F., and Wickiewicz, T.L.: Primary surgical treatment of anterior cruciate ligament lesions, Am. J. Sports Med. **10:**103, 1982.
25. Marshall, J.L., Warren, R.F., Wickiewicz, T.L., et al.: The anterior cruciate ligament: a technique of repair and reconstruction, Clin. Orthop. **143:**97-106, 1979.
26. McDevitt, C.A., and Muier, H.: Biochemical changes in the cartilage of the knee in experimental and natural osteoarthritis in the dog, J. Bone Joint Surg. (Br.) **58:**94-101, 1976.
27. Noyes, F.R., Butler, D.L., Paulos, L.E., et al.: Intra-articular cruciate ligament reconstruction, Clin. Orthop. **172:**71-77, 1983.
28. Noyes, F.R., Butler, D.L., Grood, E.S., et al.: Biomechanical analysis of human ligament grafts used in knee-ligament repair and reconstruction, J. Bone Joint Surg. (Am.) **66:**344-352, 1984.
29. Odensten, M., and Gillquist, J.: Functional anatomy of the anterior cruciate ligament and a rationale for reconstruction, J. Bone Joint Surg. (Am.) **67:**257-261, 1984.
30. Paulos, L.E., Butler, D.L., and Noyes, F.R.: Intra-articular cruciate ligament reconstruction. II. Replacement with vascularized patellar tendon, Clin. Orthop. **172:**78-84, 1983.
31. Roth, J.H., Kennedy, J.C., Lockstadt, H., et al.: Polypropylene braid augmented and nonaugmented intra-articular anterior cruciate ligament reconstruction, Am. J. Sports Med. **13:**321-336, 1985.
32. Scapinelli, R.: Studies on the vasculature of the human knee joint, Acta Anat. **70:**305-331, 1968.
33. Torg, J.S., Conrad, W., and Kalen, V.: Clinical diagnosis of anterior cruciate ligament instability in the athlete, Am. J. Sports Med. **4:**84-91, 1976.
34. Wirth, C.J., and Artmann, M.: Ist die lange der patellarsehne fur die vordere kruzbandplastik aurreichend? Arch Ortop. Unfall-Chir. **79:**149-152, 1974.
35. Zarins, B., and Rowe, C.R.: Combined anterior cruciate ligament reconstruction using semitendinosus tendon and iliotibial tract, J. Bone Joint Surg. (Am.) **68:**160-177, 1986.

13

Anterior cruciate ligament allografts

TIMOTHY M. SIMON
DOUGLAS W. JACKSON

The surgical repair and reconstruction of cruciate ligament injuries continues to challenge the surgeon. Arthroscopic and open surgical techniques have become more precise, and the use of tendon substitutes has made surgery more successful. Duplication of the anterior cruciate ligament with a biocompatible, durable, and long-lasting replacement that is readily available remains in the developmental stages.

The criteria for an ideal anterior cruciate ligament substitute are as follows: (1) the substitution should duplicate the physiologic function of the anterior cruciate ligament; (2) the graft should be non-immunogenic to the host; (3) the graft should present no increased susceptibility to infection; (4) there should be an absence of associated hyperplastic or malignant transformations; (5) the substitution should restore immediate stability and allow immediate motion; (6) the graft should be readily available in the necessary sizes and have ease of implantation; and (7) the graft material should be amenable to long-term storage.

Although a prosthetic ligament offers many potential advantages, current synthetic materials have yet to demonstrate the long-term success met by autologous biological counterparts. The use of the patients own tissue has been preferred in anterior cruciate ligament repairs since its immunogenicity is essentially nonexistent and graft incorporation has been quite predictable. A potential advantage in the use of the patellar tendon as a graft is that it can be transferred with some of its blood supply still intact. It still remains controversial whether or not this enhances or is any advantage over the usual ingrowth into a totally devascularized tissue. However, the use of patellar tendon with bony attachments at each end enhances the fixation of the autograft in the osseous tunnel.

When any autograft bone is transferred from the donor to the tend to support observations made in animals. Fresh allografts are capable of inducing human antibody formation.[13,14] Studies by Friedlander demonstrated that freeze-dried bone receptors (determined but not matched for implant) stimulated anti-HLA antibodies to these receptors in 20% of the recipients.[9] It has been documented that an allograft can stimulate an immune response that in turn could impair the healing of the allograft.[1,6,7] However, no adverse clinical results have been ascribed to an allograft-elicited immune response in the size of bone used with the ligament complexes needed for knee reconstructions. Clearly, immune responses to allografts have not been completely explored and will continue to be an area of research in the future.

Methods of reducing immune responses to allografts

Fresh allografts, in particular bone, present predictable immunogens. A method that appears to significantly decrease the immunologic reactivity and increase the rate of incorporation of the graft consists of freezing the allograft bone before implantation. Freeze-drying the graft further blunts the immunogenicity to a level below the detection limits of most assay techniques. This technique renders the graft devoid of viable cells but maintains the biological usefulness of the graft as a scaffold for infiltrating cell growth. Although bone healing may be augmented by the presence of viable osteogenic cells, bone healing and graft survival are not dependent on the presence of these cells. It appears that the nature of the preservation technique that reduces the immunogenicity of soft-tissue–bone allografts does not clinically detract from its use even though there are no viable cells. The size of the bony grafts used in knee surgery make the consideration less significant.

Immunosuppressive drugs

The potential impact of immunosuppressive drugs on the immune response to allografts has been typically demonstrated in animal studies using freeze-dried osteochondral allografts. The healing was less than optimal in these studies. When azathioprine was administered, the healing process was enhanced.[2] This led to the assumption that immune response can influence the rate of graft healing. However, the rationale for using these potent cytotoxic agents for small bone-ligament or tendon allografts must be questioned at this time, especially when the association of immune response and poor clinical outcome has not been documented.

Types of allografts for anterior cruciate ligament repair

Soft-tissue allografts used for anterior cruciate ligament repair include freeze-dried fascia lata, Achilles tendon, bone-patellar tendon-bone, and bone-anterior cruciate ligament-bone complexes (Fig. 13-1).

Our experience has been with fascia lata, patellar tendon-bone, and anterior cruciate ligament-bone complexes in the goat model and with fascia lata and patellar tendon-bone complexes in humans.

Fascia lata allografts provide a collagen fiber matrix lattice for ingrowth with minimal immunogenicity. Multilayered fascia lata passed through the osseous tunnels has not demonstrated bony

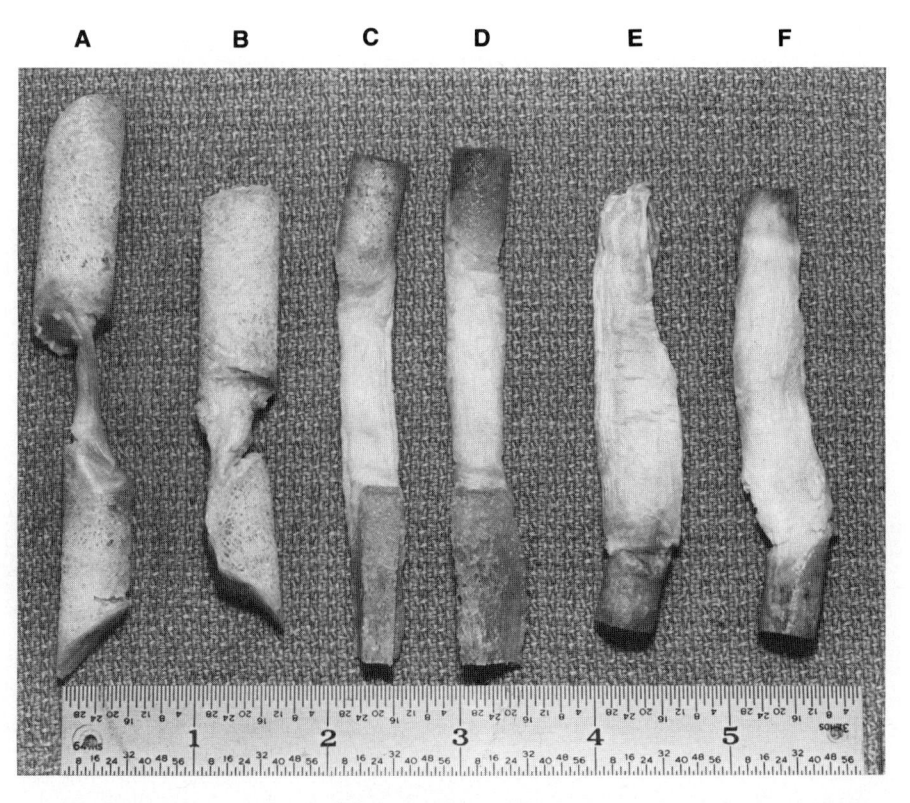

Fig. 13-1 *Typical harvest of six allografts obtainable from one knee. **A**, Anterior cruciate ligament; **B**, posterior cruciate ligament; **C** and **D**, bone-patellar tendon-bone; **E** and **F**, quadricep tendon-bone.*

ingrowth and subsequent permanent biological fixation. Random fiberous tissue ingrowth generally occurs around and through the osseous tunnels providing only soft-tissue fixation strength. Although isometric placement minimizes motion in the osseous tunnels, it allows for the potential of less rigid fixation than bone to bone healing. During our preliminary work, two cases with multilayered fascia lata and biodegradable augmentation material had necrosis and liquefaction of the graft in the tunnels. These two problems in our limited clinical experience (8 human cases) led us to explore soft-tissue–bone complexes further. Allografts of patellar tendon-bone complexes have been used over the past 1½ years in excess of 50 patients. The patellar tendon grafts are shaped with a 1 to 2.5 cm bony attachment (Fig. 13-2). They represent parallel fibers and vary in length. The bone is placed in the bony tunnel at one side (tibial or femur) and recessed depending on its length on the other.

It is our desire to duplicate the anatomical twisting of the anterior cruciate ligament fibers. This potentially can be duplicated with the use of an anterior cruciate ligament allograft. The important biomechanical effect the anterior cruciate ligament has on rotation as well as translation of the tibia could be addressed better when

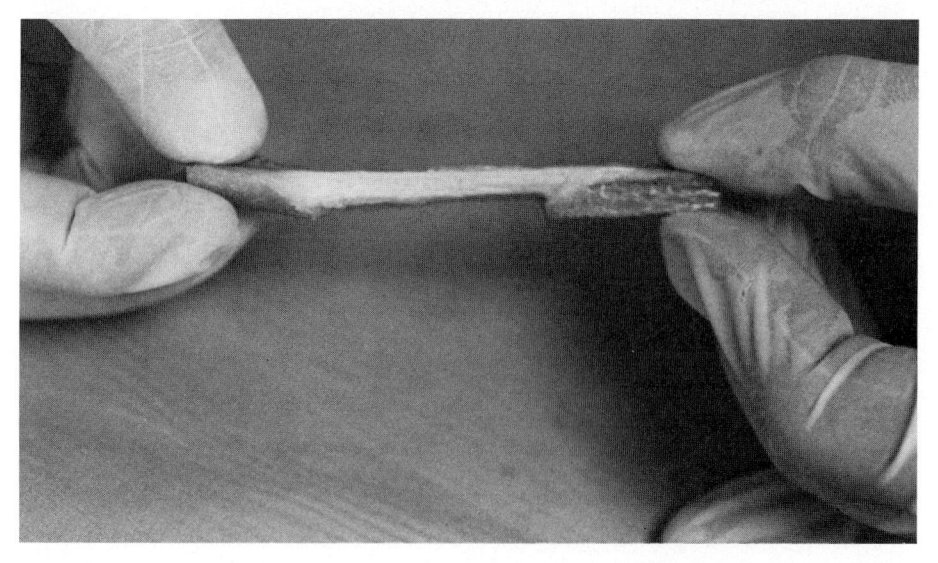

Fig. 13-2 *Patellar tendon allograft with circular patellar bone plug* (left) *and tibial bone block* (right). *In these allografts the collagen fiber bundles are parallel with no inherent twist. The patellar bone plug is harvested as a half circle so surface fiber bundles are not disturbed. New harvesting instrumentation allows circular cores to be obtained for both bony ends.*

anterior cruciate ligament physiology is duplicated. It is for this reason that anterior cruciate ligament-bone complex allografts were explored in the animal model (goat).

Anterior cruciate ligament allografts, consisting of anterior cruciate ligament and their bony insertions, are the subject of current research (Fig. 13-3). As with other bony grafts, the biological response to the bony portions of these grafts applies. The ligament portion of the graft is essentially devoid of cells, leaving only the structural collagen fiber bundles. These grafts offer a complex structure, providing physiological function, a means for rapid bone healing, and a support lattice for biological ingrowth. Revascularization progresses in a manner similar to autografts in the goat model. The biomechanical testing of these replacements still needs further documentation.

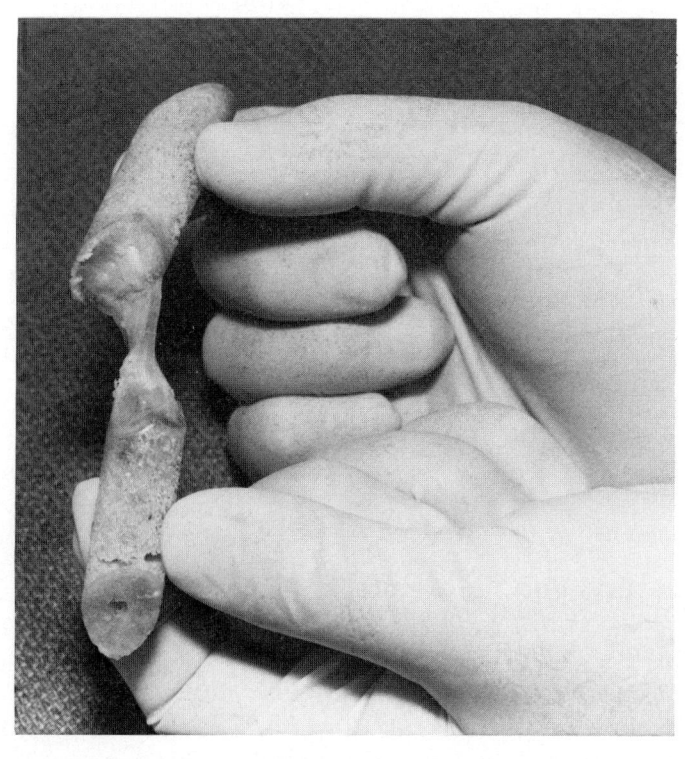

Fig. 13-3 *Anterior cruciate ligament allograft complex with its "hour glass" twist collagen fiber bundles and bony insertions. The broad femoral insertion (top) is intact in this 15-mm plug, and a 13-mm plug encompasses the entire tibial insertion. Core sizes would vary with donor knee size but would not be expected to exceed 15 mm.*

Conceptually, an anterior cruciate ligament allograft consisting of a donor anterior cruciate ligament with its bony tibial and femoral insertions is more appealing than a bone-patellar tendon-bone graft. It is more appealing because of the fiber bundle orientation, that is, twisting fiber (anterior cruciate ligament) rather than the parallel fiber (tendon), and because the sizing for the soft-tissue osseous junction can be more precise. The actual graft length more closely approximates the natural conditions, providing maximal bony plug exposure to the osseous tunnels for rapid bone healing and biological fixation. It also allows for the oblique orientation of the fibers into the bony end plate. This reduces some of the problems with bending fatigue and allows more variation in obliquity and sizing of the bony tunnels. Allograft harvesting instruments allow precise removal of the anterior cruciate ligament along with its femoral origin and tibial insertion, providing dimensionally uniform bone plugs that closely appose the recipients osseous tunnels.

Our studies to date have been limited to goat models in which the anterior cruciate ligaments are removed and replaced with freeze-dried-bone anterior cruciate ligaments-bone allografts from donor goats. Within 24 hours the goats were able to move around their pen with weight bearing, although favoring of the leg was evident for 3 to 4 days. At 6 months, the goats were functionally able to move freely and run without limping or favoring the leg. The results of forthcoming mechanical testing and revascularization studies will address the important issues: Do the fibers remain oriented and functional as they are replaced? Does the revascularization result in loss of the orientation of the anterior cruciate ligament fibers in its substance and their bony attachment? If the graft loses this orientation, then it is weaker than the original anterior cruciate ligament, and a stronger graft with parallel fibers may be more desirable.

Procurement, preservation, and storage of allografts

Tissue banks will play an increasingly important role in the development of anterior cruciate ligament allografts. It will be the responsibility of the tissue bank to provide grafts with optimal biological potential and predictable biomechanical properties for the intended clinical application. The donor selection process is an important aspect of responsible tissue banking. Stringent guidelines must be followed to eliminate donors with potentially transmittable diseases. Furthermore, selection of donor tissues with the best biological potential must be made. For example, allografts of anterior cruciate ligament or patellar tendon should come from young, not elderly, donors. Fortunately, procurement and processing of tissues for transplantation is becoming more standardized through the efforts of the American Association of Tissue Banks.

Tissues should be collected under operating room conditions with the donor skin scrubbed and draped as for a surgical procedure. For most osteoallografts sterile procurement has been considered ideal. The burden of proof that the tissue is suitable for transplantation resides in the liberal use of cultures to document that the tissue is indeed sterile. Most knee structures can be removed by mid-line joint incisions. With careful dissection it is possible to remove the joint with the capsule intact. The entire structure may then be aseptically wrapped and transported to the tissue bank facility for further processing. The specimen should be reprepared, and any subsequent processing is done under strict aseptic conditions. Liberal use of cultures document the absence of microbial contamination. Sterile procurement of allograft material is considered ideal, since no further manipulation or exposure to chemical sterilization agents or radiation is necessary.

Although aseptic collection of tissue may be ideal, this may not always be possible. Secondary sterilization provides the means to salvage such tissue and increases the potential number of grafts. Secondary sterilization is more applicable in small allografts. All methods of sterilization considered must provide effective microbial killing of bacteria, spores, fungi, and viruses. Furthermore, these agents must not leave residual elements that may interfere with biological or biomechanical function of the allograft or be toxic to the surgeon or the recipient. Preservation techniques that have been applied to osteochondral allografts range from simple refrigeration, alcohol treatment, autoclaving, antibiotic washes, and irradiation, to involved methods that preserve functional osteogenic factors. An example of the latter is the antigen extracted surface demineralization method described by Urist.[19] In this method allograft bone is chemosterilized, glycoproteins are chemically extracted, antigenic determinants are removed, the bone is demineralized by acid, and reactive molecules are stabilized with sulfhydryl reagents. All of this is followed by freeze-drying for final preservation.

It has been claimed that some secondary sterilization techniques may adversely affect the biological potential of the graft—most notably in this respect is gamma radiation. Gamma radiation tends to weaken the structural integrity of bone and can leave reactive radicals that may interfere with the grafts biological potential. Although irradiated bone is associated with decreased ability to sensitize the host,[10] the usefulness of gamma radiation for soft-tissue sterilization remains to be determined. Weakening of the collagen fiber bundles in an allograft make it less suitable to handle the initial loads it will encounter within the joint.

Of the variety of methods and chemicals used for secondary sterilization, ethylene oxide treatment has proved effective in terms of penetrating smaller bone grafts. Removal of its residual by-products is relatively easy by aeration or sterile washes. The depth of ethylene oxide penetration in bone is approximately 1 cm. Accordingly, it is suitable for small bone and soft tissues but may not be effective in large bony grafts.

Effective long- and short-term preservation and storage of tissues will be necessary to make allograft transplantation successful and practical. Once the tissue bank has procured the tissue under the appropriate conditions, the graft must be preserved and stored in a manner suitable for its ultimate application. Two methods are currently employed as optimal storage procedures: freezing at $-70°$ C or below and freeze-drying. In general, frozen grafts are more practical when the tissue bank is close to the institution where the implant will take place and when there will be no problem in maintaining the frozen state during transport of the graft. Alternatively, freeze-drying and storage of allografts in vacuum-sealed containers enables the grafts to be maintained at room temperature for years, and distribution and shipping are made significantly easier. Freeze-drying offers the immediate availability of large numbers of sizes and shapes of grafts in the operating room setting.

Freezing can significantly reduce the allograft-induced immune response, and freeze-drying can reduce this reactivity still further. Freeze-drying is a process in which water is removed from the specimen by sublimation of ice. In sublimation, ice is converted to water vapor directly without passing through its natural liquid state. It has also been demonstrated that the type of cryoprotectant can influence immune reactivity.[17] Dimethylsulfoxide (DMSO) cryopreserved bone fails to elicit an immune response from the host, whereas polyvinylpyrrolidine (PVP) sucrose does not impair immune responsiveness. This suggests a selective effect that may be exploited in future clinical applications. The cellular destruction that occurs in freezing or in freeze-drying is considered important in reduction of cell surface antigens. It has been argued that although most of the transplantation antigens are destroyed, sufficient quantities should still persist in freeze-dried allografts to preserve immunogenicity. Although it is technically correct that freeze-drying will preserve certain histocompatibility antigens, the immune reactivity predicted on this basis has not been observed clinically. This is either because current immunolgic testing techniques can not demonstrate the phenomenon or because the host provides some interaction to mask the antigenic components (blocking antibody)[12] or provides a means of disposal of the remaining antigenic fragments. Mammalian cells, under proper cryoprotective techniques and a controlled freezing rate, can be frozen and stored for long periods of time. The only living cells that can survive freeze-drying as generally practiced now are microorganisms—notably bacteria and fungi. The potential for the survival of viruses also exists. Viruses are a real concern because of the potential transmission of hepatitis or acquired immune deficiency syndrome (AIDS) through a frozen or freeze-dried allograft. The current approach to this problem is for the procurement agency to follow stringent screening guidelines for donor selection. Secondary sterilization methods for AIDS virus (HTLV-III) inactivation are currently under study.

One of the key features to the successful application of allograft transplantation will be the standardization of collection of tissues with optimal storage. An essential part of responsible tissue banking is record keeping, including a detailed procedure manual, a record of all processing steps, and a record of all adverse reactions. The ability to scrutinize records of adverse reactions and/or procedures involved with reactions will enable alterations or modifications in processing techniques or surgical procedures to ensure successful transplantation for future recipients. Tissue banks are operating with state-of-the-art technology, and this technology will certainly improve as biological, immunological, and biomechanical considerations become more clearly understood.

Once the technical considerations of procurement, storage, and processing have been met, there is an underlying problem that adversely impacts on the availability of tissues—the lack of suitable donors. The short supply of transplantable tissues and organs requires a new effort at education of the public, individual physicians, and hospital personnel. It is important that community education be provided so that becoming a donor becomes the rule rather than the exception.

Surgical considerations

Better anterior cruciate ligament allografts resulting from improvements in harvesting will require parallel improvements in surgical techniques for positioning, testing, and final drilling of the osseous tunnels (Figs. 13-4 and 13-5). Like the current total knee replacements, anterior cruciate ligament allograft repair will require improved precision in surgical technique, particularly when done arthroscopically. Ultimately, graft survival is also dependent on more precise placement and fixation. The disadvantage of using a biological tissue is the period of revascularization. Biological tissue needs time to become viable and able to maintain integrity in face of the loads to which it is exposed. Mechanical and biological enhancement of allografts will help to improve some of their present limitations. These will either be permanent, biodegradable, or removable

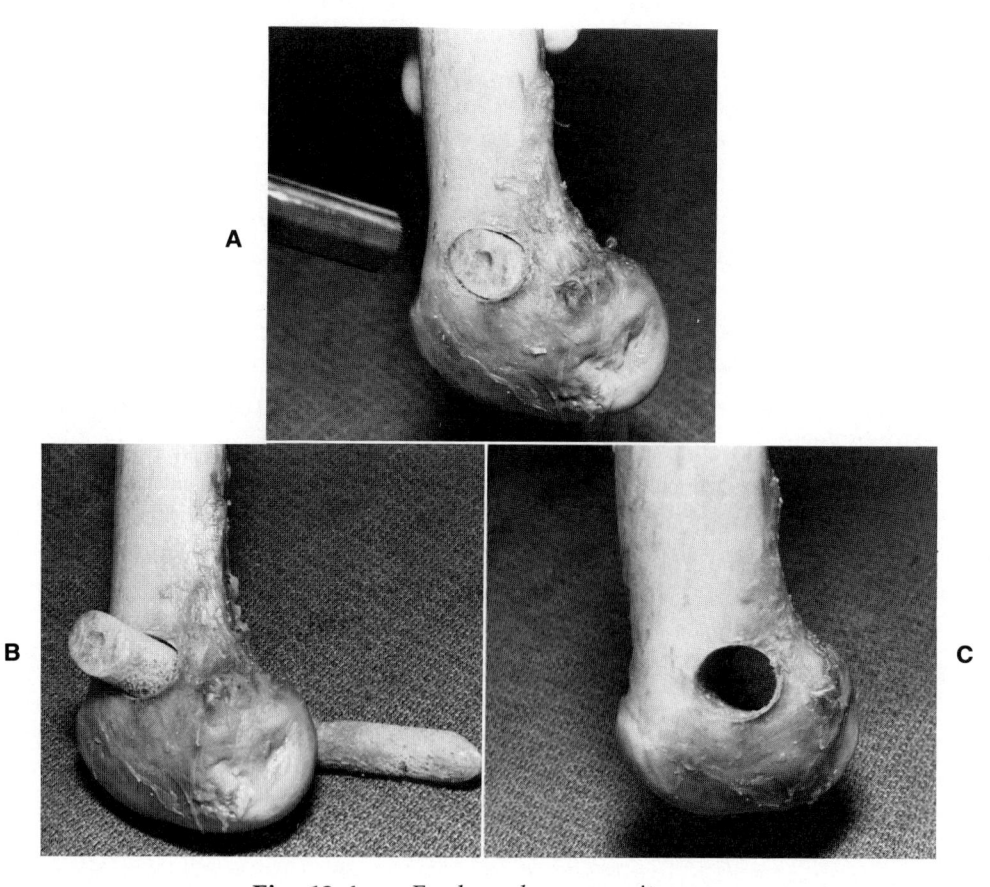

Fig. 13-4 *For legend see opposite page.*

Anterior cruciate ligament allografts

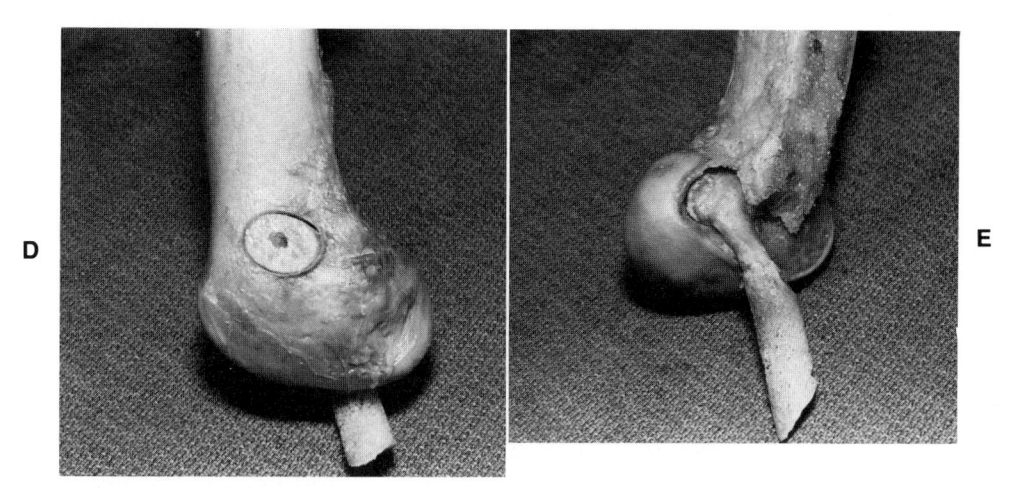

Fig. 13-4, cont'd. **A,** *Harvest of the femoral insertion. The angle of donor bone anterior cruciate ligament harvest should approximate the angle used for recipient implant surgery.* **B,** *Removal of complete anterior cruciate ligament allograft. The uniformity of these bone cores aids in their removal and insertion into the recipient.* **C,** *Appearance of the osseous tunnel after harvest. The same size plug cutter or equivalent drill bit would be used in the recipient.* **D,** *Anterior cruciate ligament allograft reinserted in osseous tunnels as it might appear in the recipient.* **E,** *Intracondylar notch view of anterior cruciate ligament allograft. The entire anterior cruciate ligament femoral insertion is intact.*

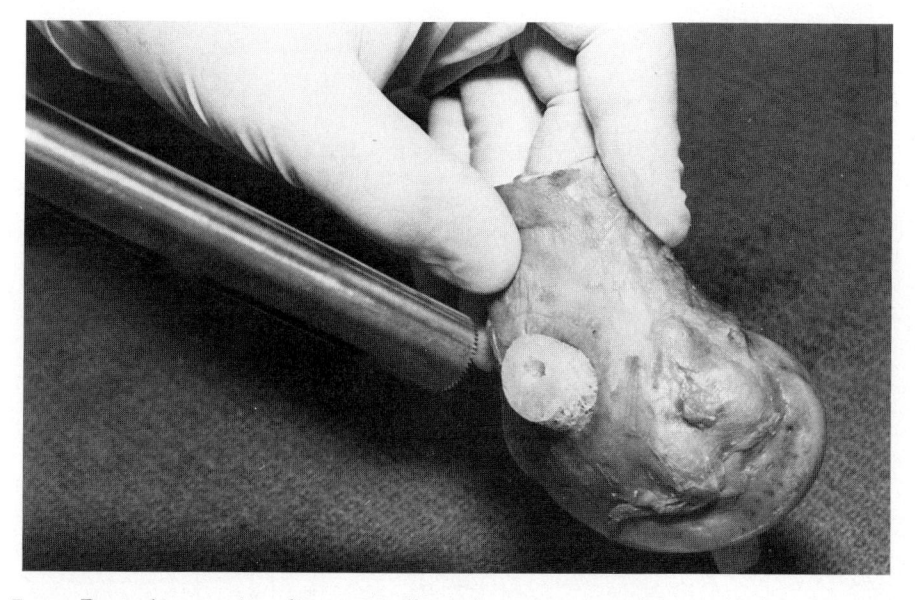

Fig. 13-5 *Posterior cruciate ligament allografts are procured in a similar manner to anterior cruciate ligament allografts. Care is taken to match the angles of harvest to those used for implant surgery.*

augmentations. Stress shielding of the graft and the length of the protection of the allograft will be the bases of ongoing studies.

Summary

Anterior cruciate ligament substitution using allografts is still in its infancy but will play an increasing role over the next 5 to 10 years in the ongoing effort to duplicate anterior cruciate ligament function and anatomy. Some biological and mechanical enhancements may be required to achieve early protection and still allow immediate motion and function while healing occurs. The use of allografts as anterior cruciate ligament substitution will play some part in the evolving history of anterior cruciate ligament surgery, and its role in the future remains to be determined.

REFERENCES

1. Bos, G., et al.: The immunogenicity of frozen bone grafts in inbred rats, Transact. Orthop. Res. Soc. **6:**97, 1981.
2. Burchardt, H., Glowczewskie, F.P., and Enneking, W.F.: Allogeneic segmental fibular transplants in axathioprine immunosuppressed dogs, J. Bone Joint Surg. (Am.) **59:**881, 1977.
3. Burchardt, H., et al.: Freeze-dried allogenic segmental cortical bone grafts in dogs, J. Bone Joint Surg. (Am.) **60:**1082, 1978.
4. Cracchiolo, A., III, et al.: The occurrence of antibodies to collagen in synovial fluids, Clin. Immunol. Immunopathol. **3:**567, 1975.
5. Elves, M.W.: Newer knowledge of the immunology of bone and cartilage, Clin. Orthop. **120:**232, 1976.
6. Friedlaender, G.E.: Immune response to preserved bone allografts in humans. In Friedlaender, G.E., Mankin, H.J., and Sell, K.W., editors: Osteochondral allografts: biology, banking and clinical applications, Boston, 1983, Little, Brown & Co., Inc.
7. Friedlaender, G.E.: Immune responses to osteochondral allografts: current knowledge and future directions, Clin. Orthop. **174:**58, 1983.
8. Friedlaender, G.E., Strong, D.M., and Sell, K.W.: Studies on the antigenicity of bone. I. Freeze-dried and deep-frozen bone allografts in rabbits, J. Bone Joint Surg. (Am.) **58:**854, 1976.
9. Friedlaender, G.E., Strong, D.M., and Sell, K.W.: Donor graft specific anti-HLA antibodies following freeze-dried bone allografts, Transact. Orthop. Res. Soc. **2:**87, 1977.
10. Friedlaender, G.E., Sell, K.W., and Strong, D.M.: Tissue banking and bone allograft immunology. In Phillips, G.O., Tallentire, A., and Triantfyllou, N., editors: Radiation sterilization: irradiated tissues and their potential clinical use, Clwyd, U.K., 1978, The North E. Wales Institute, p. 1-25.
11. Friedlaender, G.E., Ladenbauer-Belles, I., and Chrisman, O.D.: Cartilage marix components as antigenic agents in an osteoarthritis model, Transact. Orthop. Res. Soc. **5:**170, 1980.
12. Langer, F., Czitrom, A., and Pritzker, K.P.: The immunogenicity of fresh and frozen allogeneic bone, J. Bone Joint Surg. (Am.) **57:**216, 1975.
13. Langer, F., et al.: The immunogenicity of allograft knee joint transplants, Clin. Orthop. **132:**157, 1978.
14. Lee, E.H., et al.: The immunology of osteochondral and massive bone allografts, Transact, Orthop. Res. Soc. **4:**61, 1979.
15. Musculo, D.L., Kawai, S., and Ray, R.D.: Cellular and humoral response analysis of bone-allografted rats, J. Bone Joint Surg. (Am.) **58:**826, 1976.
16. Schachar, N.S., et al.: A feline model for the study of frozen osteochondral allografts. II. Development of lymphocytotoxic antibodies in allograft recipients, Transact. Orthop. Res. Soc. **3:**130, 1978.
17. Sell, K.W., Friedlaender, G.E., and Strong, D.M.: Immunogenicity and freeze drying, INSERM **62:**187, 1976.
18. Trentham, D.E., et al.: Humoral and cellular sensitivity to collagen in type II collagen induced arthritis in rats, J. Clin. Invest. **61:**89, 1978.
19. Urist, M.R., Mikulske, A.M., and Boyd, S.D.: A chemosterilized antigen extracted autodigested alloimplant for bone banks, Arch. Surg. **110:**416, 1975.

14

Synthetic augmentation of biological anterior cruciate ligament substitutions

CRAIG L. VAN KAMPEN

H. VINCENT MENDENHALL

GREGG K. McPHERSON

The natural anterior cruciate ligament has unique mechanical properties.[2,3,8] It is a very strong tissue designed to resist excessive deformations; however, in its normal, working load range it is somewhat compliant. In addition, the natural anterior cruciate ligament is capable of withstanding virtually unlimited load cycling. No currently available synthetic material can reproduce the biomechanics of the normal anterior cruciate ligament; therefore biological grafts are generally used for these reconstructions.

Biological grafts, however, undergo postoperative necrosis when the vascular supply to the tissue is disrupted by the transplantation procedure.[1] Several weeks are required for revascularization of the graft.[1] Anterior cruciate ligament reconstruction therefore is generally accompanied by an initial period of immobilization and by prolonged rehabilitation. In addition to the necrosis caused by devascularization of the graft, the period of immobilization itself contributes to further weakening of the tissue.[9] Postoperative immobilization also appears to have a detrimental effect on the joint cartilage.[11]

Basic principles of augmentation

Synthetic augmentation of biological grafts has been proposed as a means to protect the graft tissue from excessive stress during early healing.[5] Synthetic augmentation devices are designed to be used in conjunction with biological grafts in order to enhance the strength of the graft. The ability of an augmentation device to enhance the strength of a biological graft lessens the risk of the graft breaking or stretching during the time when the tissue is regenerating and in a weakened state. Augmentation devices also enable greater flexibility in selecting the tissue to be used as the graft source. Tissues that might otherwise be considered too weak to use for anterior cruciate ligament reconstruction may be of adequate strength when augmented with a synthetic device. Thus the enhanced strength provided by a synthetic augmentation device protects the biological graft from stretching or breaking and results in an improved reconstruction.

A critical aspect of synthetic augmentation of a biological graft is the recognition that long-term remodeling of the biological graft is dependent on the tissue carrying a portion of the load. Biological tissues remodel according to the loads that they carry, and therefore the biological graft must be subjected to appropriate loading in order to develop a strong biological reconstruction. It is very important that some load sharing occur between the augmentation device and the biological graft in order to stimulate proper reorganization of the tissue during healing. Two basic principles are suggested for successful augmentation of a ligament reconstruction with a synthetic device.

First, a composite graft must be prepared, consisting of the synthetic augmentation device and the biological tissue. Both components must be mechanically coupled so that load sharing between them can occur. The coupling of the two components to form a composite graft may be achieved by securely suturing the synthetic augmentation device to the biological graft.

Second, the synthetic augmentation device must not be anchored directly to bone at both ends of the device. Such a configuration could excessively shield the biological graft from stress by creating a parallel load path. This would have a detrimental effect on the reorganization of the biological tissue. The synthetic augmentation device should be anchored directly to bone at one end only; the other end of the device should be attached to soft tissue.

Biomechanics of augmentation

The following hypothesis is suggested to describe the function of a synthetic augmentation device. During early healing the tissue is weak and the augmentation device carries the majority of the load, thus protecting the tissue from excessive stress. However, the tissue is subjected to a safe level of loading as a result of the mechanical coupling between the synthetic augmentation device and the biological graft. Although the initial load on the biological graft is small, it is sufficient to stimulate proper reorganization of the tissue. As the biological graft reorganizes it becomes stronger and capable of carrying greater loads. The nature of the mechanical coupling between the synthetic augmentation device and the biological graft permits the tissue to carry greater loads as it becomes stronger. Therefore a gradual transfer of load from the augmentation device to the biological graft takes place as the strength of the tissue increases. Because of the gradually increasing load carried by the biological graft, the tissue eventually develops a ligamentous structure. Both the level of load on the biological graft and the rate at which the load is transferred from the synthetic augmentation device to the tissue appear to be important factors in the performance of the composite graft. It is suggested that the long-term outcome of proper augmentation of a ligament reconstruction with a synthetic device will be that the majority of the load in the composite graft is carried by the biological tissue.[6]

The preceding hypothesis has been analyzed by a simple mechanical model in which the components of an augmented ligament reconstruction are represented by spring elements. As shown in Fig. 14-1, the biological graft, the synthetic augmentation device, and the suture connection between them can each be assigned a spring constant, K, which approximates the relative stiffness of these components. The load transmitted from the femur to the tibia is distributed between the augmentation device and the biological graft by the sutures along the length of the reconstruction. An important aspect of this model is that at one end of the composite graft, in this case the tibial end, the augmentation device is not anchored directly to bone. Therefore a short length of unaugmented tissue is present.

The application of basic spring theory to the model in Fig. 14-1 gives the following mathematical expression for the ratio of forces in the biological graft and the synthetic augmentation device:

$$\frac{F_{graft}}{F_{device}} = \frac{K_g}{K_a K_s / (K_a + K_s)}$$

This simple analysis indicates that the ratio of forces is dependent only on the relative stiffness of the components. Assumptions may

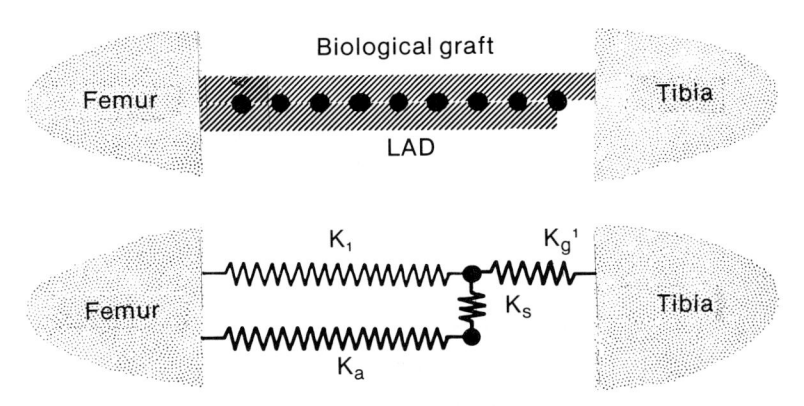

Fig. 14-1 *Spring model of the components in an augmented ligament reconstruction. Relative stiffness of the biological graft, the ligament augmentation device (LAD), and the suture connection between them are given by K_g, K_a, and K_s, respectively.*

now be made regarding the relative stiffnesses in order to analyze load sharing in the composite reconstruction. First, assuming that the tissue is relatively compliant during early healing, the following values may be assigned to the spring constants:

$$K_g = K$$
$$K_a = 10K$$
$$K_s = 10K$$

Using these spring constants, the ratio of forces in the composite reconstruction can be calculated:

$$\frac{F_{graft}}{F_{device}} = \frac{1}{5}$$

Thus the augmentation device is carrying approximately 5 times the load of the biological graft. This appears to be reasonable level of stress protection.

Assuming that the biological graft is loaded sufficiently for appropriate tissue remodeling, as healing progresses the regenerating graft will become stronger and stiffer. Now assuming the stiffness of the graft has doubled such that $K_g = 2K$, the ratio of forces can be recalculated:

$$\frac{F_{graft}}{F_{device}} = \frac{2}{5}$$

At this stage of the healing process the augmentation device is carrying only about 2.5 times the load of the biological graft.

With time the increasing loads carried by the biological graft stimulate further reorganization of the tissue. This stronger, stiffer tissue is then capable of carrying further increased loads. A positive feedback system is thus established for remodeling of the tissue, and the biological graft eventually develops a ligamentous structure capable of functioning as the primary load-carrying component of the composite graft.

Further analysis of the expression for the ratio of forces between the graft and the device indicates the importance of secure suturing for successful augmentation. If the mechanical coupling provided by the suturing is compliant, such that $K_s = K$ instead of 10K, then the loads would be almost evenly distributed between the biological graft and the synthetic augmentation device. This would have the potential to overload the biological graft in the early postoperative healing phase.

A similar mechanical model may be used to demonstrate the effect of anchoring the augmentation device directly to bone at both ends of the device. Such a configuration would result in two separate, parallel pathways for carrying the load. The following expression describes the ratio of forces in this situation:

$$\frac{F_{graft}}{F_{device}} = \frac{K_g}{K_a}$$

In the case where $K_g = K$ and $K_a = 10K$, the ratio of forces in the biological graft and the synthetic augmentation device would be calculated as follows:

$$\frac{F_{graft}}{F_{device}} = \frac{1}{10}$$

Thus, if the augmentation device is fixed to bone at both ends of the device, it would be carrying 10 times the load of the biological graft. This degree of stress shielding may be too great to allow for proper tissue reorganization. In addition, the higher level of load on the augmentation device may overload the synthetic material.

Material requirements for synthetic augmentation

The material used for a synthetic augmentation device must be strong and flexible in order to withstand the loading and bending of an anterior cruciate ligament reconstruction. In addition, the material must be resistant to creep, fatigue, and abrasion under cyclical loading. A conservative estimate of the typical working loads on the anterior cruciate ligament during normal activities is approximately

500 newtons (N).[3,7] The ultimate strength of the anterior cruciate ligament is approximately 1700 N.[3] The number of cycles the knee joint is exposed to during a year of normal activity is estimated at 3.5 to 4 million.[2] Thus an anterior cruciate ligament reconstruction must be able to withstand hundreds of millions of load cycles at 500 N without stretching or breaking.

The material requirements for a synthetic augmentation device are not as stringent as for a total anterior cruciate ligament prosthesis. The reason for this is that as the biological graft heals, the augmentation device will gradually carry less and less load, as the hypothesis suggested earlier. Assuming that the biological graft heals completely in 12 to 18 months, the synthetic augmentation device must withstand approximately 5 million load cycles. During the initial healing period, the load carried by the augmentation device would be substantially less than 500 N since the patient would be protecting the operated knee to some extent. When the patient returns to normal daily activities, the synthetic augmentation device would carry the majority of the load, but as healing progresses, the augmentation device would gradually carry less and less load as a result of load sharing. Thus a synthetic augmentation device must withstand loads of less than 500 N for 12 to 18 months or about 5 million cycles. In contrast, a total prosthesis must withstand the full 500 N load for 60 years or 250 million cycles.

Although the issues of material creep and fatigue are less critical for synthetic augmentation devices than for total prostheses, these properties cannot be ignored. The material for an augmentation device must have reasonable creep resistance in order to avoid being stretched out before the biological tissue has healed substantially. Similarly, the fatigue strength of the material must be adequate to prevent the device from breaking. Another important material characteristic is abrasion resistance. Rubbing of the device against bone or of fibers against one another may lead to failure of the augmentation device unless the material possesses good abrasion resistance.

Polypropylene is an example of a material that possesses the properties necessary for a ligament augmentation device. A flat braid of high-tenacity polypropylene yarn has been evaluated for augmenting biological anterior cruciate ligament reconstructions in animals and humans.[5,6,10]

The mechanical properties of the polypropylene braid were tested to determine its tensile strength, fatigue properties, and cyclical creep behavior. Details of the testing methods and results have been published previously.[6] The ultimate tensile strength of the polypropylene braid is approximately 1700 N, which is similar to the strength of the natural anterior cruciate ligament.[4,8] Dynamic loading to 500 N results in 9% strength loss and 3% creep after 1 million cycles.

Most of the animal and human investigations of this polypropylene braid have used the central one third of the patellar tendon, the prepatellar periosteum, and a strip of the quadriceps tendon as the source of the biological graft. The polypropylene braid is sutured to the transplant along its length with interrupted sutures to form a composite graft. The patellar tendon is left attached at its normal insertion on the tibia and the augmented graft is routed through a tibial bone tunnel and over the top of the femoral condyle for fixation to the lateral femur.

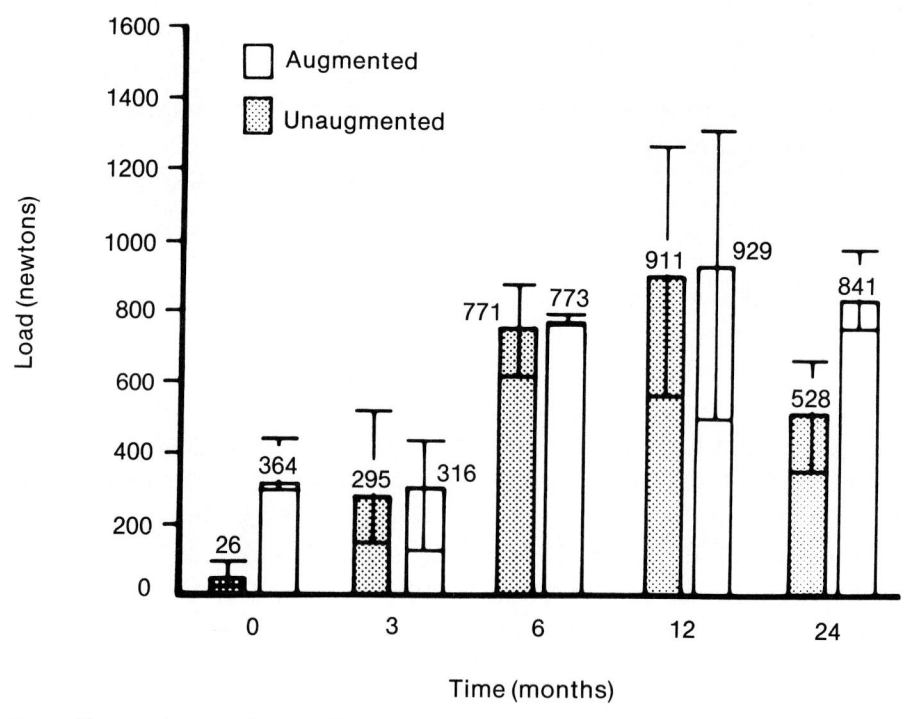

Fig. 14-2 *Comparison of the tensile strength of augmented and unaugmented anterior cruciate ligament reconstructions in goats. The range of measured values in each group is indicated by the error bars. (From McPherson, G.K., et al.: Clin. Orthop. Rel. Res. **196**:186, 1985.)*

A study that compared augmented and unaugmented grafts in goats was carried out with 6 weeks postoperative immobilization. At the time of surgery the augmented grafts had substantially higher tensile strengths (Fig. 14-2), which enabled adequate tensioning without fear of rupturing the transplant. At 3, 6, and 12 months the graft strengths in both groups were similar, but at 24 months the augmented grafts were somewhat stronger. Failure analysis following mechanical testing showed that the unaugmented grafts always failed by midsubstance rupture, and the augmented grafts failed as the composite graft pulled out of the tibial bone tunnel (Fig. 14-3).

Histology from both groups showed revascularization and remodeling taking place at 3 months and collagen organization similar to that of a normal ligament taking place at 24 months.[6] Occasional wear particles from the braid were observed at 12 and 24 months, but wear was confined to the surface of the individual braid filaments and no ruptured braid filaments were observed.

Another study was conducted on goats to evaluate the effect of anchoring both ends of the polypropylene braid to bone. Grafts in which the augmentation device was anchored at one end only were approximately 30% stronger than the grafts with the device anchored at both ends (see Table 14-1). In addition, the polypropylene braids anchored at both ends were noticeably abraded and failed

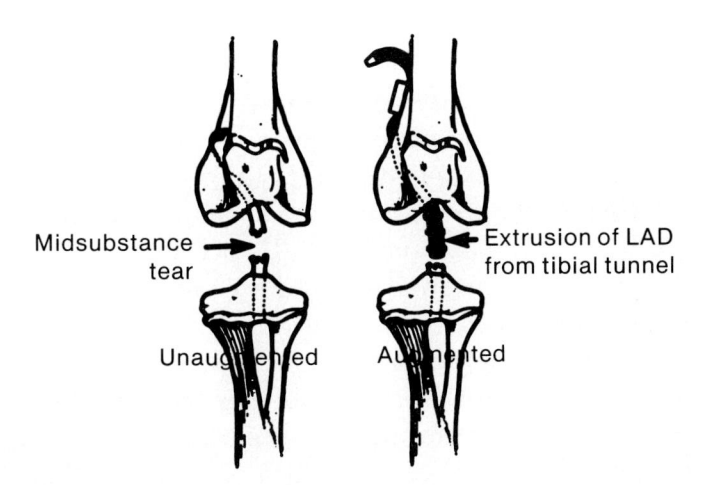

Fig. 14-3 *Comparison of the failure mode of augmented and unaugmented MacIntosh transfers in goats. The use of an augmentation device protects the graft from intra-articular failure during mechanical testing.*

TABLE 14-1 / Effect of anchoring both ends of an augmentation device directly to bone*

ANIMAL NUMBER	TIME POSTOPERATIVE	FAILURE LOAD
GAL-56L	18 months	458 N
GAL-56R	24 months	658 N

*The tensile strength of augmented anterior cruciate ligament reconstructions in goats is significantly lower when both ends of the device are anchored directly to bone. Compare to failure loads shown in Fig. 14-1 for reconstructions anchored directly to bone at one end only: 12 months = 929 N; 24 months = 841 N.

during mechanical testing by midsubstance rupture rather than by pulling out of the bone tunnel.

Clinical evaluation of polypropylene augmentation devices has been carried out using the extensor mechanism as the graft source and comparing results to a similar unaugmented group.[5,10] At 3 years mean follow-up, improved stability and better subjective patient evaluation were demonstrated in the augmented group.[10] The device has also enabled retensioning of grafts loosened by reinjury.

Alternative augmentation methods

Most of the experiments using high-tenacity polypropylene as a synthetic augmentation device for biological anterior cruciate ligament reconstruction have been performed as described earlier. However, it appears reasonable to assume that alternative methods of augmentation may be used as long as the basic principles of augmentation are followed. The goal of synthetic augmentation of biological grafts is to provide enough stress shielding during early healing to protect the tissue from stretching or breaking while not providing so much stress shielding that the tissue lacks a stimulus for proper regeneration. Optimal load sharing is achieved by anchoring the synthetic augmentation device to bone at only one end and by suturing the augmentation device to the biological tissue to form a composite graft.

When a synthetic augmentation device is used with a biological graft that has an inherent weak spot, such as the prepatellar section of an extensor mechanism graft, the device bridges the weak section and clearly provides enhanced strength. However, the value of using a synthetic augmentation device with a strong biological graft that does not have any weak spots is often questioned on the grounds that even if the device enhances the strength along most of the length of the graft, an unaugmented weak link exists where the tissue alone is attached to bone. This is true, but the value of the augmentation device in this case must be viewed in terms of preventing stretching not breaking. A strong, unaugmented biological graft may be capable of functioning without breaking, even if it loses 50% or more of its strength during regeneration. Although, the forces on the graft may not be sufficient to cause the graft to break, these forces may be sufficient to cause the graft to stretch. Use of an augmentation device in this instance would protect the graft from stretching, except at the unaugmented attachment to bone. If the loads were great enough to cause the tissue to stretch 10%, a 10 cm unaugmented graft would stretch 1 cm, and an augmented graft with only 1 cm of unaugmented tissue at the bone attachment site would stretch only 1 mm. Thus better stability would be achieved with the augmented graft, even though the unaugmented graft was not in danger of breaking. It appears therefore that synthetic augmentation of biological grafts may be beneficial regardless of the tissue selected as the source for the transplant.

Synthetic augmentation of autografts has been the focus of almost all augmentation research to date. However, some investigators have become interested in augmenting allograft tissues with a synthetic device. Allografts apparently go through a period of revascularization similar to autografts and therefore would similarly benefit from augmentation. The same principles of augmentation apply to allografts. Long-term remodeling of the allograft tissue will depend on the loads to which the allograft is exposed. Therefore a load sharing situation must be established by creating a composite graft and by anchoring only one end of the synthetic device to bone.

In the event that the biological tissue selected for the anterior cruciate ligament reconstruction is too short, it may be possible to use the synthetic augmentation device as a leader to provide extra length to the reconstruction. It appears that insertion fibers form between the biological graft and the bone in the drill hole and in the over-the-top region. Therefore it may not be necessary for the tissue to extend all the way to the bone fixation site, as long as the biological graft extends from the tibial tunnel to the over-the-top region. The basic principles of augmentation should still be adhered to in such cases, and the biological graft should at least extend through the joint and make contact with bone at both ends.

The methods for suturing the composite graft and for bone fixation may also be varied within the basic concept of augmentation. The studies described here have primarily used a series of interrupted sutures along the length of the graft to prepare the composite. Analysis of load sharing and stress distribution in the composite indicate that the sutures near the soft-tissue–bone attachment carry the highest loads. Therefore an alternative suturing method currently in use is to place 4 pairs of interrupted sutures at the soft-tissue attachment end of the device and form the remainder of the composite with a running absorbable suture. Various methods may be used to anchor the augmentation device and biological tissue to bone. In the animal studies described earlier, bone fixation was achieved with a screw and spiked bushing, wherein the bushing penetrates the center of the polypropylene braid and protects the braid from the screw threads. In humans spiked staples have generally been used for bone fixation, wherein the staple is oriented perpendicular to the braid. In some cases staples have been oriented longitudinally with the legs of the staple penetrating the braid. Screws and plastic washers have also been used for bone fixation, but care must be taken not to allow the screw threads to damage the braid or the tissue.

Another variation on the basic augmentation concept is the use of an absorbable material for the synthetic augmentation device. Interest in such an approach stems from concern for leaving a foreign material in the knee joint for possibly 50 years or longer. Although polypropylene has been demonstrated to be stable and to not have any detrimental effect on the joint in its 6-year history, it appears reasonable to want the device to do its job and then disappear to avoid the question of potential long-term complications. Absorbable augmentation devices might eliminate this unknown, and as appropriate absorbable augmentation devices become available this concept will be investigated.

Augmentation advantages and disadvantages

Synthetic augmentation of biological grafts serves to protect the tissue from excessive stress during early healing and establishes appropriate load sharing for proper long-term remodeling of the regenerating tissue. However, the enhanced strength provided by the synthetic augmentation device does not work miracles. An augmentation procedure still relies on healing of the biological graft, which takes a number of weeks with or without augmentation. The benefit of the augmentation device is in reducing the risk of the biological graft either stretching or breaking. Thus early passive motion can be approached with greater confidence, but return to normal activities the day after surgery cannot be expected.

The principal drawbacks of augmentation relate to the morbidity associated with harvesting the graft and the time required during surgery to prepare the composite. The current trend in augmentation procedures is aimed at decreasing morbidity through the use of tissues such as the semitendinosus or gracilis tendons and by routing the graft through the joint arthroscopically. Such procedures combined with alternative suturing methods decrease surgery time and patient morbidity significantly. Patients often feel well enough to be discharged from the hospital the day after surgery. In such cases it is critical that the need for gradual rehabilitation be emphasized with the patient. The patient must recognize that even though the knee might feel well, the tissue still takes time to heal and that returning to activity too soon will likely result in greater instability than might be the case with gradual rehabilitation.

The fact that augmentation procedures use biological tissue is a disadvantage in terms of morbidity and healing time, but it is also a significant advantage. The long-term result of augmentation is the development of a ligamentous structure in the biological graft. This regenerated tissue is then capable of functioning as a ligament replacement for the lifetime of the patient. It may not be as strong as the original ligament, but near normal joint kinematics can be expected as the tissue reorganizes to resemble a normal ligament. Such a long-term result is not possible with any currently available synthetic materials used as total anterior cruciate ligament prostheses because these materials lack the normal ligament stress-strain properties and are subject to creep and fatigue failure.

The long-term presence in the joint of a permanent augmentation device, such as the polypropylene braid described earlier, is a concern. No detrimental effects have been observed for polypropylene devices in the 6-year history, but the effect of the device on the tissue over 60 years can only be speculated. All evidence to date indicates that the polypropylene braid is well tolerated by the tissue; thus there is little reason to believe that any long-term problems will develop. According to the hypothesis for augmentation, the device carries little load long-term, and therefore the potential for fatigue failure is unlikely. A potential long-term benefit of the presence of the augmentation device relates to the ability to use the device for retensioning in the event of reinjury.

Summary

Synthetic augmentation of biological grafts provides enhanced graft strength that decreases the risk of the graft stretching or breaking during early motion and rehabilitation. Proper use of an augmentation device requires that a load sharing situation be established so that the tissue will have a stimulus for reorganization. This is achieved by preparing a composite graft in which the augmentation device is directly anchored to bone at one end only. Both human and animal investigations using a high-tenacity polypropylene braid as an augmentation device have demonstrated improved results of anterior cruciate ligament reconstruction associated with synthetic augmentation of biological grafts.

REFERENCES

1. Arnoczky, S.P., Tarvin, G.B., and Marshall, J.L.: Anterior cruciate ligament replacement using patellar tendon, J. Bone Joint Surg. (Am.) **64**:217, 1982.
2. Chen, E.H., and Black, J.: Materials design analysis of the prosthetic anterior cruciate ligament, J. Biomed. Mater. Res. **14**:567, 1980.
3. Grood, E.S., and Noyes, F.R.: Cruciate ligament prosthesis: strength, creep, and fatigue properties, J. Bone Joint Surg. (Am.) **58**:1083, 1976.
4. Kennedy, J.C., Hawkins, R.J., and Willis, R.B.: Strain gauge analysis of knee ligaments, Clin. Orthop. Rel. Res. **129**:225, 1977.
5. Kennedy, J.C., Roth, J.H., Mendenhall, H.V., et al.: Intra-articular replacement in the anterior cruciate ligament-deficient knee, Am. J. Sports Med. **8**:1, 1980.
6. McPherson, G.K., Mendenhall, H.V., Gibbons, D.F., et al.: Experimental mechanical and histologic evaluation of the Kennedy Ligament Augmentation Device, Clin. Orthop. Rel. Res. **196**:186, 1985.
7. Morrison, J.B.: Bioengineering analysis of force actions transmitted by the knee joint, Biomed. Engr. **4**:573, 1969.
8. Noyes, F.R., and Grood, E.S.: The strength of the anterior cruciate ligament in humans and rhesus monkeys, J. Bone Joint Surg. (Am.) **58**:1074, 1976.
9. Noyes, F.R., Torvik, P.J., Hyde, W.B., et al.: Biomechanics of ligament failure. II. An analysis of immobilization, exercise, and reconditioning effects in primates, J. Bone Joint Surg. (Am.) **56**:1406, 1974.
10. Roth, J.H., Kennedy, J.C., Lockstadt, H., et al.: Polypropylene braid augmented and nonaugmented intraarticular anterior cruciate ligament reconstruction, Am. J. Sports Med. **13**:5, 1985.
11. Roth, J.H., Mendenhall, H.V., Van Kampen, C.L., et al.: The effect of full thickness sectioning of the central one-third of the patellar tendon and joint immobilization on the knee joint of goats following reconstruction of the anterior cruciate ligament. Presented in part at the Annual Meeting of the ORS, Las Vegas, Nevada, 1985.

15

Biomechanics of artificial ligaments and associated problems

FRANK O. BONNARENS

DAVID DREZ, Jr.

The challenge of designing an artificial ligament is to develop a substitute that will duplicate the characteristics of the original ligament. This chapter describes the biomechanical and mechanical properties of the normal anterior cruciate ligament and some of the properties of substitutes that have been under investigation.

Mechanical properties of ligaments

There are a number of engineering terms that are used to describe the mechanical properties of ligaments. Definitions of some of the most commonly used terms follow.

Ultimate tensile strength (breaking point). The ultimate tensile strength is the point at which all components of a material fail. For the anterior cruciate ligament, the ultimate tensile strength is approximately 1700 newtons (N) (Fig. 15-1).[22]

Elastic deformation. Elastic deformation occurs when an object returns to its original resting state following removal of a load (Fig. 15-2).

Plastic deformation. Plastic deformation occurs when an object does not return to its original resting state when a load is removed (permanent deformation). Thus there has been failure of some of the components of the material (Fig. 15-3).

Yield point. Yield point is the point at which the material starts plastic deformation (i.e., some of the components of the material have failed) (see Fig. 15-1).

Fatigue strength. Fatigue strength is the ultimate tensile strength after cyclic loading. There are three common methods of fatigue testing: tension, flexion, and torsion (twisting). The anterior cruciate

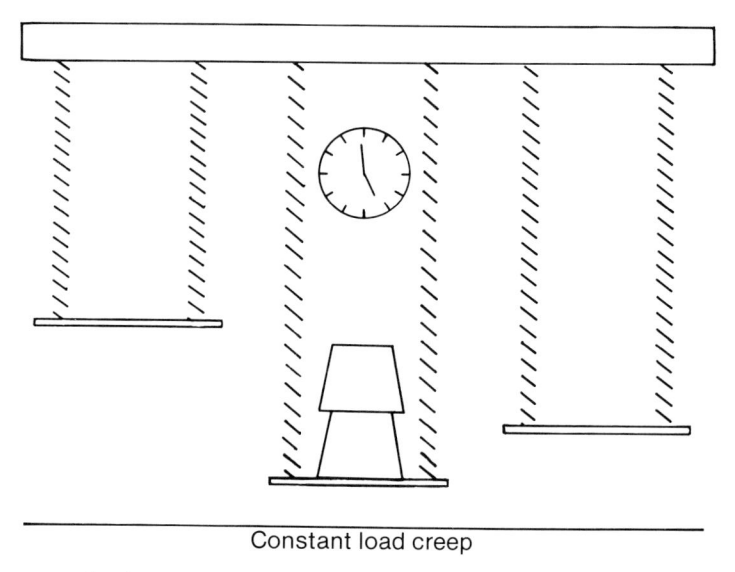

Fig. 15-4 *Constant load creep is the time dependent plastic deformation of an object subject to a static load.*

load is removed (Fig. 15-4). *Cyclic creep* occurs when a force is repeatedly applied and removed over a much longer period of time. The deformation is measured when the force is removed (Fig. 15-5).

Stiffness. Stiffness is an object's resistance to deformation as a result of a change in force. It is the amount of force required to deform a material, and is a ratio of the change in force divided by the change in length. The normal stiffness for the anterior cruciate ligament is 175 N/mm (Fig. 15-6).[22]

Compliance. Compliance is the reciprocal of stiffness and is defined as the amount of deformation that occurs from an applied load. It is the amount a material deforms when a force is applied, and is the ratio of the change in length divided by the change in force. For the normal anterior cruciate ligament, this is 0.006 mm/N (Fig. 15-7).[22]

Biological degradation. Biological degradation is an important factor to consider in artificial ligamentous structures that are used in the knee joint. It must be determined if such degradation occurs in the body's environment since this represents simulated aging of the material. Many synthetic polymers will undergo loss of strength in the synovial fluid environment.

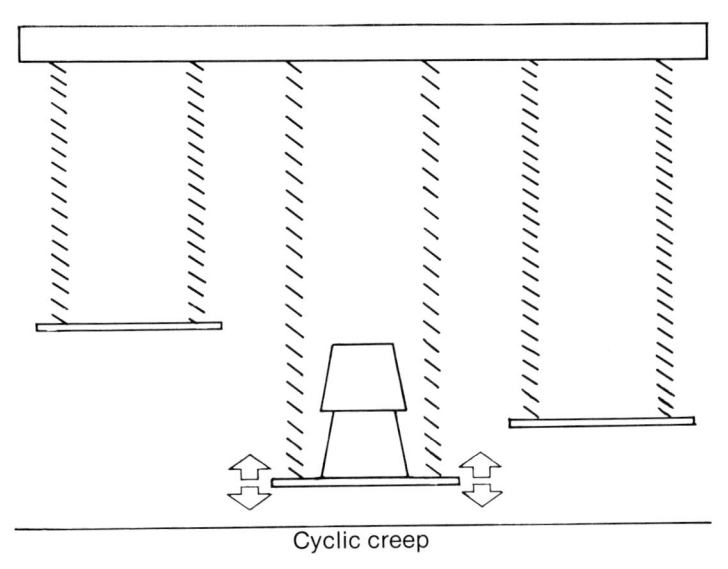

Fig. 15-5 *Cyclic creep is the plastic deformation that results from a load that is repeatedly applied and removed.*

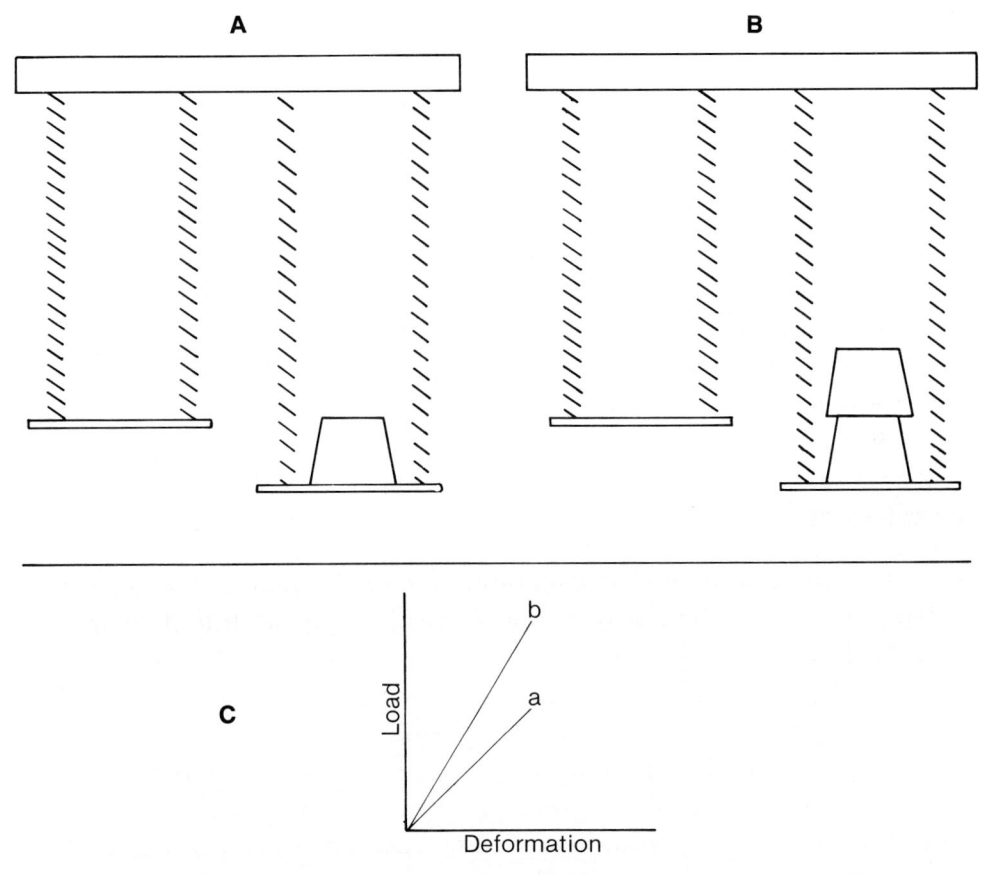

Fig. 15-6 *Stiffness is an object's resistance to deformation as a result of a change in force. The load is greater in **B** than in **A**. The resulting change in height is the same. Therefore the rope in **B** must be supplying greater resistance to the change in force. **B** is stiffer than **A**. **C**, This is shown on a load deformation curve.*

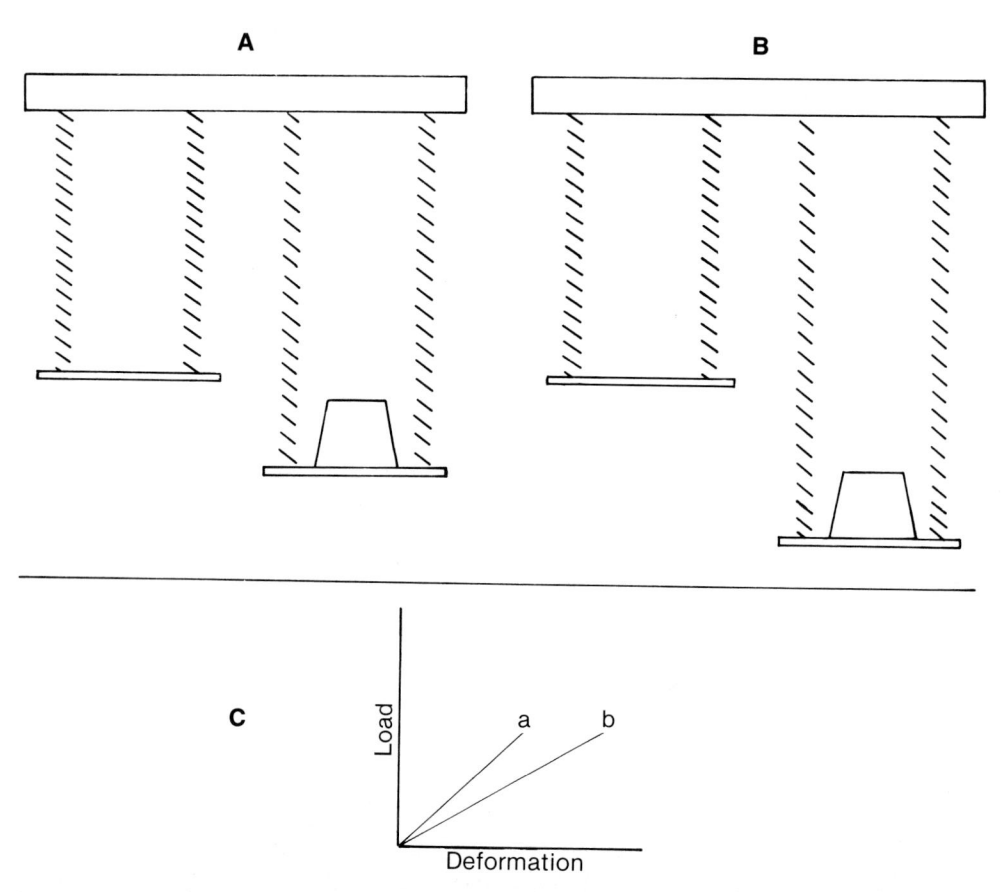

Fig. 15-7 *Compliance is a measure of how much deformation occurs from an applied load. Here the load is the same. The swing in **B** changed its height more than in **A**. Therefore the rope in **B** must have yielded more than the rope in **A**. **B** is more compliant than **A**. **C**, This is shown on a load deformation curve.*

Factors affecting success of the procedure

The successful use of an anterior cruciate ligament substitute depends not only on adequate mechanical properties but on numerous technical factors as well.

The *bone tunnels* in the tibial and femoral area must approach isometry, and sharp edges must be avoided. The need for avoiding sharp edges should be obvious, but the concept of isometry is one that has often been obscured. It is important to duplicate the natural position of the anterior cruciate ligament during reconstruction. Isometry implies that the length of the cruciate ligament would be constant throughout the range of motion. This is theoretically possible for only a small portion of the ligament. The natural ante-

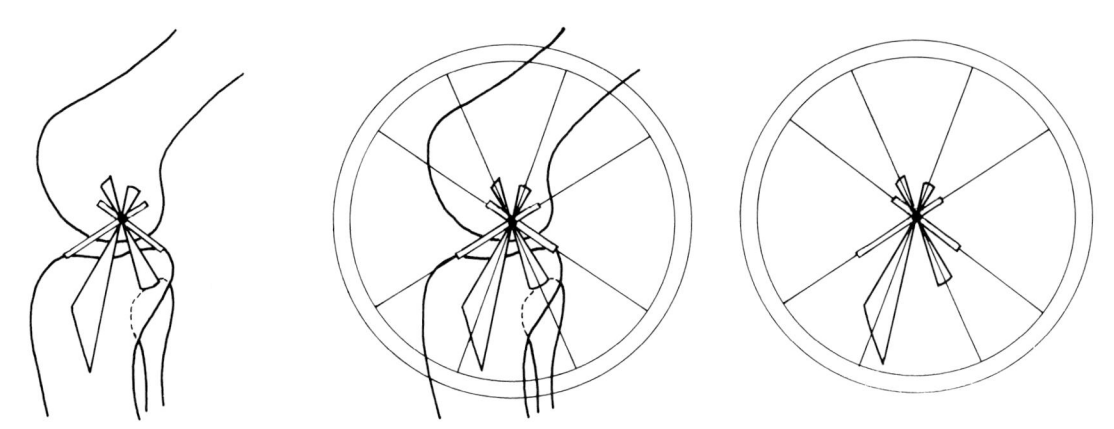

Fig. 15-8 *The spokes of a wheel are superimposed on the cruciate and collateral ligaments. The axle of this wheel is the transverse flexion axis. Although the ligaments change position, they maintain this relationship for all degrees of flexion.*

rior cruciate ligament has some fibers that are tense in extension and some that are tight in flexion. The natural rotation of the anterior cruciate ligament as it travels from its tibial to its femoral attachment allows for a maximal number of fibers to be taut as the knee moves. The relationship between the cruciate ligaments and the collateral ligaments has been described as similar to the spokes of a wheel[21] (Fig. 15-8). The ideal lines formed by each of the ligaments always intersect at the center of rotation. This is the transverse flexion axis. If one of the ligaments is not in its proper location, it will alter the kinematics of the joint just as surely as when a spoke is fixed to a point off of the hub of a wheel (Fig. 15-9).

It has been said that the ligaments must be tangent to the hole in the femur and the tibia.[1] This is possible only through a very limited arc of motion since these holes are constantly changing their relationship to each other (Fig. 15-10).

The *initial fixation* as well as the *ultimate fixation* must be considered. Daniels has shown that screw fixation with either a spiked washer or ligament fixation plate is superior to staples or suturing.[8] Ultimate fixation that relies totally on mechanical means is doomed to failure. Biological fixation is necessary with bony ingrowth being the most desirable.

An *intercondylar femoral notchplasty* not only provides better visualization when placing the femoral drill hole but reduces the possibility of notch impingement on the anterior cruciate ligament graft.

Proper tensioning of the artificial ligament is important to restore

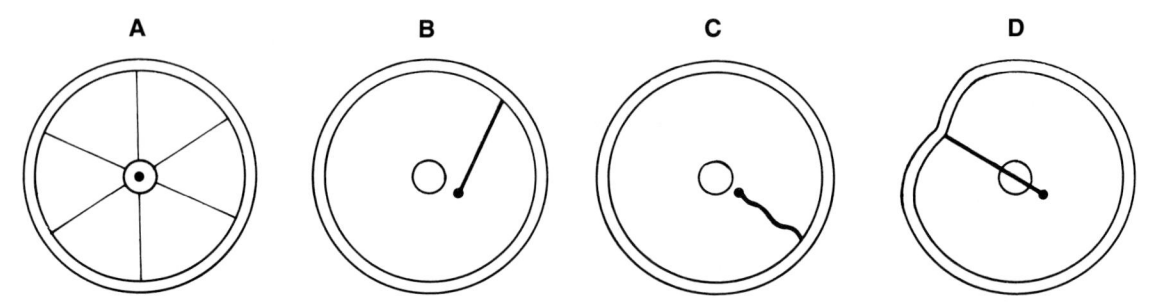

Fig. 15-9 In *A* the wheel is normal. *B, C,* and *D* a spoke is fixed to a point off of the axle. In *B* the spoke is its normal length. As the wheel rotates it becomes too long *(C)* and is lax. If it rotates further it becomes too short and will deform the wheel *(D)*. In the knee, *C* causes abnormal laxity, and *D* will result in a rupture or stretching out of the ligament as a result of the great strength of the bone.

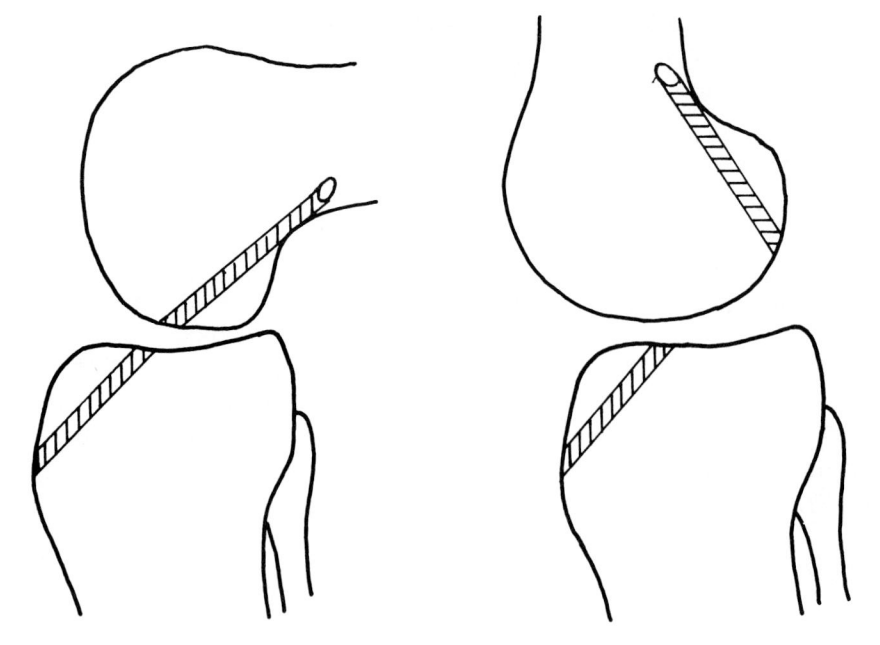

Fig. 15-10 The changing relationship of drill holes is immediately obvious at the extremes of motion.

normal laxity to the knee. The amount of tension needed in absolute terms cannot be given. Proper tensioning is best achieved by duplicating the laxity existing in the contralateral knee.

Matching the bone tunnel size to the graft size allows better incorporation of the material and prevents fistula formation.

A problem that ligament replacement will probably never overcome is the loss of the proprioceptive and sensory feedback provided by the normal anterior cruciate ligament. Mechanoreceptors have been demonstrated in the anterior cruciate ligament, and reestablishment of these neurosensory fibers may not be possible.[28,29]

Types of artificial ligaments (Table 15-1)

The artificial ligaments that have been and are under investigation can be placed into three major categories:
  I. True prosthetic devices
     a. Gortex
     b. Leids Keio
     c. Meadox
     d. Polyethylene
     e. Proplast
     f. Xenotech
 II. Collagen scaffolding devices—carbon fiber
III. Augmentation devices
     a. Biodegradable—Dexon
     b. Non-biodegradable—Kennedy LAD

Gortex

The Gortex graft is made from a single fiber of expanded polytetrafluoroethylene.[3,4] The fiber is folded into bundles that are then braided in a way that forms an eyelet at each end of the graft. The braid allows more even load distribution through the prosthesis. The eyelets are for mechanical fixation by screws. This graft is designed to restrain subluxation not to duplicate the normal anterior cruciate ligament. Its strength and stiffness make the technical aspects of placement very important. The procedure uses over-the-top positioning and is recognized not to be isometric. This over-the-top position will reduce the stresses of rotation and tension on the graft but does allow anterior laxity of the joint when it is flexed more than 45 degrees. Immediate mobilization is possible. The graft material is biocompatible, and the ultimate fixation is bony. Early reports on its use in humans is promising.

TABLE 15-1 / Characteristics of artificial ligaments

CHARACTERISTICS	NORMAL ANTERIOR CRUCIATE LIGAMENT[9,22]	GORTEX[3,4]	LEEDS-KEIO[16,30]	MEADOX[23]	POLYETHYLENE RICHARDS[6,9]
Ultimate strength (N)	1730	4830	2100	3045	420
Stiffness (N/mm)†	175	219	a‡	420	a
Cyclic creep (# cycles)	0% 1.6×10^8	3% 3.4×10^7	a	1% 1.0×10^6	3% 2.5×10^5
Elongation at failure	15%	8.9%	a	15%	10%
Fatigue strength‖	61%	100%	100%	95%	62%
Cycles	1.6×10^8	3.7×10^7	b	1.0×10^6	8.1×10^7
Load	0-500	111	b	100-1000	364
Mode	Bending, tension, torsion	Bending	b	b	Bending
Resistance to abrasion	Excellent	Fair	Poor	Poor	a
Attachment	Bone	Bone	Bone	Bone	Mechanical

*By 5 weeks the prosthesis is absorbed and provides no support. These data are for prosthesis at implantation.
†Normalized; 25 mm specimen.
‡a, Data not available.
§b, Test conditions not specified.
‖As percent of original strength.
¶Two of six ligaments tested failed at the clamp site at less than 5.0×10^5 cycles. The remaining four ligaments were within one standard deviation of expected strength when tested in tension.

Leeds-Keio

The Leeds-Keio ligament is made of a polyester fiber that is woven into a tube that is 1 cm in diameter.[16,30] The tube is slit on one end, and the other end has a loop built in to facilitate passage of the graft. Placement is isometric through femoral and tibial drill holes. Each end is secured in the holes with a bone plug. The technical factors concerning placement and site preparation are important for graft survival. The graft is said to stimulate tissue production along its course in the joint. When observed during arthroscopy in humans, this tissue was reported to be well vascularized but no biopsies were taken for tissue typing. Polyester has recently been shown to be degraded by the body in a time-dependent manner.[14]

PROPLAST II[11,12]	XENOTECH[2,17,18]	CARBON FIBER[32,33]	DEXON[5]	KENNEDY LAD[14,20,25]
1500	3000	1600	910*	1700
1900	527	230×10^9	3100	360
0%	0%	0%	a	3%
2.5×10^6	b§	b	a	b
16%	10%	1%	22%	22%
100%¶	100%¶	a	a	91%
2.5×10^6	1×10^6	a	a	1×10^6
200	0-900	a	a	50-500
Bending	Tension	a	a	Tension
Poor	Poor	Poor	Poor	Poor
Bone	Fibrous cartilage	Soft tissue	Absorbed by 5 weeks	Fibrous tissue

The long-term survival of this graft in vivo has not been determined. Clinical use is still too limited for any conclusions to be drawn.

Meadox

The Meadox graft is composed of dacron (polyester) that has been formed into four woven dacron tapes surrounded by dacron velour.[23] Velour is a shag carpet type weave that is used to enhance fibrous tissue ingrowth. The woven tapes provide strength. The prosthesis can be inserted by either an over-the-top or drill hole technique. Both ends of the graft are fixed with staples. The procedure is augmented with an iliotibial band lateral tenodesis (Mac-

Intosh). Ultimate fixation is to bone. The mechanical properties of the graft are good, and the dacron is biocompatible. Intra-articular tissue ingrowth has been shown to be disorganized collagen. This prosthesis may be subject to slow chemical degradation. The disorganized collagen has little strength so the graft really functions as a true prosthesis. The 2 year data on the clinical trials is very good.

Richards Polyflex

The Richards Polyflex ligament was made of ultra high-molecular weight polyethylene shaped into a solid rod.[6,9] Each end of the rod was threaded. The rod was placed through femoral and tibial drill holes that were rarely isometric. The ligament was fixed in place with nuts that screwed onto either end of the rod and this was supplemented with polymethylmethacrylate cement. These ligaments virtually always failed in use. There were many reasons for this, including the inability of a solid rod to distribute stress within itself, inadequate strength, inadequate fatigue characteristics, and anisometric placement. It has been withdrawn from the market.

Proplast

The Proplast ligament is a stent made of many polyaramid fibers imbedded in fluorinated ethylene propylene copolymer.[11,12] The stent is then coated with proplast (a vitreous carbon fiber and polytetrafluoroethylene composite) to facilitate tissue ingrowth. Placement is through tibial and femoral drill holes placed isometrically. Initial fixation is by staples at each end. Ultimate fixation is to bone. All of the anterior cruciate ligament procedures were combined with extra-articular repairs. There were multiple technical problems during the clinical trials. These problems, combined with the inherent stiffness of the prosthesis, led to the failure of the majority of the anterior cruciate ligament grafts.

Xenotech

The Xenotech prosthesis is a Y-shaped tendon of bovine origin.[2,17,18] It is chemically treated for preservation and to maintain compliance. It is stored in glutaraldehyde. Placement is isometric through tibial and femoral tunnels. There has been no evidence of an immune response or sensitization using a wide variety of immunological testing procedures. There have been no infections that can be attributed to the graft by the designers. However, some investigators have reported infection and graft breakdown.[10,31] Early problems with cyst formation have been eliminated by matching graft and tunnel sizes. Reports have been varied, and no definite conclusions can be drawn at this time.

Carbon fiber

The carbon fiber ligament prosthesis has generated more literature, pro and con, than any of the other ligament prostheses.[7,13,19,33] It was originally a tow of pure carbon fibers. The prosthesis fibers are extremely friable, and are now coated with a resorbable copolymer of polycaprolactone and polylactic acid. This coating facilitates intraoperative handling. The fibers are woven into a fascial band that is then tubed to enclose the graft. The reinforced tendon with its bone plug at one end is then used for a MacIntosh over-the-top reconstruction. The femoral end is not fixed. The bone plug and a special carbon fastener hold the carbon fibers and are used to secure the tibial end. The mechanical properties of the ligament prosthesis are said to be unimportant by the clinical investigators.[32] They believe that the collagen ingrowth is so rapid that a strong prosthetic device is not needed. In most studies this collagen has been shown to be oriented. Collagen typing has been done on this tissue. It was 60% Type I and 40% Type III collagen. This resembles more the scar tissue of healing tendon; normal anterior cruciate ligament is 85% Type I and 15% Type III collagen. Additionally, carbon fiber debris has been reported by some investigators on follow-up arthroscopy.[24] Judicious use has been advised.[19]

Dexon

The Dexon graft is made of braided polyglycolic acid. It was used by Cabaud et al.[5,25] in animal experiments. The hope was that it would provide strong initial support and then allow progressive load sharing as it was resorbed. Unfortunately, pure Dexon grafts are degraded too quickly to be of use. Later experiments using Dexon-coated dacron were also disappointing.

Kennedy

The 3M/Kennedy Ligament Augmentation Device (LAD) is made of high-tenacity polypropylene yarn.[14,20] The LAD consists of 9 tows and 180 fibers braided into a band 6 mm by 1 mm in size. It is used in a modified MacIntosh/Marshall procedure. The LAD is sutured inside the tubes autogenous tissue graft, starting at the origin of the patellar tendon and ending at the terminal portion of the rectus femoris. The augmented tissue is then stapled for initial fixation on the femoral side. The augmentation device is designed to protect the graft from excessive stress during early healing and to allow progressive load sharing during healing. Ultimate fixation is fibrous. Initial reports are good. It is our opinion that when the results are closely analyzed they are no better than when a graft of high initial strength is used.

Summary

In this chapter we have defined the biomechanical properties of the anterior cruciate ligament and of those materials used in clinical trials as substitutes. In addition, a brief statement about the results of some of these clinical trials was given.

The ideal anterior cruciate ligament substitute should be easily inserted, allow immediate joint motion, and restore normal laxity. If such a substitute is to act as a prosthesis, it must show little or no degeneration with time. However, if an augmentation device were to be developed, it must allow for progressive load sharing.

The use of such a substitute would significantly reduce the morbidity of the anterior cruciate ligament deficient knee requiring operative treatment.

REFERENCES

1. Abbink, E.P., Kramer, F., Bom, P.: Assessing bovine xenograft knee ligament reconstructions. Presented at The American Academy of Orthopaedic Surgeons Fifty-third Annual Meeting, New Orleans, Louisiana, 1986.
2. An, K.N., Hein, T.J., and Okuda, Y.: Mechanical evaluation of Xenotech bioprosthesis. Progress report to Xenotech Laboratories, Inc., November 8, 1985.
3. Bolton, C.W., and Bruchman, W.C.: The Gore-Tex expanded polytetrafluoroethylene prosthetic ligament, Clin. Orthop. **196:** 202-213, 1985.
4. Bruchman, W.C., Bolton, C.W., and Bain, J.R.: Design considerations for cruciate ligament prosthesis, W.L. Gore & Associates Laboratories, Flagstaff, Arizona, 1985.
5. Cabaud, H.E., Feagin, J.A., and Rodkey, W.G.: Acute anterior cruciate ligament injury and repair reinforced with a biodegradable material device for repair and reconstruction of injured tendons, Am. J. Sports Med. **13:**242-247, 1985.
6. Chen, E.H., and Black, J.: Materials design analysis of the prosthetic anterior cruciate ligament, J. Biomed. Mater. Res. **14:**567-586, 1980.
7. Claes, L., and Neugebauer, R.: In vivo and in vitro investigation of the long term behavior and fatigue strength of carbon fiber ligament replacement, Clin. Orthop. **196:** 99-111, 1985.
8. Daniels, D.: Personal communication, October 1985.

9. Grood, E.S., and Noyes, F.R.: Cruciate ligament prosthesis: strength, creep and fatigue properties, J. Bone Joint Surg. (Am.) **58**:1083-1088, 1976.
10. Guilquist, J.: Anterior cruciate ligament reconstruction using a bovine xenograft prosthesis: a two-year followup. Presented at The International Knee Society Meeting, Salzburg, Austria, 1985.
11. Homsy, C.A., Prewitt, J.M., and Woods, G.W.: Proplast ligament implants: design and in vitro testing in alloplastic ligament replacement. In Burri, C., and Claes, L., editors: Alloplastic ligament replacement, Bern, 1985, Hans Huber.
12. James, S.L., et al.: Cruciate ligament stents in reconstruction of the unstable knee, Clin. Orthop. **143**:90-96, 1979.
13. Jenkins, D.H.R.: The repair of cruciate ligaments with flexible carbon fibre, J. Bone Joint Surg. (Br.) **60**:520-522, 1978.
14. Kennedy LAD Investigational Plan, Orthopedic Products Division, 3M, St. Paul, Minnesota, 1985.
15. King, M.W., et al.: Degradation of polyester arterial prosthesis: a physical or chemical mechanism. In Fraker, A.C., and Griffin, C.D., editors: Corrosion and degradation of implant materials. Second symposium, Philadelphia, 1985, pp. 294-307, ASTM STP 859, American Society for Testing and Materials.
16. Lynch, D.: Howmedica. Personal communication, November 1985.
17. McKibbin, B.: Carbon fibre as a surgical implant, J. Bone Joint Surg. (Br.) **66**:157-158, 1984.
18. McMaster, W.C.: A histological assessment of canine anterior cruciate substitution with bovine Xenograft, Clin. Orthop. **196**:201, 1985.
19. McMaster, W.C.: Personal communication, December 1985.
20. McPherson, G.K., et al.: Experimental mechanical and histologic evaluation of the Kennedy ligament augmentation device, Clin. Orthop. **196**:186-195, 1985.
21. Müller, W.: The knee: form, function and ligament reconstruction, Berlin, 1983, Springer-Verlag.
22. Noyes, F.R., and Grood, E.S.: The strength of the anterior cruciate ligament in humans and rhesus monkeys, J. Bone Joint Surg. (Am.) **58**:1074-1082, 1976.
23. Park, J.P., et al.: A high strength dacron augmentation for cruciate ligament reconstruction, Clin. Orthop. **196**:175-185, 1985.
24. Parsons, J.R., et al.: Carbon fiber debris within the synovial joint, Clin. Orthop. **196**:69-76, 1985.
25. Rodkey, W.G., et al.: A partially biodegradable material device for repair and reconstruction of injured tendons, Am. J. Sports. Med. **13**:242-247, 1985.
26. Roth, J.H., et al.: Polypropylene braid augmented and nonaugmented intraarticular anterior cruciate ligament reconstruction, Am. J. Sports Med. **13**:321-336, 1985.
27. Rushton, N., Dandy, D.J., and Naylor, C.P.E.: The clinical arthroscopic and histological finding after replacement of the anterior cruciate ligament with carbon fibre, J. Bone Joint Surg. (Br.) **65**:308-309, 1983.
28. Schultz, R.A., Miller, D.C., Kerr, C.S., et al.: Mechanoreceptors in human cruciate ligaments, J. Bone Joint Surg. (Am.) **66**:1072-1076, 1984.
29. Schutte, M.: Personal communication, January 1984.
30. Seedhom, B.B., Fujikawa, K., and Atkinson, P.J.: The Leeds-Keio artificial ligament for replacing the cruciates, I Mech E, **C200**:99-110, 1984.
31. Teitge, R.A.: Anterior cruciate ligament reconstruction using bovine xenograft prosthesis. Presented at The American Orthopaedic Society for Sports Medicine Annual Meeting, Nashville, Tennessee, 1985.
32. Weiss, A.B.: Personal communication, 1985.
33. Weiss, A.B., et al.: Ligament replacement with an absorbable copolymer carbon fiber scaffold: early clinical experience, Clin. Orthop. **196**:77-85.

16
Design considerations for cruciate ligament prostheses

WILLIAM C. BRUCHMAN

C. WILLIAM BOLTON

JAMES R. BAIN

For the past 8 years we have been actively involved in the development of a prosthetic cruciate ligament. During that time, we have reviewed the history of autogenous and prosthetic cruciate ligament substitution and have developed a battery of tests applicable to the evaluation of new designs.[4] The primary purpose of this article is to present the issues we consider important in cruciate ligament substitution and to describe fundamental criteria for the assessment of the adequacy of a ligament prosthesis. This discussion addresses only intra-articular prosthetic replacement of the anterior cruciate ligament, although many of the principles extend to replacement of the posterior cruciate ligament as well.

Ideally, an anterior cruciate ligament prosthesis would provide:
- Ease of insertion with minimal trauma (e.g., arthroscopic placement)
- Immediate joint mobility, thus avoiding the degenerative events within the joint associated with immobilization
- Exact reproduction of the physical restraint system provided by the natural anterior cruciate ligament (including stiffness)
- An average lifetime (or success rate) greater than existing methods of reconstruction using autologous tissue
- Long-term biological compatibility with the intraarticular and intraosseous environments

The following are critical questions that arise in the consideration of a prosthetic ligament:
- Should the device ultimately rely on intra-articular healing for strength, or should it be a true prosthesis?

- If a given device is successful in anterior cruciate ligament replacement in laboratory animals, will it necessarily be successful in humans? Also, what are the criteria by which "success" in an animal model should be gauged, and what animal models, if any, are appropriate for the functional evaluation of cruciate prostheses?
- What are the required mechanical properties? Specifically, how strong should the device be? (Is strength equal to that of the natural anterior cruciate ligament adequate?)
- Should the prosthesis be inserted anatomically in an attempt to mimic the function of the natural anterior cruciate ligament as closely as possible?

These questions are addressed to the extent that answers are available.

Ultimate tensile strength

Understanding the tensile strength (i.e., ultimate break strength) needed to replace the anterior cruciate ligament requires a knowledge of the creep properties of a device. Establishment of this specification without creep testing should be considered arbitrary at best. Examples of anterior cruciate ligament prostheses that have failed as a result of inadequate resistance to creep are well documented.[3,7,15,31]

Creep can be defined as the permanent, time-dependent deformation of a structure under load. Elongation of the ligaments of a patient whose leg is placed under excessive traction for long periods is a graphic illustration of this phenomenon. Both natural tissue and synthetic polymers exhibit mechanical behavior that is influenced by time under load and by load magnitude. This behavior is termed *viscoelasticity*. Within normal working limits, metals can be modeled as a spring (Fig. 16-1). The elongation that results when a tensile load is applied is completely recovered when the load is removed. Viscoelastic materials are better modeled by a combination of spring and fluid elements (Fig. 16-2). Each time a natural or synthetic polymer is placed under load, three components of elongation occur:

1. A recoverable "elastic" deformation like that in metals (element A).
2. A time-dependent, recoverable deformation (element B).
3. A non-recoverable fluid deformation (element C).

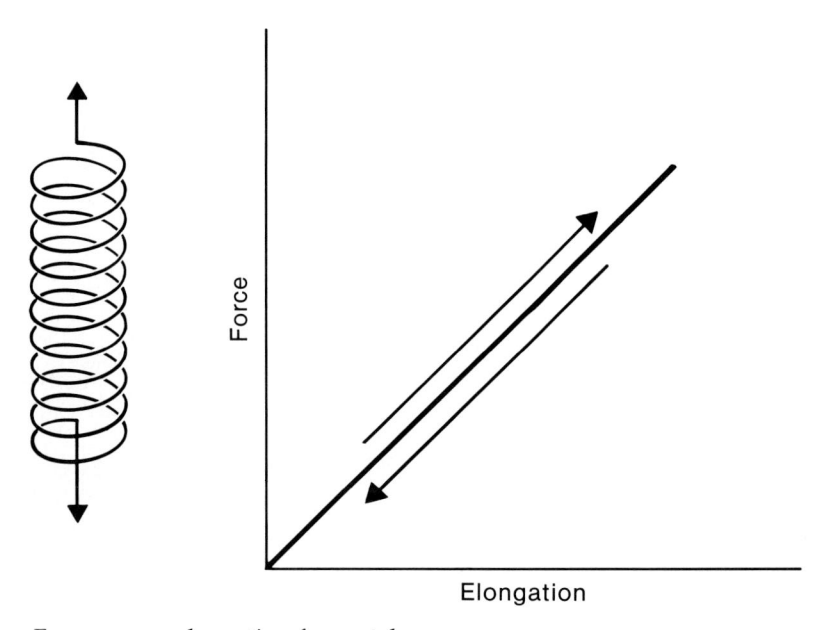

Fig. 16-1 *Force versus elongation for metals.*

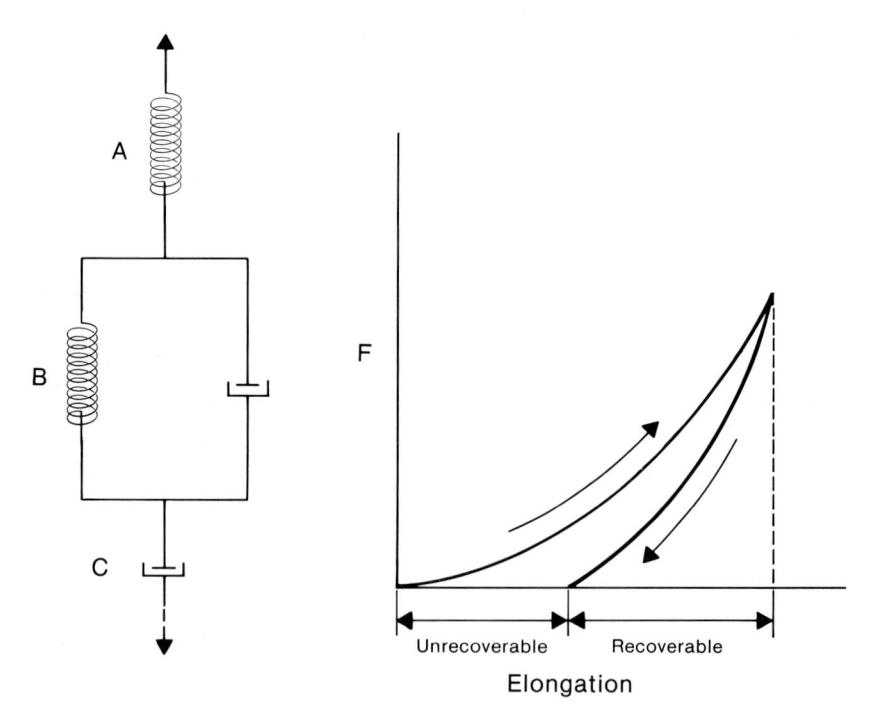

Fig. 16-2 *Force versus elongation for viscoelastic materials.*

Under cyclic loads such as those imposed on an anterior cruciate ligament replacement, this time-dependent behavior can have a significant effect on the elongation occurring with a given number of load cycles. If a load is of sufficient magnitude to produce a residual elongation after removal, and if the next load occurs before this elongation has recovered, permanent elongation will result.

Using methods previously reported,[4] we developed a cyclic creep model that addresses the question of how long a prosthesis will last before it ruptures or elongates under load conditions simulating those in the human. A prosthesis intended to last many years cannot practically be tested under real time conditions. Our test model uses load magnitude as the accelerating factor since failure will occur more rapidly under greater than physiological loads. Prostheses are subjected to cyclic loads at various multiples of the anticipated mean anterior cruciate ligament load. Previous authors have estimated both the force magnitude and the numbers of cycles to which an individual subjects the anterior cruciate ligament each year.[7,22] For purposes of this test, we have elected to use 285 newtons (N) as the mean of the force produced in the anterior cruciate ligament when weighed for activity level.[4] This approximation of the mean value is supported by the observations of Noyes et al.[26] and Henning et al.[17]

The profile of force applied to the prosthesis is illustrated in Fig. 16-3. Maximum load is applied at the position representing full extension, with the force falling to zero for one-half of the cycle. For ease of test control, we selected a constant temperature of 40° C and a rate of one cycle per second.

Elongation of the device under each test load is expressed as a function of the number of cycles necessary to produce that elongation (Fig. 16-4). Adequate samples must be tested to ensure the statistical validity of results. For each test group, some degree of scatter will exist in the elongation data. This variability should be estimated to a 95% confidence level. Using linear regression, a line is fitted to the points representing the upper limit of elongation at a given number of cycles. This equation provides an estimate of the maximal likely elongation at any load condition.

For most polymer constructions, this relationship can typically be expressed as:

$$\ln(\% \text{ elongation}) = k_1 + k_2 \ln(\text{force}) + (k_3 + k_4 \text{force}) \times \ln(\text{no. of cycles})$$

where: ln is the natural logarithm and k_1, k_2, k_3, and k_4 are constants unique to the construction.

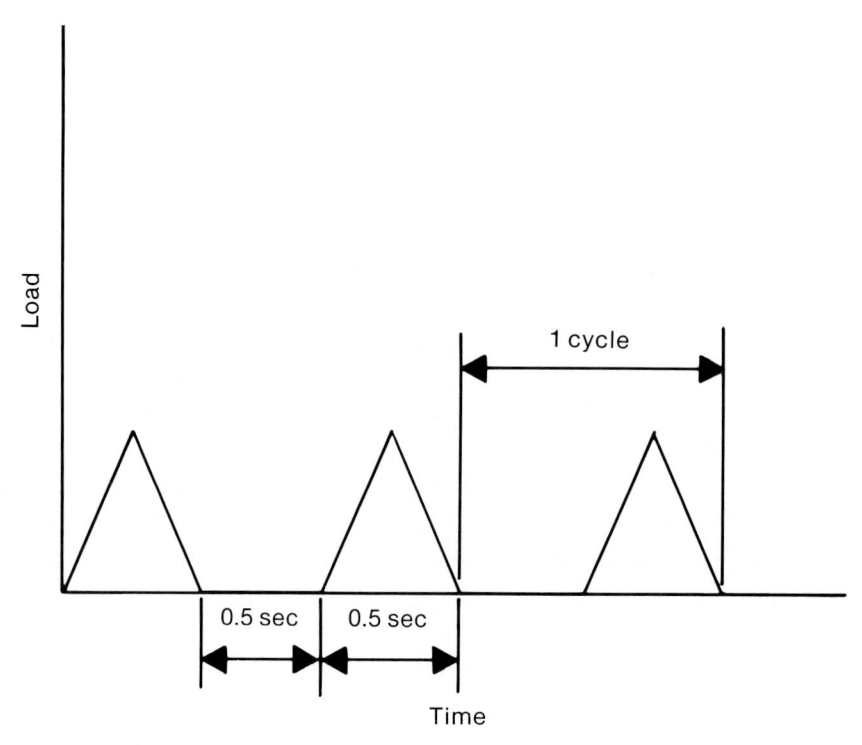

Fig. 16-3 *Load imposed versus time in cyclic creep testing.*

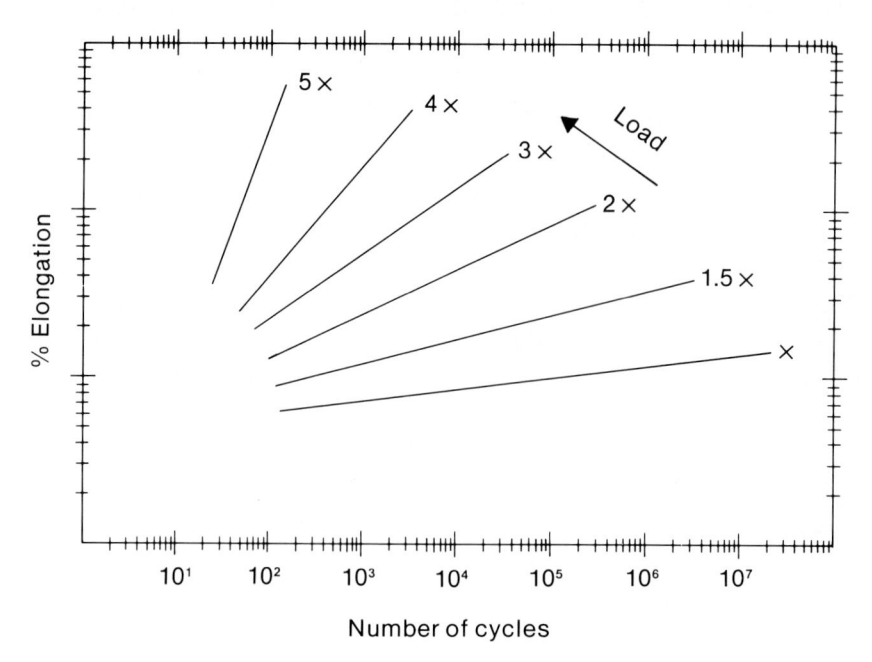

Fig. 16-4 *Elongation versus cycles in cyclic creep testing.*

This equation describes the elongation caused by a given force at a specified number of cycles. For our purposes, we have assumed a 10% elongation to represent clinical failure of the device. This elongation would allow approximately 7 mm of anterior tibial laxity.

By substituting the desired conditions (285 N load and 10% elongation) and the values of the constants, this equation can be solved for the projected lifetime of the device:

$$\ln(\text{no. of cycles}) = \frac{\ln(10\%) - k_1 - k_2 \ln(285)}{(k_3 + k_4\, 285)}$$

Creep testing need not be carried out to the full equivalent of desired life. It is accepted engineering practice to extrapolate the results for the last factor of 10 (one logarithmic decade) or to within one tenth of the total number of cycles that constitute the desired life. For example, if the desired life is 10 years, the required number of cycles is then somewhat greater than 4×10^7, and testing to more than 4×10^6 cycles is required. At one cycle per second, this requires less than 2 months of continuous testing.

Creep rupture is another mode of failure. Using the ruptures that result from greater multiples of the anticipated mean *in vivo* load, a relationship can be developed that predicts time to rupture under this load (Fig. 16-5). This must be done to ensure that rupture will not precede 10% elongation. For most constructions, this should not be the case.

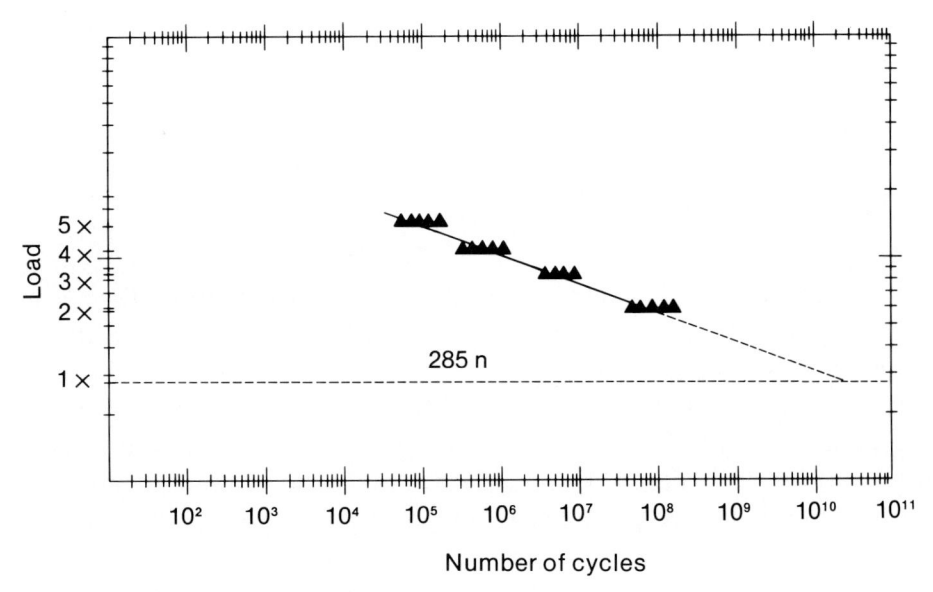

Fig. 16-5 *Rupture curve for cyclic creep testing.*

The precise empirical relationships thus derived are not applicable to all prostheses. The material and structural properties of an artificial ligament have profound effects on its elongation under load. Each device must be treated as unique, and its behavior must be determined accordingly. The first equation is generally applicable to all constructions, but the values of constants k_1, k_2, k_3, and k_4 will vary.

What, then, are the strength requirements for a synthetic anterior cruciate ligament? As previously mentioned, strength requirements are determined by the construction, the polymer, and the polymer's susceptibility to creep. In our own experience with a cruciate prosthesis constructed from threads of expanded polytetrafluoroethylene, we have determined that the minimal ultimate tensile strength is more than twice that of the normal young human anterior cruciate ligament. Although other constructions may not require as great a multiple as this, it is clearly inappropriate to assume adequacy of a device merely because the ultimate tensile strength is similar to that of the human anterior cruciate ligament.

This method of accelerated testing is not the sole means of determining required strength or longevity. Temperature or combinations of temperature and load are equally useful as accelerating factors. One problem with the method described here is worth mention. For the sake of simplicity, we have assumed a constant peak magnitude of cyclic loading for the anterior cruciate ligament. This does not represent the true in vivo loading situation. Greater and lesser forces are imposed, depending on the activity; so an assumption that the behavior of the device under average loads approximates that occurring under the wide variation of actual in vivo loads is required.

Fatigue

A second critical design requirement for a cruciate prosthesis is resistance to fatigue. Fatigue refers to material changes that occur as a result of dynamic internal stresses generated within the device. These changes can ultimately result in failure. The stresses producing fatigue can be induced in several ways, including bending and torsional loading. Bending can occur at both the tibial and femoral insertions during the flexion-extension cycle. Torsional loading (i.e., twisting) can occur during flexion as the tibia is rotated.

Of primary concern are the flexural stresses induced during

flexion and extension. To model this, we developed a method that simulates the bending that takes place at the tibial insertion as the knee bends from full extension to 90 degrees of flexion. We elected to model only the bending at the tibial end of the prosthesis since our own development employed an over-the-top placement of the device. This femoral placement results in a very mild bending over the large radius of the posterior intercondylar fossa. If the device is inserted at the anatomical femoral origin of the anterior cruciate ligament, severe bending over a small radius must also be taken into account (Fig. 16-6).

Typically, polymers respond to testing of this nature with relatively little change in mechanical properties until catastrophic failure occurs. For this reason, testing should be conducted to the equivalent of the desired life. Since the combined stresses imposed by both tensile loading and bending are more severe than the stresses imposed by either alone, this test should also include a static (i.e., constant) tensile load on the device. The load should be the static force that produces the same elongation per cycle as the 285 N

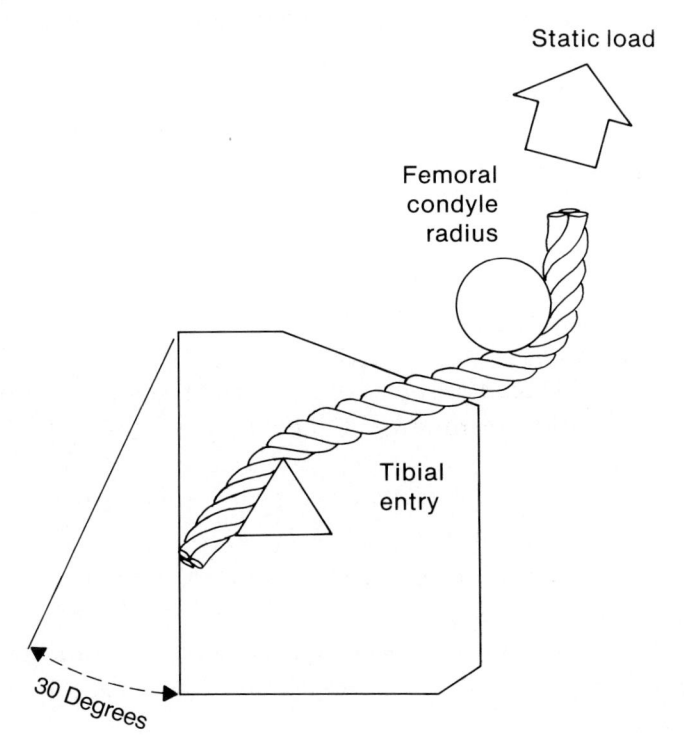

Fig. 16-6 *Fatigue test station.*

periodic load applied in the cyclic creep test. If this information is unavailable, a suitable rule of thumb is to statically apply the weighted mean anticipated load (285 N).

Given an anticipated rate of 4.2 million cycles per year, the required number of test cycles for a life of 10 years is approximately 4.2×10^7. To imply adequacy of a prosthesis after 50,000 cycles (0.1% of 10 years) or even 1 million cycles (2.4% of 10 years) is unjustifiable.

It is entirely possible to create a prosthesis with adequate strength and creep resistance but with inadequate resistance to fatigue. An example of this would be a simple steel wire, which could possess a very large ultimate tensile strength but suffer fatigue failure after only a few cycles of this test. Indeed, any device in which substantial stresses are induced during bending is unlikely to provide suitable lifetime as an anterior cruciate ligament prosthesis.

Other mechanical considerations

After creep and flexural fatigue, the mechanical phenomena next most likely to cause failure of a prosthesis are abrasion and stresses at sharp edges. Abrasion is wear produced through rubbing contact of surfaces. This will inevitably occur when the prosthesis is routed through a narrow anterior intercondylar fossa ("notch"). High-stress levels can also occur at sharp edges (for example, osteophytes or the bone entry sites). In general, the response of natural or synthetic polymers is localized creep ("cold flow") at these areas. This is not abrasion, but can occur simultaneously with abrasion. In either case, the effect is reduction in the load capacity of the prosthesis, potentially leading to failure.[10,14,16,23,29]

Failure of anterior cruciate ligament prostheses has been noted to be related to abrasion and stress concentration, both in experimental animals and in humans.[1,18] These appear to occur primarily in three areas:

1. The anterior rim of the femoral intra-articular bone entry site (when anatomical routing is employed)
2. The posterior rim of the entry site on the tibial plateau
3. The region of the intercondylar notch; an excessively narrow notch, osteophytes or other bony edges can impinge on the device; also, if the device exits the tibia anterior to the natural insertion of the anterior cruciate ligament, the notch will be forced against the prosthesis in extension.

Design considerations for cruciate ligament prostheses

Of materials that can be considered for this application, those that are more resistant to abrasion are also those that are harder. This presents a dilemma. One of the fundamental requisites of a cruciate prosthesis is that the stresses imposed on the bone adjacent to the prosthesis remain low. Bone loss through abrasion or high local compressive loads is a likely outcome with the use of hard polymer constructions.[19,29,30] For this reason, we believe the problem must be addressed through the surgical routing of the graft.

Surgical routing

Positioning of the tibial attachment has a significant effect on stresses induced in the graft as it enters the bone. Excessively anterior placement of the entry into the tibial plateau (Fig. 16-7) can promote early failure. If the resulting graft course is so far anterior that impingement by the anterior portion of the notch occurs in full extension (where maximal loads occur), severe local load concen-

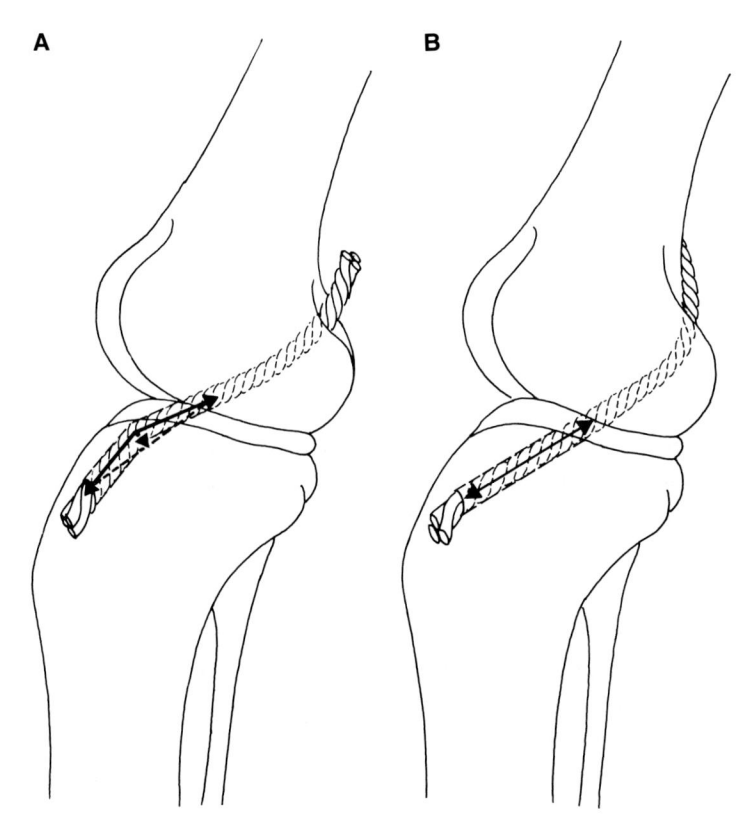

Fig. 16-7   *A and B, Anterior tibial placement versus anatomical tibial placement.*

A modified over-the-top placement (i.e., through the posterior intercondylar fossa—Fig. 16-9) reduces stresses induced in the graft in several ways. Most importantly, the concentrated stresses that occur at the drill hole edge (at the anatomical femoral origin of the natural anterior cruciate ligament) are essentially eliminated because the compressive load is distributed over the large radius formed by the posterior intercondylar fossa. Secondly, bending occurs over this large radius and is separated from stresses imposed at the more proximal fixation site. Additionally, rotational movement of the graft relative to the femur is reduced, thereby reducing the possibility for abrasion.

An "over-the-top" placement will enhance graft longevity. Although the geometric restraint system provided by the natural anterior cruciate ligament is not reproduced with this approach, our observations suggest no resulting functional deficit.

Animal model

Humans are the only true bipeds among the living species of mammals. Over the years, researchers have used rats, cats, rabbits, rhesus monkeys, dogs, goats, sheep, pigs, and cattle to assess methods of anterior cruciate ligament repair.

In our search for a suitable animal model for the functional evaluation of anterior cruciate ligament prostheses, we have progressed from dogs to sheep and are now using goats. All three of these animals share a common limitation as test subjects in their inability to attain 0 degrees extension. Furthermore, the sheep has a propensity for osteoarthritic degeneration with osteophyte proliferation. Another limitation of these animals is an extremely narrow notch when compared to that in humans. The canine (greyhound) model also has the limitation of small bone size relative to body weight. Small bone size precludes proper anatomical insertion into the tibial plateau. In this regard, the goat appears to be superior to the dog or the sheep. To obtain an adequate tibial tunnel length, the graft must be placed such that a significant posterior deflection results as the graft enters the tibial plateau. This, in conjunction with the flexed posture of the hindlimb in these quadrupeds, creates excessive stresses at the posterior rim of the tibial intra-articular exit site. In this respect, all of these animal models impose excessively severe conditions on prosthetic cruciate ligaments.

Strength of the cruciate ligaments appears to be a good indicator

TABLE 16-1 / Tensile strength of natural anterior cruciate ligament of three domestic mammals

ANIMAL	N	MEAN WEIGHT (KG)	MEAN BREAK STRENGTH (N)
Greyhound	24	29.5	1362
Goat	10	27.0	1550
Sheep	30	68.6	1912

of the loads imposed during activity. Noyes et al.[24,26] speculated that normal loads constitute approximately 10% to 26% of anterior cruciate ligament strength. We studied the tensile strength of the natural anterior cruciate ligament of several domestic animals, using strain rates of 25% to 40% sec^{-1} (see Table 16-1). These data, along with a review of the literature on anterior cruciate ligament strength in mammals, support the hypothesis of Noves and Grood[24] that anterior cruciate ligament strength in mammals is directly proportional to body mass raised to the two-thirds power.

Although the relationship of anterior cruciate ligament strength to body mass in these animals appears to approximate that in humans, each species has one or more unique features that render it less than ideal for in vivo testing of anterior cruciate ligament prostheses. The loads imposed by these quadrupeds, with their unique joint geometries, are uncertain, so longevity of a device in humans should not be inferred from these tests. Longevity is more appropriately estimated from the accelerated in vitro tests previously described.

The value of animal testing is in the observation of the biological response to the device. With any anterior cruciate ligament prosthesis, it is of paramount importance that the compatibility of the device with bone, synovium, and other tissues about the knee be evaluated in a suitable healing model before use in humans. Such studies are also of great use in determining the potential for fixation by tissue ingrowth and for evaluating postoperative strength.

Postoperative strength

To assess the performance of a cruciate substitute, whether it be a natural or synthetic polymer, a knowledge of tensile strength at various postoperative durations is required. Gross and histological observations notwithstanding, tensile testing is essential to accurately measure the effects of all the previously described phenomena on reconstruction strength; characterizing a reconstruction through its appearance alone is a poor substitute for biomechanical tests of the anterior cruciate ligament replacement and its fixations.

Upon sacrifice, the specimen should be rapidly tested (or frozen) to avoid artifactual results stemming from autolysis. We remove all muscles and their tendinous insertions and sever the other ligaments of the knee. We test the knee at 45 degrees of flexion since previous workers have shown this angle to produce the greatest strength values[12,24]; it presumably imposes maximal simultaneous tension on the primary bundles of the natural anterior cruciate ligament. The effects of knee flexion on the length-tension relationships in the cruciates of humans and other mammals remain somewhat controversial.[2,9,21,27]

The femur-prosthesis-tibia preparation is oriented so that the intra-articular portion of the graft is on the same axis as the load cell of the tensile tester (Fig. 16-10); if the preparation is oriented in this way, the values recorded by the instrument represent the force imposed by a given elongation. The strain rate should be a minimum of 30% $\sec^{-1}$ to approximate the physiological conditions.

Using these methods, the immediate surgical fixation strength can be measured. One of the primary potential advantages of a cruciate prosthesis is the immediate mobility provided to the patient. The prolonged immobility traditionally employed after autogenous repair results in muscle atrophy and degenerative changes within the joint. Immediate mobility requires a fixation strength approaching the strength of the natural anterior cruciate ligament. In our laboratory, initial fixation through knots, sutures, or staples has proved marginal at best. To provide initial strength approaching that of the natural anterior cruciate ligament, we have found it necessary to use bone screws with bicortical fixation.

The use of an anterior cruciate ligament prosthesis should avoid the early degeneration that takes place in autogenous substitutes placed within the joint. This degeneration appears to occur whether or not the tissue maintains or reestablishes a vascular supply.[20,25] Substantial degradation in mechanical properties of autogenous grafts has been documented, but the amount of strength ultimately regained by the implant remains a subject of discussion.[6,8,20] Even healing of a primary repair of a ruptured natural anterior cruciate ligament results in tissue of questionable tensile properties.[5,11,28] In view of these observations, we concur with Frank et al.[13] that meth-

Design considerations for cruciate ligament prostheses

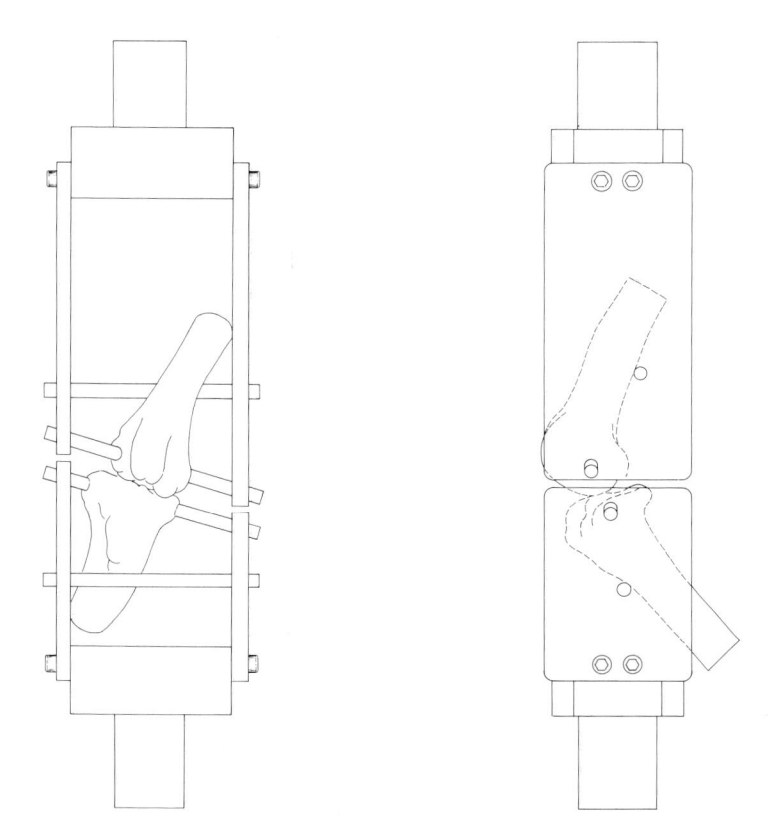

Fig. 16-10 *Vertical orientation of the tibia-prosthesis-femur preparation under the load cell.*

ods of ligament replacement relying on healing for strength augmentation can result in only limited success.

Ideally, long-term fixation of the device would be achieved through biological means. Since the ends of a reconstruction terminate in the osseous and extrasynovial environment, tissue fixation can occur. Biological fixation of the anterior cruciate ligament substitute occurring through bony attachment appears to be preferable because of superior viscoelastic properties of bone and the implied permanence of the bond. The most important aspect is the strength of tissue fixation. Tensile testing is the only objective method of quantifying this value.

Throughout this discussion, biochemical degradation of the device has been ignored. As with natural tissues, many synthetic polymers also undergo a loss of strength in the synovial environment.

Summary

Numerous device configurations have been proposed for use as cruciate prostheses. These can be categorized into those constructions that rely on intra-articular tissue healing (biodegradable or augmentation devices) and those that do not (permanent prostheses). This discussion has addressed primarily the latter. The accelerated mechanical tests we have devised are suitable only for devices that do not undergo degradation during testing. Such tests are therefore not applicable to devices intended to degrade and become composites of new host tissue. Our investigations have dealt exclusively with permanent prostheses because of three considerations:

1. Avoidance of immobilization
2. Vagaries of intra-articular healing among patients
3. Inability to assess the adequacy of a composite or biodegradable device through accelerated in vitro testing

We believe the critical requirements for permanent anterior cruciate ligament prostheses to be:

- Biocompatibility and chemical stability without genotoxic or mutagenic effects
- Creep properties providing an adequate lifetime under in vivo loads
- A demonstrated resistance to bending fatigue equivalent to the desired lifetime
- Softness, good compliance, and low bending force to minimize the possibility of bone loss
- Surgical routing that reduces the stresses imposed on the device and elimination of sharp edges that can cause failure
- A demonstrated immediate fixation strength allowing for immediate mobility of the limb
- A demonstrated biological fixation strength providing for long-term function

Although in vitro mechanical testing is valid only for permanent prostheses, the remaining requirements are applicable to all proposed methods of intra-articular cruciate substitution, including grafts of autogenous tissues. Efficacy of any prosthesis must ultimately be demonstrated through use in the human knee. Success in tests such as those discussed here should be a prerequisite to that use. The surgeon contemplating the use of an anterior cruciate ligament prosthesis should carefully examine the properties of the device in light of these requirements.

REFERENCES

1. Allen, P.R., Amis, A.A., Jones, M.M., et al.: Bovine glutaraldehyde-treated tendon as a graft material: a clinical and laboratory study, J. Bone Joint Surg. (Br.) **67**:159, 1985.
2. Arms, S.W., Pope, M.H., Johnson, R.J., et al.: The biomechanics of anterior cruciate ligament rehabilitation and reconstruction, Am. J. Sports Med. **12**:8, 1984.
3. Beauchamp, P., Laurin, C.A., and Bailon, J.-P.: Etude des proprietes mecaniques des ligaments croises en vue de leur remplacement prothetique, Rev. Chir. Orthop. **65**: 197, 1979.
4. Bolton, C.W., and Bruchman, W.C.: The GORE-TEX™ expanded polytetrafluoroethylene prosthetic ligament: an *in vitro* and *in vivo* evaluation, Clin. Orthop. **196**:202, 1985.
5. Cabaud, H.E., Rodkey, W.G., and Feagin, J.A.: Experimental studies of acute anterior cruciate ligament injury and repair, Am. J. Sports Med. **7**:18, 1979.
6. Cabaud, H.E., Feagin, J.A., and Rodkey, W.G.: Acute anterior cruciate ligament injury and augmented repair: experimental studies, Am. J. Sports Med. **8**:395, 1980.
7. Chen, E.H., and Black, J.: Materials design analysis of the prosthetic anterior cruciate ligament, J. Biomed. Mater. Res. **14**:567, 1980.
8. Clancy, W.G., Narechania, R.G., Rosenberg, T.D., et al.: Anterior and posterior cruciate ligament reconstruction in rhesus monkeys: a histological microangiographic, and biomechanical analysis, J. Bone Joint. Surg. (Am.) **63**:1270, 1981.
9. Edwards, R.G., Lafferty, J.F., and Lange, K.O.: Ligament strain in the human knee joint, J. Basic Eng. **92**:131, 1970.
10. Emery, M.A., and Rostrup, O.: Repair of the anterior cruciate ligament with 8mm tube Teflon in dogs, Can. J. Surg. **4**:111, 1960.
11. Feagin, J.A., and Curl, W.W.: Isolated tear of the anterior cruciate ligament: 5-year follow-up study, Am. J. Sports Med. **4**:95, 1976.
12. Figgie, H.E., III, Bahniuk, E.H., Heiple, K.G., et al.: The effects of tibial-femoral angle on the failure mechanics of the canine anterior cruciate ligament, Transactions of the Twenty-eighth Annual Meeting of the Orthopaedic Research Society, Abstracts, p. 309, 1982.
13. Frank, C., Amiel, D., Woo, S.L.-Y., et al.: Normal ligament properties and ligament healing, Clin. Orthop. **196**:15, 1985.
14. Gerdes, M.H., Haynes, D.W., and Nelson, C.L.: The failure of Dacron as an anterior cruciate ligament, Transactions of the Twenty-eighth Annual Meeting of the Orthopaedic Research Society, Abstracts, p. 257, 1982.
15. Grood, E.S., and Noyes, F.R.: Cruciate ligament prosthesis: strength, creep and fatigue properties, J. Bone Joint Surg. (Am.) **58**:1083, 1976.
16. Gupta, B.N., and Brinker, W.O.: Anterior cruciate ligament prosthesis in the dog, J. Am. Vet. Med. Assoc. **154**:1057, 1969.
17. Henning, C.E., Lynch, M.A., and Glick, K.R.: An *in vivo* strain gage study of elongation of the anterior cruciate ligament, Am. J. Sports Med. **13**:22, 1985.
18. James, S.L., Woods, G.W., Homsy, C.A., et al.: Cruciate ligament stents in reconstruction of the unstable knee: a preliminary report, Clin. Orthop. **143**:90, 1979.
19. Kappakas, G.S., and McMaster, J.H.: Repair of acromioclavicular separation using a Dacron prosthesis graft, Clin. Orthop. **131**: 247, 1978.
20. Kennedy, J.D., Roth, J.H., Mendenhall, H.V., et al.: Presidential address: intra-articular replacement in the anterior cruciate ligament-deficient knee, Am. J. Sports Med. **8**:1, 1980.
21. Langrana, N.A., and Bronfeld, J.: Computer-assisted analysis of ligament constraints in the knee, Clin. Orthop. **196**:42, 1985.

22. McLeod, P.C., Kettelcamp, D.B., Srinivasan, V., et al.: Measurement of repetitive activities of the knee, J. Biomech. 8:369, 1975.
23. Meyers, J.F., Grana, W.A., and Lesker, P.A.: Reconstruction of the anterior cruciate ligament in the dog: comparison of results obtained with three different porous synthetic materials, Am. J. Sports Med. 7:85, 1979.
24. Noyes, F.R., and Grood, E.S.: The strength of the anterior cruciate ligament in humans and in rhesus monkeys: age-related and species-related changes, J. Bone Joint Surg. (Am.) 58:1074, 1976.
25. Noyes, F.R., Keller, C.S., Grood, E.S., et al.: Advances in the understanding of the knee ligament injury, repair, and rehabilitation, Med. Sci. Sports Exerc. 16:427, 1984.
26. Noyes, F.R., Butler, D.L., Grood, E.S., et al.: Biomechanical analysis of human ligament grafts used in knee-ligament repairs and reconstructions, J. Bone Joint Surg. (Am.) 66:344, 1984.
27. Odensten, M., and Gillquist, J.: Functional anatomy of the anterior cruciate ligament and a rationale for reconstruction, J. Bone Joint Surg. (Am.) 67:257, 1985.
28. O'Donoghue, D.H., Frank, G.R., Jeter, G.L., et al.: Repair and reconstruction of the anterior cruciate ligament in dogs: factors influencing long-term results, J. Bone Joint Surg. (Am.) 53:710, 1971.
29. Park, J.P., Grana, W.A., and Chitwood, J.S.: A high-strength Dacron augmentation for cruciate ligament reconstruction: a two-year canine study, Clin. Orthop. 196:175, 1985.
30. Park, J.P., Arnold, J.A., Coker, T.P., et al.: Treatment of acromioclavicular separations: a retrospective study, Am. J. Sports Med. 8:251, 1980.
31. Scharling, M.: Replacement of the anterior cruciate ligament with a polyethylene prosthetic ligament, Acta Orthop. Scand. 52:575, 1981.

17
Principles of arthroscopic anterior cruciate reconstruction

DOUGLAS W. JACKSON

PAUL R. REIMAN

Arthroscopic surgical techniques for reconstruction of the anterior cruciate ligament deficient knee are in the early stages of their development. More and more surgeons are technically capable of doing this type of surgery and are guided by the desire to have smaller incisions and less morbidity, in particular pain, for their patients postoperatively. The deleterious effects on patella tracking and the extensor mechanism pain associated with open procedures are the result of capsular incisions, detachment of the vastus medialis, and patellar dislocation and can be decreased by this procedure. Early motion becomes easier and less painful to perform. The arthroscopic technique of anterior cruciate substitution is ahead of clinically tested and available substitute ligament. Certain basic principles of arthroscopic cruciate substitution have emerged from the early experiences and are common to the techniques presently used.

Diagnosis and treatment of instability and associated intra-articular injuries

The success of any ligamentous reconstructive procedure depends on many factors. Accurate diagnosis and classification of the ligament instability present is made preoperatively and confirmed with the patient under anesthesia. The examination should establish the presence or absence of the components of anterior, posterior, valgus, varus, and rotatory instability of the particular knee. The arthroscope is an important tool for expanding the diagnosis and treatment of associated injuries to the menisci, capsular structures, and articular cartilage.

Diagnostic arthroscopy with visualization of the entire joint is the first step in the operative procedure. Injuries to associated structures are documented, and those injuries amenable to arthroscopic techniques are treated. Of particular importance is visualization of the posterior horns of both menisci since they are frequently injured in association with or subsequent to injury of the anterior cruciate ligament. Arthroscopic treatment of meniscal lesions, either by repair when possible or partial excision when necessary, is performed before the anterior cruciate ligament substitution. Visualization of the posterior aspect of the joint and meniscal surgery is more difficult after the substitution procedure. The positioning required for meniscal repair and/or partial menisectomy may require stresses or motion on the anterior cruciate substitute that are greater than desired. Once the associated injuries are treated arthroscopically, attention is directed to the ligament substitution.

Ligament substitution

Preparation of the intercondylar notch

In order to ensure accurate placement of the material to be substituted, the lateral and superior wall of the intercondylar notch must be debrided of soft tissue and well visualized. The residual ligament can be used to locate the area of the anatomical femoral origin and tibial insertion of the anterior cruciate ligament. Use of a high-speed synovial resector or debrider with a large bore is useful in debriding the remnant of the anterior cruciate and associated soft tissue from the notch. It is also helpful to debride hypertrophic synovium from the notch; special care should be taken to not injure or remove the soft tissue overlying the posterior cruciate ligament. The femoral attachment of the anterior cruciate ligaments needs to be debrided posteriorly in order to visualize its bony origin on the lateral femoral condyle. This is well posterior to the anterior margin of the posterior cruciate ligament. Visualization of the posterior capsule is an indication of adequate debridement. Care must be taken not to injure the posterior cruciate ligament, the articular cartilage, or the posterior horns of the medial and lateral menisci. This is of particular concern when using the newer and more aggressive resectors and debriders. Manual use of a curette may further allow the bony architecture to be delineated. At the conclusion of this portion of the procedure the lateral wall of the notch back to the capsule and the superior margin of the notch should be well visualized.

Following soft-tissue debridement of the notch, a "notchplasty" of the lateral femoral condyle may be performed using a high-speed burr similar to the chondral abrasion instrument (Fig. 17-1).[2] Notchplasty is of particular importance in the chronically unstable knee where osteophyte proliferation and notch encroachment are common. Beginning anteriorly, the notch is enlarged from the articular surface to the roof of the notch. In many knees there is a ridge within the roof of the notch and debridement must be carried beyond this ridge to be far enough posterior to visualize the femoral origin of the anterior cruciate ligament. However, care should be taken to avoid excessive bone resection since it is possible to resect the wall too far laterally. The debridement of soft tissue and bone should allow for selection of a point high posteriorly and laterally in the notch (Fig. 17-2). After placement of an anterior cruciate ligament substitute, direct visualization of the ligament during range of motion of the knee is necessary to confirm that the femoral condyle does not impinge on the substitute.[2] If the intercondylar notch impinges on the graft, whether superiorly or laterally and particularly in extension, further debridement is necessary.

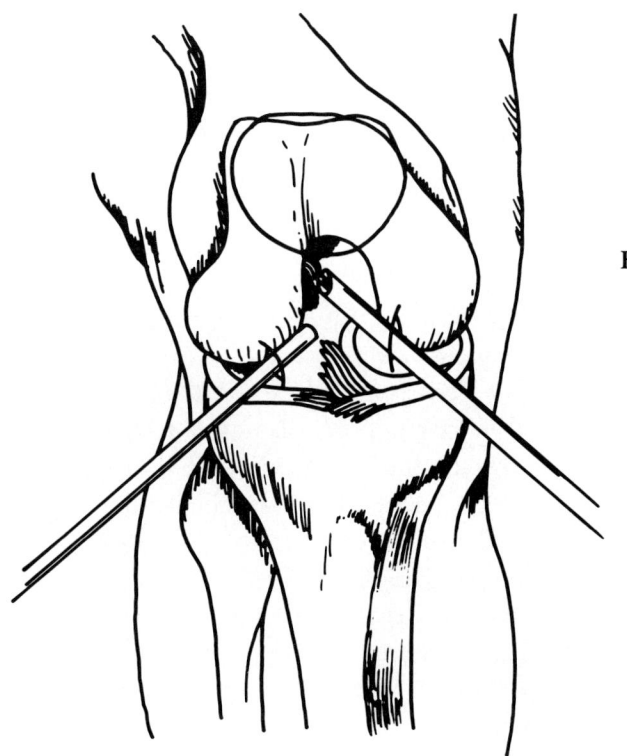

Fig. 17-1 *Debridement of notch. Use of a high-speed burr to debride and widen the intercondylar notch. (Adapted from Rosenberg, T.: Arthroscopic technique for anterior cruciate ligament surgery, Technical Bulletin, Acufex Microsurgical, Inc., Norwood, Mass., 1984.)*

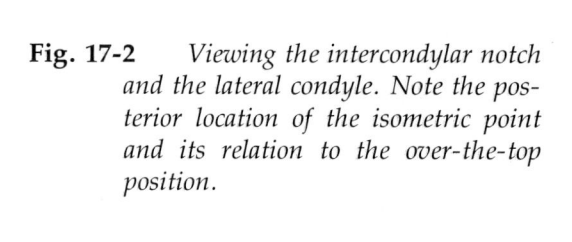

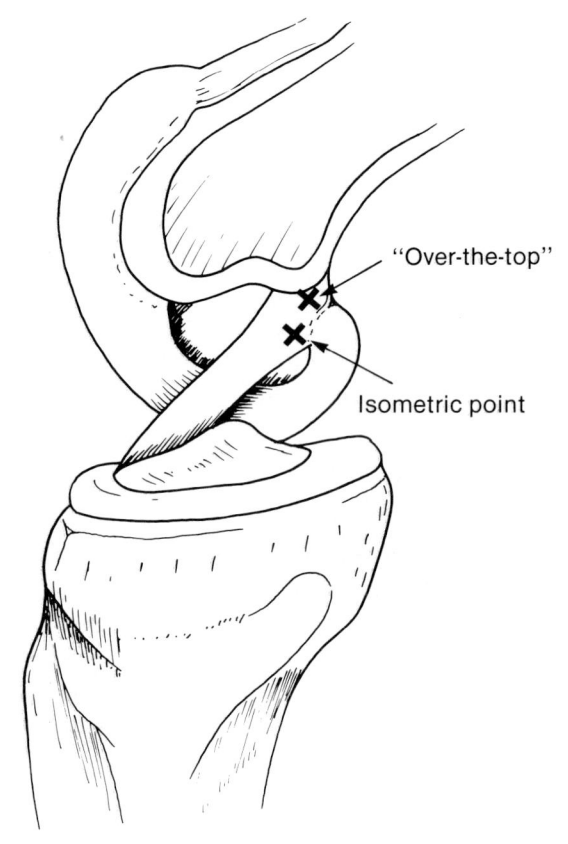

Fig. 17-2 *Viewing the intercondylar notch and the lateral condyle. Note the posterior location of the isometric point and its relation to the over-the-top position.*

Irrigation is an important part of the visualization and control of bleeding. Adequate visualization is usually not a problem but may require several liters of irrigant solution or an irrigation pump during this portion of the procedure.

Selection of extra-articular osseous tunnel sites

A lateral incision is made directly along the lines of the femoral shaft and carried distally to the level of the lateral condyle. The area to be exposed is just proximal to the junction of the shaft of the femur and the lateral femoral condyle. The fascia is split at the junction of the iliotibial band and the fascia of the vastus lateralis. The vastus lateralis musculature is then reflected subperiosteally to expose the lateral cortex of the femoral shaft. The lateral superior geniculate arteries and veins are encountered in the dissection and should be coagulated. An oblique femoral tunnel, directed from the lateral metaphysis to the intercondylar notch, makes it easier to pass a graft. Bending fatigue and other problems with sharp corners are minimized. Care must be taken to place the osseous tunnel anterior to the linea aspera to avoid any posterior neurovascular structures. The osseous tunnel in the proximal tibia is prepared through a small second incision, that is 4 cm in length, made over the proximal medial tibia, and approximately 3 cm below the joint line.

Selection of the isometric point

The selection of the location of bony tunnels or of the over-the-top position is a most critical portion of the procedure. Although the composite fibers of the anterior cruciate ligament have no single isometric point, each individual fiber has an origin and insertion. Substitution with a graft of parallel fibers requires accurate placement at a functional isometric point for the center of the graft to prevent undue stresses on the graft during range of motion. The most common error is to place the center too far anteriorly, causing tension to be placed on the graft in flexion. Conversely, placing the graft too far posteriorly produces tension when the knee is extended.

Placement of guide pins

The femoral guide pin is placed using one of two methods. The guide pin may be drilled from the inside out using an anteromedial portal with the knee in a figure-four position. Under arthroscopic control, a point is selected and the pin is drilled obliquely toward the lateral femoral shaft (Fig. 17-3). Care must be taken not to injure the articular cartilage of the medial femoral condyle. The angle of drilling should be selected so that the pin will exit in the exposed area on the distal femur laterally. This should be anterior to the linea aspera to protect the neurovascular structures and should allow for over drilling from the outside into the notch.

A second and the authors' preferred method is to use a commercially available drill guide. The tip of the guide is placed at the desired location in the intercondylar notch, and under direct visualization and arthroscopic control, the guide pin is drilled from the lateral femoral condyle into the intercondylar notch (Figs. 17-4 and 17-5). The drill guide, depending on its shape, can be placed either through an anterolateral or anteromedial portal with visualization of the tip by the arthroscope through a separate portal.

Before the skin incision is made, the drill guide is placed against the lateral thigh to estimate the optimal location for the incision. This minimizes the size of the incision needed to attain the desired exposure.

Fig. 17-3 *Placement of the guide wire into the femoral isometric point from the anteromedial portal.*

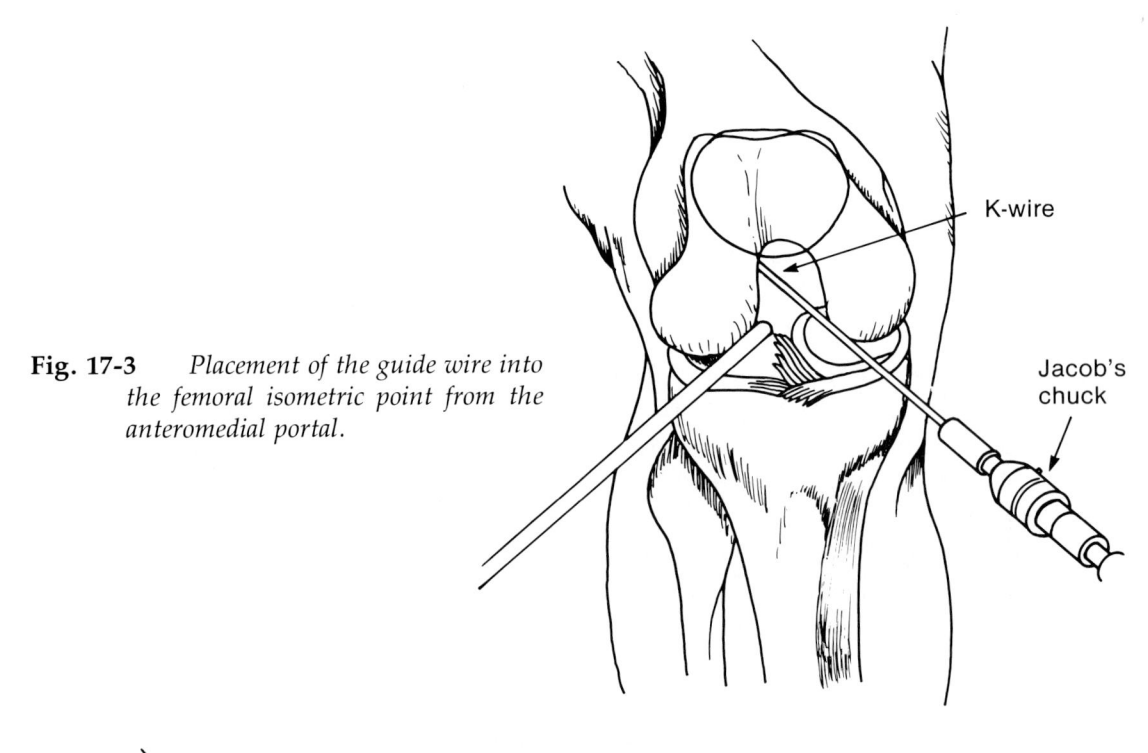

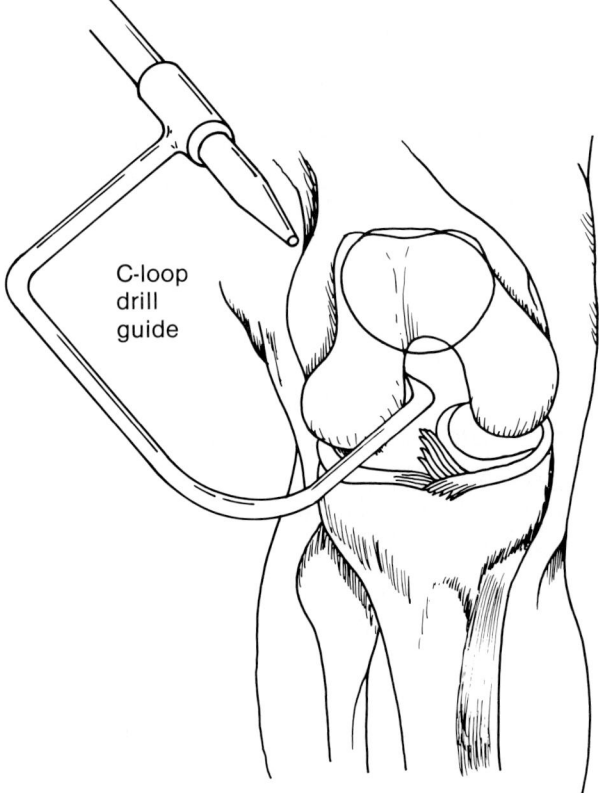

Fig. 17-4 *Use of a C-loop drill guide facilitates accurate placement of the osseous tunnels. This figure illustrates using a drill guide for the femoral tunnel.*

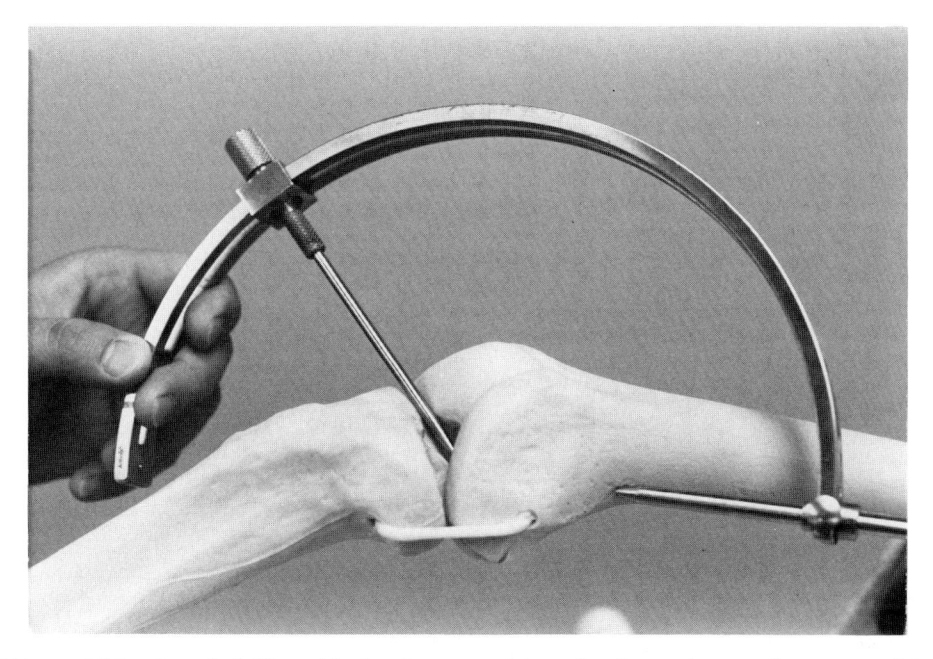

Fig. 17-5 *This slotted drill guide is shown making the femoral tunnel on a model femur. The "bow and arrow" design is common to several manufacturers.*

Some of the prosthetic ligaments require a modified femoral placement. Some use an over-the-top placement, in which a rasp is used to debride the area at the junction of the lateral femoral condyle and the femoral shaft, and some use the technique of passing the ligament through the posterior capsule. In order to achieve an isometric point in the over-the-top method, a fair amount of bone, up to 5 mm, needs to be removed posteriorly (Fig. 17-2).

The tibial insertion point is then selected to reflect the anatomical insertion. This is usually anterior and medial to the tibial spine (Fig. 17-6). As with the femoral origin, the remnant of the anterior cruciate is a helpful landmark (Fig. 17-7).

The drill guides should be tightly anchored against the cortical bone before the guide wire is drilled. Trochar pointed tip guide pins are used. The pins tend to "walk" because of the oblique angle used to approach the cortices. On occasion it is helpful to predrill the lateral femoral condyle with a 3 or 4 mm drill to prevent deflection on the lateral femoral cortex as the pin moves toward the intercondylar notch. The tip must be sharp and must be inserted at a slow speed to prevent deviation of the pin as it tries to penetrate the cortex of the lateral femoral condyle and the cortex of the inter-

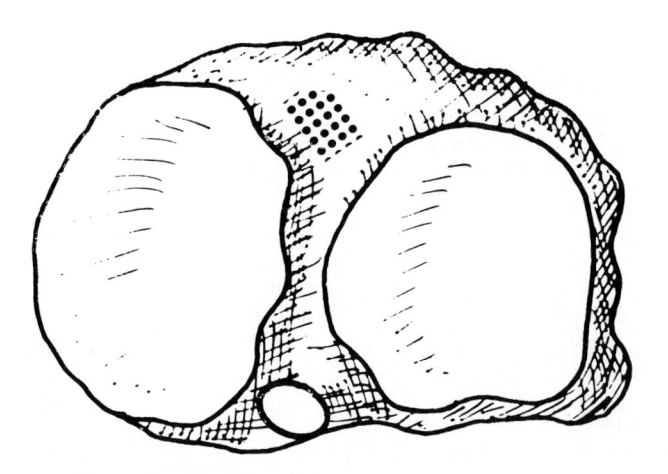

Fig. 17-6 *The area of the tibial isometric point is within the dotted area.*

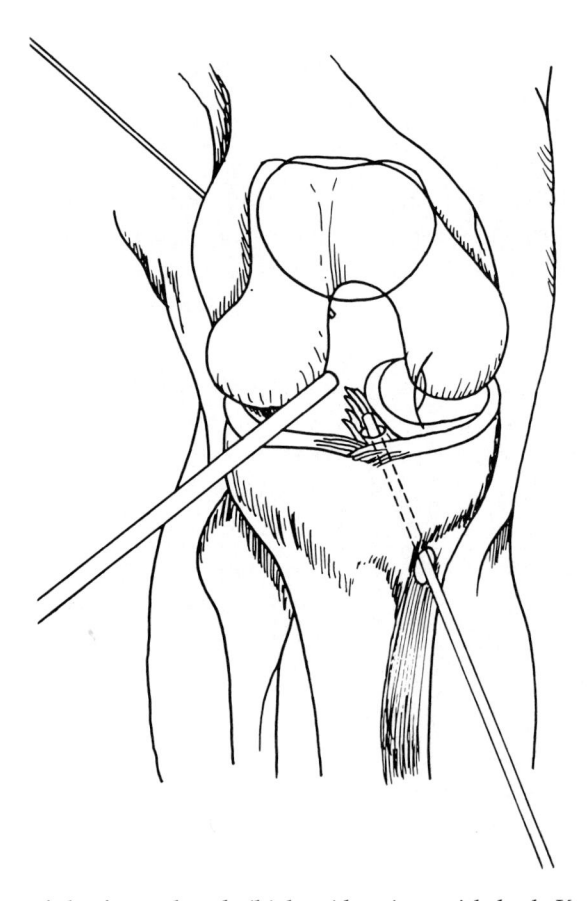

Fig. 17-7 *Placement of the femoral and tibial guide wires with both K-wires in place.*

condylar notch.[1] It has been our experience that in the numerous guides available, this "walking" may be a significant problem.

Familiarity with the anatomy of the intercondylar notch and awareness of the possible problems with placement are important in establishing reproducibility. The use of a single large drill with the drill guide decreases the deviation problem but makes changes in tunnel position after the initial placement difficult. The accuracy of the drill guide placement must be reproducible in the individual surgeon's hands.

The "inside out" method has the advantage of being more accurate with direct intercondylar notch placement of the guide pin. However, the variation of the location where the pin exits on the lateral femoral condyle may be considerable. Care must be taken to aim the pin so that it does not exit posteriorly to the linear aspera, placing the posterior neurovascular structures at risk. It is sometimes difficult to overdrill the guide pin when posterior placement on the lateral femoral cortex occurs.

Determining the isometry of the guide pin placement

After femoral and tibial points have been selected with guide pins, the accuracy of the placement needs to be checked. It has been our experience that even with direct visualization, the isometric point can be misjudged. The development of a spring loaded tension device (Acufex, Inc.) has been an important addition to ante-

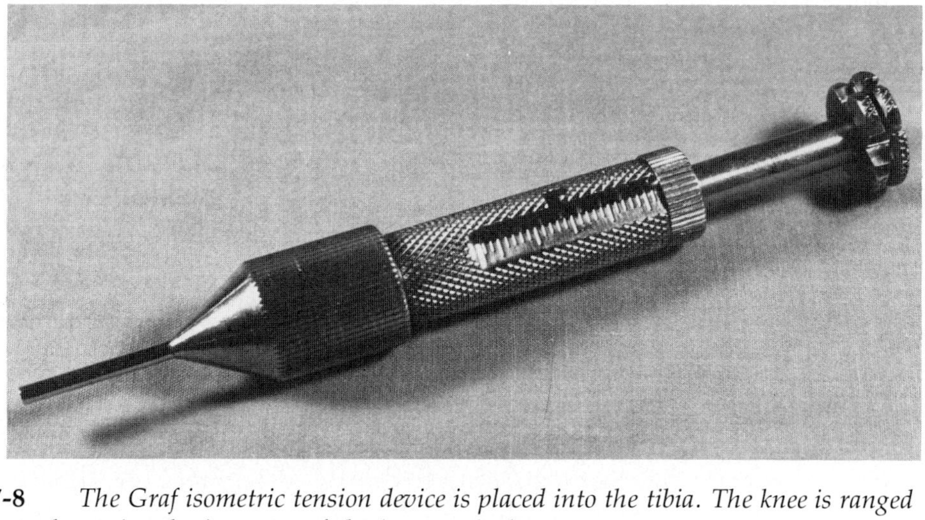

Fig. 17-8 *The Graf isometric tension device is placed into the tibia. The knee is ranged to determine the isometry of the intra-articular suture.*

rior cruciate ligament instrumentation. The functional isometry of the placement is checked by passing a heavy suture through the holes made by the guide wires in the femur and tibia. The suture is anchored against the lateral femoral cortex and the tibial end is passed through the tension device. After anchoring the tibial end to the device, the joint is passed through a range of motion (Fig. 17-8). An acceptable placement is isometric, if a change in length of less than 2 mm on the tension device is observed during the range of motion between 0 and 90 degrees. The most commonly observed error is placement of the femoral point too far anteriorly. With this placement, the tension device will show an increase in length when the knee is flexed. If the anterior cruciate ligament substitute is placed in this anterior location, it will be stretched, it will rupture, or the patient will not regain flexion. Conversely, if the graft is too far posterior, it will lengthen in extension or prevent full extension. Observation of the suture during flexion and extension also suggests if the notch has been adequately debrided. For further explanation concerning isometric placement and the use of the Graf tension device see Chapter 7.

Preparation of the bony tunnels

Following confirmation of their isometric placement, the guide wires are overdrilled using a cannulated reamer or drill (Fig. 17-9). We prefer overdrilling from the outside into the notch. The skin and articular cartilage need to be protected during the reaming portion of the procedure. The articular surfaces are best protected by inserting a large curette through the anteromedial portal in order to cover the tip of the guide wire. This is of particular importance when overdrilling the tibial guide wire.

The diameter of the bony tunnel depends on the material to be used for the anterior cruciate ligament substitution. The reaming or drilling is performed at slow speed to decrease the amount of bone necrosis at the tunnel margins. Avoiding damage to the bone enhances bone ingrowth into the substitute or its bony attachments. Sharp drill bits are important. Starting with a smaller-sized drill bit or reamer and then enlarging the tunnel in increments may facilitate this procedure.

The intra-articular edges of the bony tunnels should then be smoothed using a curette, rasp, or burr to prevent damage to the anterior cruciate ligament substitute during placement or subsequent range of motion. Any remaining soft tissue around the tunnels should also be debrided to facilitate passage of the substitute.

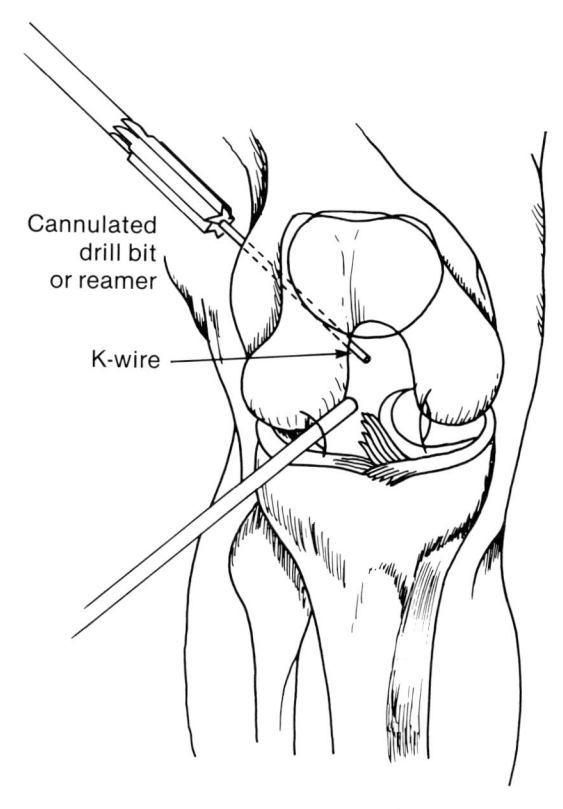

Fig. 17-9 *Reaming over K-wires. The guide wires are overdrilled using a cannulated reamer or drill. Care should be taken to protect the articular surfaces when penetrating the inner cortex.*

Placement and fixation of the anterior cruciate ligament substitute

The anterior cruciate ligament substitute is then prepared for placement into the bony tunnels and the joint. Our preferred method is to pass a rubber catheter through both tunnels and to attach the substitute to the catheter by heavy suture. The catheter is pulled through the joint, guiding the ligament substitute first through the tibial tunnel. Arthroscopic visualization and guidance is then used to place the substitute into the femoral tunnel. The substitute is then held taut manually while the knee is placed through a range of motion under arthroscopic visualization to determine if an impingement exists. The substitute is then anchored to the femur and tibia with the knee in 20 degrees of flexion. If the center of the graft has been placed at the isometric point, the knee flexion is not critical; however, the bulk of the anterior cruciate ligament usually is taut in extension. The substitute must be securely anchored to allow for early range of motion. Screw fixation is preferred over staples in order to decrease the amount of tenderness at the fixation points postoperatively. A properly positioned graft allows movement easily through a full range of motion. The desired stability must be present at this point.

Extra-articular reconstruction

If the surgeon prefers, extra-articular surgery may be performed after the substitute is anchored. We use an iliotibial band tenodesis, which is usually performed through the same lateral incision needed to perform the cruciate substitution procedure. It is important that the extra-articular procedure not require a large incision or immobilization if one is to benefit from the arthroscopic anterior cruciate ligament surgery.

The tourniquet, if used, should be deflated so that the bleeding can be controlled. Drains are placed in the lateral incision, if necessary, and the postoperative care depends on the type of substitute used. If possible, early postoperative motion should be encouraged in order to decrease adhesions and enhance articular cartilage nutrition. Early active quadriceps exercises in the last 45 degrees of extension are usually avoided in the biological graft; however, passive motion should be tolerated if the center of the graft is isometric.

Summary

The technique of arthroscopic substitution of the anterior cruciate ligament is rapidly evolving. The technique at this time is demanding, and the surgeon should be experienced in arthroscopic techniques before undertaking the anterior cruciate substitution. Patient morbidity is decreased with a technically well done arthroscopic procedure. This is primarily the result of the use of smaller skin incisions and of not disturbing the extensor mechanism.

The principles of the technique should be followed in a stepwise fashion. An accurate diagnosis of the instability and injuries to associated structures should be established before any surgical intervention. Meniscal and articular cartilage lesions should be addressed first. The intercondylar notch requires adequate debridement and enlargement. The isometric point must be accurately determined and the bony tunnels made in the femur and tibia to reflect the isometric points. The substitute material should be anchored securely to the femur and tibia to allow for early range of motion. Early motion helps prevent postoperative arthrofibrosis and associated extensor mechanism pain syndrome.

Techniques and instrumentation for arthroscopic reconstruction of the anterior cruciate ligament will continue to improve in the future. The technology for placement of the substitute is currently quite satisfactory, but the decision as to which substitute is best is still to be determined. Only after long-term follow-up studies will this determination be possible.

REFERENCES

1. Hewson, G.F.: Drill guides for improving accuracy in anterior cruciate ligament repair and reconstruction, Clin. Orthop. **172**:119-124, 1983.

2. Rosenberg, T.: Arthroscopic technique for anterior cruciate ligament surgery, Technical Bulletin, Acufex Microsurgical, Inc., Norwood, Mass., 1984.

18
Knee braces

DAVID DREZ, Jr.

A *brace* can be defined as a device that functions to clasp or connect objects firmly together so they can resist deforming forces as well as provide support for weakened structures. Many braces have been and are being manufactured in hopes of performing these functions for the knee joint. Prior to the seminar report on knee braces by the American Academy of Orthopaedic Surgeons in 1985,[1] limited objective data was available regarding the ability of knee braces to perform these functions.

This chapter discusses the role knee braces have in *preventing* injuries to the anterior cruciate ligament, how they can be used in *rehabilitating* the knee after repair or reconstruction of the anterior cruciate ligament, and the role they may play in *controlling the laxity* that results from injuries to the anterior cruciate ligament in active individuals. Much of the material presented is data obtained as a result of the American Academy of Orthopaedic Surgeon's 1985 seminar report on knee braces.[1]

Prophylactic knee braces

A prophylactic knee brace is one that is designed to prevent or reduce the severity of injuries to the ligaments of the knee. There is considerable controversy on how effective these braces are in preventing such injuries.

Clinical studies have been presented by Hewson,[3] Rovere,[7] and Taft[8] that evaluate the use of prophylactic knee braces in college football players. Despite the fact that these studies show disagreement regarding the effectiveness of prophylactic braces in reducing injuries to the medial collateral ligament, there was no data pre-

Address request for reprints to: David Drez, Jr., M.D., 2615 Enterprise Boulevard, Lake Charles, LA 70601.

sented showing any protection of the knee against injuries to the anterior cruciate ligament.

Biomechanical investigations performed by Baker[2] and Paulos[5,6] demonstrated that a straight lateral bar brace in varus aligned extremities could produce preloading of the medial and cruciate ligaments. Such preloading would make these ligaments more susceptible to injury by reducing the energy required for them to fail. If these data are clinically significant, there should be an increase in ligament sprains (medial and cruciate) in varus aligned extremities when the straight lateral bar brace is used.

It can thus be concluded that prophylactic knee braces have not been shown to prevent or reduce the severity of injuries to the anterior cruciate ligament. Furthermore, if biomechanical data prove clinically applicable, some prophylactic braces may result in an *increased* incidence of anterior cruciate ligament injuries.

Rehabilitative knee braces

A rehabilitative knee brace is designed to allow protected and controlled motion of knee joints that have been treated operatively or nonoperatively following a ligamentous injury. The rewards of maintaining motion in any joint are understood. The concerns regarding rehabilitative braces are whether they can effectively control passive motion and the joint displacing forces that active knee motion creates. If such motion and forces are not controlled, loads will be provoked that can stretch out or disrupt healing ligamentous tissue. Rehabilitative knee braces have been designed in hopes of controlling such loads while allowing beneficial joint motion.

After a repair or reconstruction of the anterior cruciate ligament, it is necessary to prevent active knee extension past 40 to 60 degrees. Limiting extension in this range would eradicate the anterior tibial displacement produced by active quadriceps contraction. Moynes[1] presented a preliminary study showing that the knee joint extended 15 to 20 degrees more than the setting on the rehabilitative knee brace hinges.

Whether or not rehabilitative knee braces can effectively resist anteroposterior tibial motion is unresolved. Hoffman[4] reported that one of the rehabilitative knee braces he tested was better than the others in providing stability to static anterior forces. This study is subject to error because there was no control over the tightness of brace application.

There is little disagreement that rehabilitative knee braces are more convenient for both the patient and the surgeon. They are easily applied and adjusted, are light weight, and provide easy access to the skin. Stops on the hinges permit active and passive motion to be limited. However, caution must be exercised when allowing motion in rehabilitative knee braces since more knee joint motion than expected will occur and since there is little static anteroposterior control obtained.

Functional knee braces

Functional knee braces are those braces designed to provide stability for knees rendered unstable by injuries to their ligamentous structures. These braces provide static knee stability to control the excessive laxities resulting from these ligamentous injuries.

Clinical studies[1] have been performed to evaluate the effectiveness of functional knee braces in patients with excessive laxity secondary to incompetence of the anterior cruciate ligament. Such patients reported increased knee joint stability and fewer or no episodes of giving way with the use of functional knee braces. The greatest benefits were in those individuals with less severe degrees of laxity and in those who placed less severe demands on their knee joint.

Biomechanical studies[1] evaluating the ability of functional knee braces to provide static stability in anterior cruciate deficient knees have also been performed. These studies showed that under low loading conditions the majority of functional knee braces did limit excessive anterior tibial translation. However, under conditions of high loading that more closely simulate high activity levels, little or no control of anterior tibial translation occurred.

Functional knee braces may have a place in the treatment of patients with excessive laxity secondary to an injury of the anterior cruciate ligament. It must be remembered that these braces do not restore normal laxity to the anterior cruciate deficient knee and that they are best used in a program that combines proper rehabilitation with activity modification that avoids twisting and cutting activities.

Summary

Many braces have been designed to restore normal stability to the knee with excessive laxity secondary to an injury of the anterior cruciate ligament. Braces for short-term use (i.e., rehabilitative knee braces) are designed to control anterior tibial translation in the anterior cruciate deficient knee that has undergone operative treatment. Braces for long-term use (i.e., functional knee braces) are designed to control anterior tibial translation in the anterior cruciate deficient knee of individuals engaging in various activities. None of these braces have been shown capable of restoring normal laxity to the anterior cruciate deficient knee.

Prophylactic knee braces have been designed to prevent or reduce the severity of injuries to the ligaments of the knee. None of these braces have been proved effective in protecting the knee against injuries to the anterior cruciate ligament. If biomechanical testing proves clinically significant, such lateral braces in varus aligned extremities may result in an increased incidence of cruciate ligament injuries because of preloading of the ligaments.

There is indeed a great deal of clinical and biomechanical research needed to evaluate the effectiveness of currently available knee braces. In addition, such research is also needed to develop braces for the knee that may be more effective in preventing and controlling excessive laxities.

REFERENCES

1. American Academy of Orthopaedic Surgeons: Knee braces. Seminar Report, 1985, The Academy.
2. Baker, B.E., et al.: A biomechanical study of the static stabilizing effect of knee braces used for medial stability. Presented at the American Academy of Orthopaedic Surgeons Annual Meeting, New Orleans, Louisiana, February 1986.
3. Hewson, G.F., Mendini, R.A., and Wang, J.B.: Prophylactic knee bracing in college football. Presented at the Eleventh Annual Meeting of American Orthopadic Society for Sports Medicine. Nashville, Tennessee, July 1985.
4. Hoffmann, A.: Am. J. Sports Med. **12**(5):371-374, 1984.
5. Paulos, L., France, P., and Rosenberg, T.: The biomechanics of lateral knee bracing for prevention of valgus ligamentous injuries. Presented at the Eleventh Annual Meeting of the American Orthopaedic Society for Sports Medicine Nashville, Tennessee, July 1985.
6. Paulos, L., et al.: Preventive lateral braces in football: do they really work? Presented at the Annual Meeting of the American Academy of Orthopaedic Surgeons, New Orleans, Louisiana, February 1986.
7. Rovere, G.D., Haupt, H.A., and Yates, C.S.: Prophylactic knee bracing in college football. Presented at the Eleventh Annual Meeting of American Orthopaedic Society for Sports Medicine, Nashville, Tennessee, July 1985.
8. Taft, T.N., Hunter, S.L., and Funderburk, C.H.: Preventative lateral knee bracing in football. Presented at the Eleventh Annual Meeting of American Orthopaedic Society for Sports Medicine. Nashville, Tennessee, July 1985.

19

Rehabilitation after anterior cruciate ligament surgery

LONNIE E. PAULOS

FRANK CORRY PAYNE III

THOMAS D. ROSENBERG

A successful outcome from the surgical correction of anterior instability in the knee is a team approach that includes the physician, a physical therapist, and the patient. A chain of treatment decisions based on the skills, knowledge, and cooperation of these individuals must be orchestrated in a manner that will produce the optimal result (Fig. 19-1). This chain of treatment decisions begins with patient assessment and selection and ends with rehabilitation. Each link in this chain of treatment decisions is vitally important to the final outcome, and the consistency of the treatment protocol will be based on the weakest link in the chain. It is for this reason that postoperative rehabilitation must be considered equally important to the other aspects of treatment.

There are many causes for failure after knee ligament surgery; however, complications such as residual laxity, articular cartilage degeneration, knee contracture, and permanent muscle atrophy can all be directly related to the rehabilitation prescription employed.

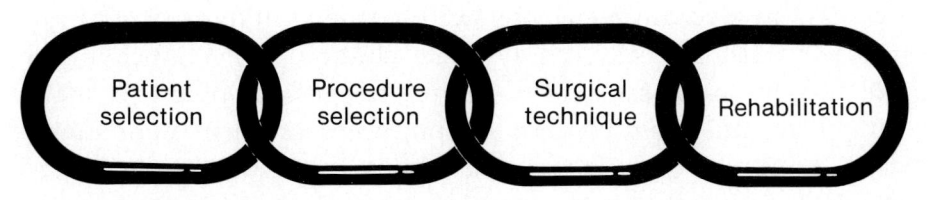

Fig. 19-1 *Rehabilitation is a critical link in the chain of treatment decisions regarding knees with anterior instability.*

Rehabilitation principles

There are two basic principles that govern the prescription for the rehabilitation link in our chain of treatment decisions. The first principle is: immobility effects must be minimized. The second principle is: healing tissues must never be overloaded. These two principles should be properly balanced, one against the other, to help achieve the optimal result.

Immobility effects

The adverse effects of prolonged immobility and disuse on the supporting structures of the knee can be significant. Not only do these effects begin immediately after injury, but the changes produced can be irreversible. Because of the extended time required for ligament healing and maturation, it is an absolute necessity that the rehabilitation program begin long before ligament healing has occurred. To begin rehabilitation *after* ligament healing would guarantee permanent disuse effects. The exercise prescription must be designed to minimize immobility and yet protect against overloading the healing tissues.

Immobility can lead to joint contracture secondary to changes in the periarticular tissues. Little change occurs before 4 weeks of immobility; however, beyond 6 weeks both mechanical and histochemical changes occur. Noted is a decrease in glycoaminoglycans, a decrease in water content, and an increase in collagen cross linking.[1-4,41] These changes are manifested mechanically in that the torque required to move the knee joint is increased up to ten times over the normally required force.

Concomitant changes occur in the cartilaginous surfaces of the joint and in their supportive subchondral bone. This "chondral unit" requires motion for nutrition and weight bearing stresses to maintain biomechanical integrity. Once this mechanical stress and/or motion is prevented, there is an alteration in cartilage fluid dynamics. Histochemically this leads to a decrease in metachromasia, a decrease in glycoaminoglycans, and a change in hydration of the cartilage.[38] Histologically, chondrocyte clumping and subchondral bone atrophy are observed.[16,19] These changes are noted to begin within days of the initiation of immobility and are permanent after 8 weeks of immobility. In laboratory studies, these early ground substance changes can be reversed through the initiation of motion.[16,17,35] If, however, overloading secondary to inappropriate rehabilitation creates disruption of the "chondral unit" microstructure, then irreversible, permanent, and progressive cartilage degeneration begins.

The ligament-bone complex reacts to immobility as a unit also. Not only does the ligament weaken, but its bone attachment site does as well. It has been demonstrated that after 8 weeks of total immobility of the knee there can be a 40% decrease in strength of normal ligament-bone units as well as a 30% decrease in stiffness. Even more alarming is the fact that before a 90% return of strength for a normal ligament unit can be expected, the joint must be reconditioned for at least 1 year.[30]

Equally impressive are the changes that can be observed in the periarticular musculature secondary to disuse and immobility. By 5 weeks of immobility there is a decrease in oxidative enzymes such as succinyldehydrogenase, and there appears to be a selective atrophy of Type I (slow twitch or red) muscle fibers. Accurate calculations of muscle mass reveal a 30% to 47% decrease in total mass.[14,15,21] Interestingly, other parameters affecting the rate of muscle atrophy after knee surgery have been noted. For example, joint position has been determined to play a role. Muscles immobilized in a shortened position actually atrophy more quickly. Also, joint distention, which leads to neuromuscular inhibition, can lead to an increased rate of atrophy.

Healing parameters

To prevent overloading of healing tissues it is imperative that the rate of healing as well as the forces associated with various levels of activity be understood. Unfortunately, a great deal of information is still necessary before these questions can be totally answered.

We now know that ligament healing time is extraordinarily longer than originally supposed. We know this by extrapolating experimental results from animal studies. As can be seen in Table 19-1, no study to date has shown a return to normal strength of grafted or repaired ligament tissue. Although graft strength and mechanical properties do improve with time, there appears to be a great reduction in mechanical strength and stiffness in collagen tissues, especially when used intra-articularly. These studies represent various animal models, all of which have higher metabolic rates than humans. Assuming that the metabolic rate is directly associated with collagen turnover and maturation, it can be concluded that the anterior cruciate ligament in the human requires at least 24

TABLE 19-1 / Return of anterior cruciate substitute strength*

AUTHOR	ANIMAL MODEL	EXPERIMENTAL FOLLOW-UP TIME (MONTHS)	MAXIMAL LIGAMENT STRENGTH (% OF ORIGINAL)
Alm[5]	Dog	6	50
Cabaud[9]	Dog	8	52
Clancey[10]	Primate	12	52
Gelberman[18]	Dog	3	40
Hirsch[26]	Rabbit	6	50
Kennedy[27]	Dog	6	40
Noyes[30]	Dog	4	50

*To date, no experimental study has shown more than a 52% return of substitute strength after anterior cruciate ligament replacement.

months to reach maturity and that it probably never returns to full strength.

A number of surgical and rehabilitative modifications have been developed in the past decade that enable patients to accelerate their recovery before maturation of the healing ligament. Cast braces, neuromuscular stimulators, variable speed dynometers, and functional braces, all contribute to a faster and safer recovery for the patient. Surgical modifications have also occurred in which the actual healing time may be reduced such as with the use of vascular pedicle grafts or initial ligament strengths increased by using biological or synthetic stents. Improved surgical techniques that use stronger grafts that are more securely fixed and in an isometric position allow a safer and more complete range of motion to be obtained early. Even more exciting is the ability to completely obviate the need for healing by using synthetic substitutes.

In the early rehabilitation phases three modes of mechanical failure must be avoided to prevent ligament disruption. The first is excessive overload associated with abnormal joint displacements (i.e., a fall or twist). A second form of failure is secondary to cyclic forces that create a fatigue-like failure at points of high stress. Avoiding repetitive, extreme motions until ligament-osseous healing has occurred is important here. The third form of failure, overelongation (i.e., stretching past the elastic limit) must also be avoided. Although surgical technique is probably the most important aspect of preventing this type of failure, high forces over an

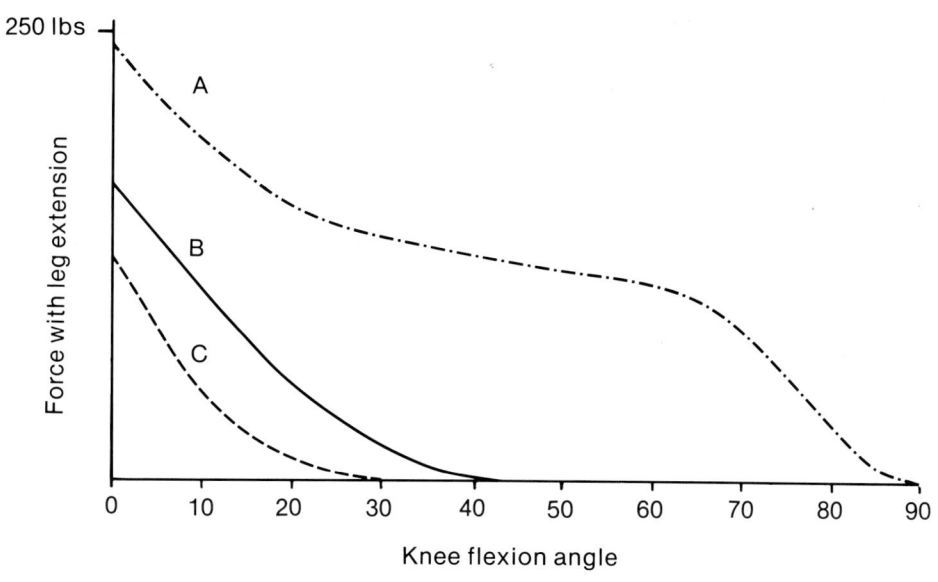

Fig. 19-2 *The anterior cruciate ligament resists anterior drawer forces beginning at approximately 40 degrees of flexion. These forces increase dramatically near complete knee extension and with the addition of distal leg weights. (A, Quadriceps force; B, anterior cruciate force with 7 pound weight on foot; C, anterior cruciate force during active leg extension.)*

extended period of time can also produce this effect even if the ligament repair is isometric. For example, leg extension exercises create an effective anterior tibial drawer.[6,20,33] Fig. 19-2 shows that anterior cruciate ligament strain increases rapidly when extending the knee from 30 degrees of flexion to full extension.

Very little is known about the forces and strains placed on the anterior cruciate ligament during various activities. Changes in knee positions associated with quadriceps function have been shown to change strain rates dramatically.[6,20,33] Others have calculated resultant forces that may be seen during running, jumping, and ramp walking.[28,39] Given weaker tissues with limited healing potential, it is understandable how various exercise modalities and activities may lead to eventual graft deformation and resultant pathological joint laxity (Fig. 19-3).

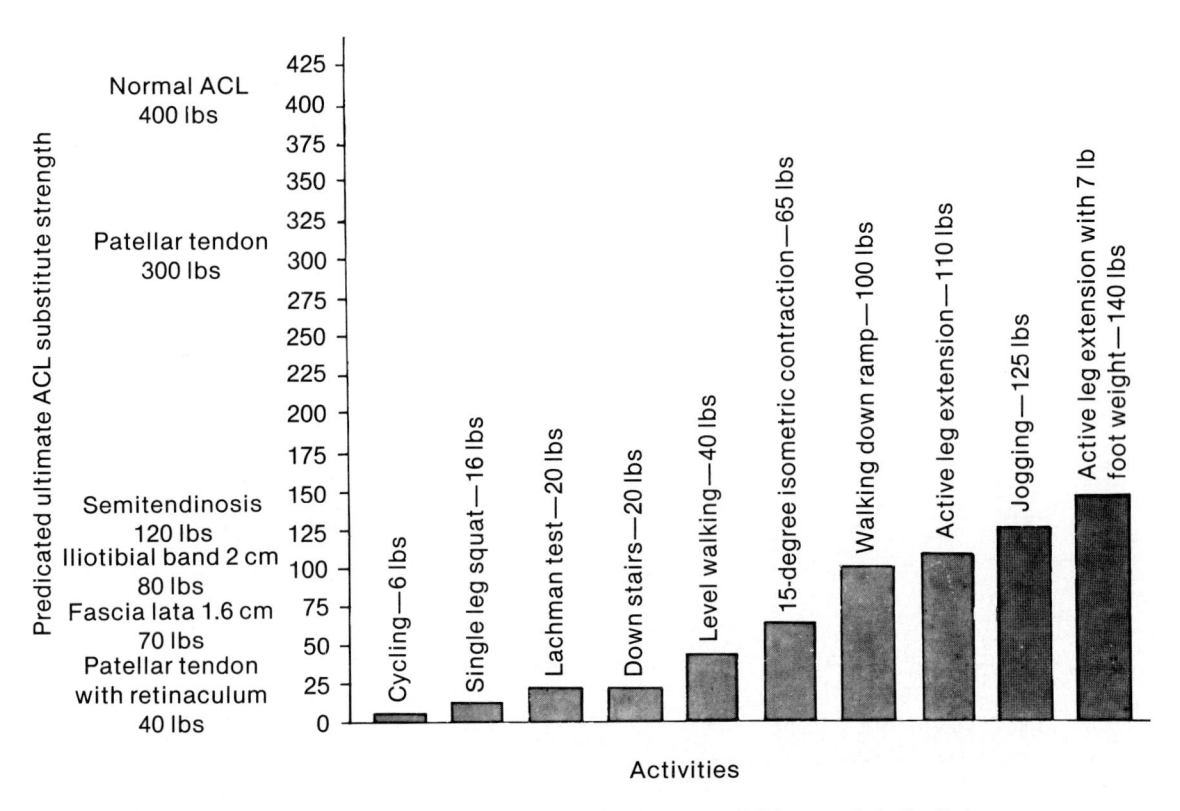

Fig. 19-3 Anterior drawer forces are constantly present with normal daily living activities. This figure compares the expected ultimate anterior cruciate ligament graft strengths for commonly used replacement tissues (50% of original strength at time of insertion) to anterior drawer forces that represent calculated and or measured forces on the anterior cruciate ligament during specific activities. Calculations are based on a person weighing 150 pounds. Anterior cruciate ligament substitute strengths are based on published data by Noyes, et al.[23] Anterior drawer forces on the anterior cruciate ligament are based on published work by Morrison et al., Smidt et al., Henning, and Paulos et al.[25]

Variables influencing the rehabilitation prescription

It is vitally important that the surgical procedure employed and the surgical techniques used be considered along with a number of other variables when prescribing the rehabilitation protocol.

Anterior cruciate ligament substitution

The type of procedure used in achieving anterior stability establishes the foundation on which the rehabilitation prescription is written. The difference in tissue healing capacities between intra-articular and extra-articular substitution is tremendous. Also, when the joint is not violated, such as in an extra-articular substitution, the effects of immobility are better tolerated. The healing capacity of peri-articular tissues secondary to a ready reservoir of vascular supply is greatly enhanced over intra-articular tissues. In contrast, intra-articular substitution demands a number of rehabilitation and surgical modifications in order to protect the repair during the prolonged healing and remodeling phases. After violating the interior of a knee joint, adverse immobility effects appear more frequently. The higher incidence of chondromalacia patellae, knee contracture, and adhesions are well documented when comparing intra-articular to extra-articular surgical results.

If a suture repair of an acutely torn anterior cruciate ligament is performed, the fixation of the remaining ligament fibers is at best tenuous and the strength of the already damaged fibers is extremely low. It is perhaps this type of repair that demands the most protection and stands the greatest risk of suffering secondary disuse and immobility effects. If a suture repair is augmented with a "stent" of either biological or synthetic tissue, then a greater overall strength is achieved immediately following surgery, usually permitting earlier and safer mobilization. Combining this type of repair with an extra-articular substitution may further enhance the capability of the ligament repair to withstand early mobilization.

A number of different biological and synthetic tissues have been employed for the direct intra-articular replacement of the anterior cruciate ligament. The mechanical properties of these substitutes have been examined in detail and offer interesting insights into graft selection.[31] Comparing graft strength and stiffness to the normal anterior cruciate ligament, tissues such as patellar retinaculum, fascia lata, and iliotibial band are extremely weak with no margin of safety. Given an initial low strength in combination with poor healing capacity, it would not be surprising to observe inconsistent surgical results when these tissues are used. Other grafts such as patellar tendon, semitendinosis, and combined substitutes such as the fascia lata plus the iliotibial band provide near normal strength with similar mechanical properties. Again, however, healing capacity will reduce the eventual strength of these tissues as well. It is our opinion that no matter which biological substitute is selected for intra-articular anterior cruciate replacement, an inordinate length of time will be necessary for healing and maturation. Also, every biological graft must undergo necrotic remodeling, thereby rendering it extremely weak sometime during the rehabilitation period. For this reason, carefully designed rehabilitation and surgical technique modifications are necessary whenever biological substitutes are used.

For reasons discussed previously, a strong emphasis has been placed on developing a ligament replacement for the anterior cruciate ligament with synthetic materials. The potential advantages of synthetics are great and include excellent strength, no harvest morbidity, and ease of placement. Initial results were extremely erratic because of poor ligament material properties; however, with recent advances in biomaterials as well as a better understanding of the biomechanics of anterior cruciate ligament function, early surgical results are improved over those reported initially. Well-fixed, high-strength synthetic grafts demand very little, if any, modification in surgical and rehabilitation techniques and provide the most favorable situation in which to avoid disuse and immobility effects.

Anterior cruciate substitute fixation

With the use of high-strength biological or synthetic anterior cruciate ligament substitutes, failures from ligament disruption or elongation will be minimized. However, fixation of these high-strength substitutes to bone emerges as the next major concern. Despite the use of high-strength anterior cruciate ligament grafts, ultimate ligament failure will occur if fixation techniques are tenous or create stress risers. Several recent studies have been conducted that look specifically at the fixation of various types of tissues to bone.[8,11] The use of sutures and buttons have proved to be the least reliable of fixation devices. Staples, although showing good fixation, actually crush tissue leading to subsequent pressure necrosis and failure. Newer devices that have increased cross-sectional areas and screw fixation have proved the most beneficial in fixing soft tissues; the use of interference bone screws have proved most beneficial in securing bone to bone. Extended protection with rehabilitation modifications would be necessary with the use of the more conventional devices such as sutures and staples.

It is a well established fact that those grafts that employ bone to bone healing or that facilitate bony ingrowth demonstrate higher pull-out strengths than those grafts that heal by slow incorporation of soft tissue around bony surfaces or through intraosseous tunnels.[40] By employing biological replacements that rely on bone to bone attachment site fixation and healing, rehabilitation modifications become less necessary. In contrast, those procedures that use tissues such as fascia lata or semitendinosis that are fixed in the over-the-top position have a slower incorporation and fixation rate and thereby require more protection.

Anterior cruciate ligament substitute placement

The use of high-strength grafts that are well secured to bone are extremely important in allowing rehabilitation techniques that will minimize disuse effects. However, regardless of how strong or well fixed the graft is, if it is placed *nonisometrically,* a subsequent ligament failure or knee contracture will occur. Nonisometric placement of weak tissues will ultimately lead to elongation and pathological laxity. Nonisometric placement of strong biological grafts or synthetic grafts will lead to "joint capture" with loss of motion and subsequent arthrosis (Fig. 19-4).

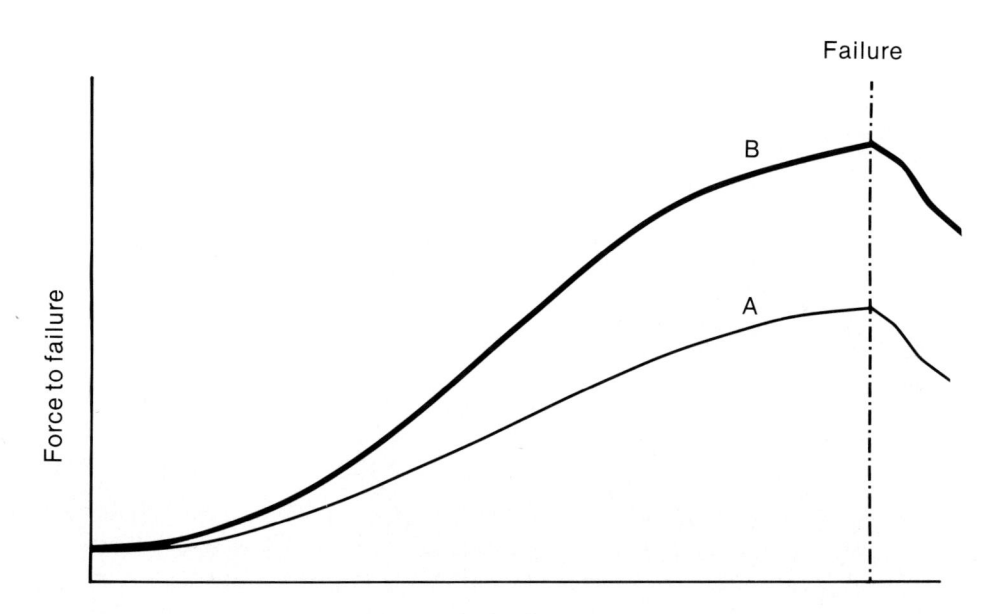

Fig. 19-4 *Although there has been an increased emphasis on using stronger tissues for anterior cruciate ligament replacements, rehabilitation can still be adversely effected if a strong replacement is secured non-isometrically. Eventual ligament failure or persistent knee contracture will result. As seen here, a strong graft (B) will fail at the same percent elongation as a weaker graft (A). Non-isometric ligament placement leads to increased graft strain and elongation, as well as increased forces necessary to achieve a normal range of motion.*

If an isometric position of the anterior cruciate ligament replacement (either intra-articular or extra-articular) is assured at the time of surgery, then the patient's ability to regain motion quickly with rehabilitation is assured. Nonisometric placement of biological tissues requires more protected motion as well as a more prolonged rehabilitation protocol that is designed to regain extension and flexion slowly. This type of repair will present more difficulties in achieving a normal range of motion and, in fact, usually requires that the patient never achieve a normal range of motion so as to maintain stability. Also, anesthetic knee manipulation, if required, may disrupt this type of repair.

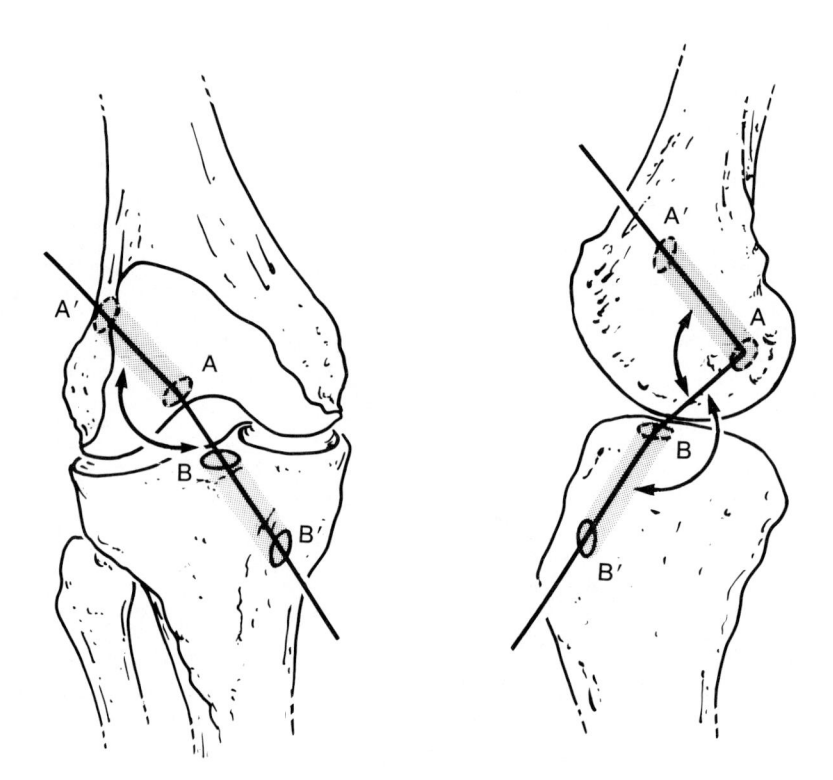

Fig. 19-5 *Excessive angulation at tunnel entrance (A and B) and exit sites (A' and B') can lead to stress concentration and ligament failure. The angle formed between A' = A and B' = B if excessive leads to stress concentration at point A or B. Tissue or bone ingrowth that dampens this effect occurs inconsistently; therefore the tunnel diversion angle must be minimized and repetitive or cyclic knee motions through a complete range of motion should be avoided early in the rehabilitation period.*

The tension under which the ligament is placed in the knee is also critical. If normal joint laxity is obliterated through excessive tension on the anterior cruciate ligament replacement, then the normal anteroposterior gliding motions necessary for flexion and extension are obliterated with an ensuing knee contracture and arthrosis. It is for this reason that the rehabilitation protocol should include passive joint motions in all planes to assure more normal joint function.

Also critical in our ability to obtan an early range of motion and perform repetitive exercises is the angle at which the anterior cruciate replacement enters and leaves the intra-articular portions of the knee and is then fixed extra-articularly to the tibia and femur. This "tunnel divergence angle" is critical early on when repetitive motions may produce stress risers at the point of contact to tunnel edges (Fig. 19-5). After incorporation of the graft in bony tunnels this concern becomes less important. However, if only fibrous union is achieved, then the tunnel divergence effect will be prolonged. Those procedures employing excessive tunnel divergence angles must be protected longer to allow bony ingrowth so as to minimize stress risers at tunnel edges or to prevent tunnel drift in the case of synthetic grafts.

Concomitant surgery

When other ligaments have been repaired concomitantly with the anterior cruciate ligament, significant modifications in the rehabilitation program must be made. In general, more prolonged immobility and protected weight bearing are necessary, thus increasing the incidence of disuse and immobility effects. Here, as in other cases, significant modifications in surgical technique and rehabilitation protocols must be made to minimize these effects. In general, if a concomitant collateral ligament repair or reconstruction can be accomplished isometrically, then an early range of motion can still be instituted. This is usually the case when the collateral ligament can be repaired by recessing the remaining tissue into the bone at the normal attachment site. If the ligament is advanced or imbricated, then an early range of motion is contraindicated. In our experience early weight bearing is not detrimental with medial collateral ligament surgery but is contraindicated with lateral collateral or arcuate ligament surgery. Our observation is supported biomechanically in that weight bearing leads to medial compartment compression (protecting the medial collateral ligament repair) but lateral compartment distraction (stretching the lateral collateral ligament repair).[39]

Concomitant meniscal repairs and patellofemoral realignment also require special modifications in the rehabilitation prescription. It is imperative that pre-existent patellofemoral instability and/or arthrosis be identified before anterior cruciate ligament reconstruction. Definite modifications in the selection of the surgical procedure, the application of surgical techniques, and the rehabilitation prescrption are necessary in this situation. Every effort must be made to use strong grafts that are fixed well and isometrically placed so as to allow an early range of motion and weight bearing.

Patient variables

Modifications in the rehabilitation prescription must also be made based on the size of the patient, intended use of the limb, and presence of hyperelasticity. Also, knee alignment as to varus-valgus position is extremely important when considering combined procedures that include anterior cruciate ligament and medial or lateral collateral ligament reconstructions. Patients who are heavier or who demonstrate hyperlaxity will require longer periods of protection (including crutch walking and bracing) than is normally the case. In combined anterior cruciate and lateral collateral ligament injuries, prolonged non-weight bearing is advised particularly when genu varum is present because of increased joint distraction forces as previously discussed.

Patients who are not available for close supervision or extensive rehabilitation should have procedures performed that are less risky from the standpoint of knee contracture or atrophy despite the fact that these procedures may produce a less stable knee.

The rehabilitation prescription

In the past, rehabilitation programs have been designed and compartmentalized based on time constraints for healing ligaments. Although this would be an ideal way in which to prescribe the rehabilitation protocol, it is arbitrary and inaccurate because of the lack of data concerning the healing parameters for ligamentous tissues. For this reason, we believe that it is more accurate to divide the rehabilitation prescription into phases or components based on performance goals with the time constraints for each phase being "approximated" by the many factors discussed earlier. To distin-

Rehabilitation after anterior cruciate ligament surgery

UNIVERSAL KNEE REHABILITATION FORM

Patient: _____ Date: _____ Physician: _____ Surgery Date: _____

Surgical Procedure: _____

Physical Therapist: _____ Post Op Week (POW): _____

PHASE I – PREOPERATIVE
A. TESTING
- ☐ Strength test
- ☐ Instrumented laxity test
- ☐ Range of motion
- ☐ Extremity girths
- ☐ Functional Brace: _____ type; Motion = _____ ° to _____ ° flexion; Other _____
- ☐ Other: _____

B. INSTRUCTIONS
- ☐ Crutch training
- ☐ % _____ weight bearing
- ☐ Neuromuscular Stimulator
- ☐ P.R.E. instructions

PHASE II – IMMOBILITY
- ☐ Postoperative brace: _____ type;   Locked flexion angle _____ °
- ☐ Immobility ends on _____ POW: ☐ Other: _____

PHASE III – MOTION
Begin Passive Range of Motion on _____ POW; Begin Active Range of Motion on _____ POW
- ☐ Passive ROM from _____ ° to _____ ° flexion; Increase _____ ° extension and _____ ° flexion per week
- ☐ Home CPM: Range _____ ° to _____ ° flexion; Frequency _____ /day; Duration _____ hrs / session
- ☐ Active ROM from _____ ° to _____ ° flexion; Increase _____ ° extension and _____ ° flexion per week
- ☐ Range of motion goal: _____ ° to _____ ° flexion; by _____ POW
- ☐ Needs Manipulation   ☐ Apply extension drop-out cast for _____ days; ☐ Other _____

PHASE IV – PROGRESSIVE WEIGHT BEARING
Begin weight bearing on _____ POW: Start with _____ % body weight; Increase _____ % per week
- ☐ Stay on one crutch (75%) until _____ POW ☐ Use functional brace on _____ POW ☐ Other _____

PHASE V – ISOMETRIC
- ☐ Isometrics   ☐ Spectrum isometrics   ☐ Straight leg raises   ☐ Patella glides and tilts
- ☐ Tens   ☐ R.O.B. program   ☐ Other _____
- ☐ Neuromuscular Stimulation: ☐ Hamstrings   ☐ Quadriceps   ☐ Frequency _____ /day; Duration _____ hrs/session

PHASE VI – ISOTONIC
Start concentric PRE on _____ POW   Start eccentric PRE on _____ POW; Body position: ☐ Supine — Prone
- ☐ Knee Extension PRE: Increase to _____ lbs.; from _____ ° to _____ ° flexion until _____ POW; then advance PRN; No limits on weight from _____ ° to _____ ° flexion. ☐ Other _____
- ☐ Knee Flexion PRE: Increase to _____ lbs.; from _____ ° to _____ ° flexion until _____ POW; then advance PRN; No limits on weight from _____ ° to _____ ° flexion. ☐ Other _____

PHASE VII – ISOKINETIC
Start on _____ POW; Pad placement: High – Low tibia; Body position: Supine — Prone
- ☐ Patellar restraining brace   ☐ Burn outs   ☐ High speed only   ☐ Eccentric work   ☐ Other _____
- ☐ ROM restriction: High speed performance from _____ ° to _____ ° flexion; Low speed from _____ ° flexion

PHASE VIII — ENDURANCE
Start cycling on _____ POW
- ☐ Stationary only   ☐ Unlimited   ☐ Adjust seat: High — Low   ☐ Patellar Restraint
Start swimming on _____ POW
- ☐ Straight leg kicks only   ☐ Pool jogging   ☐ Unlimited   ☐ Functional brace
Start stationary tract on _____ POW   ☐ Other: _____

PHASE IX – RUNNING
Begin progressive running on _____ POW (If no swelling or pain and 75% strength)
- ☐ Stretch cords   ☐ Trampoline   ☐ Functional brace   ☐ Level ground only   ☐ Pogo stick
Progressive sprints on _____ POW; Progressive cutting on _____ POW; Progressive jumping on _____ POW
- ☐ Other: _____

PHASE X – SPORTS
Begin sports participation on _____ POW
- ☐ Skills drills only   ☐ Functional brace   ☐ Sports restrictions: _____
- ☐ Other: _____

Fig. 19-6   *Universal Knee Rehabilitation Form.*

guish rehabilitation phases by unknown time constraints is not only arbitrary but confusing. Many of the phases are conducted concurrently and must be coordinated separately for each patient and specific surgery. By writing a rehabilitation prescription based on phases, individual time constraints can then be built into the exercise prescription as it applies to that particular phase and that particular patient. Depending on the variables discussed previously, these time constraints will be different for each phase and patient, and the prescription will allow an easy way to prescribe these changes without confusing the therapist or patient. A general rehabilitation outline can be employed for all patients and then modified based on the desires of the physician (Fig. 19-6). There are ten essential phases to the rehabilitation prescription that should be addressed for each patient and surgery.

Preoperative phase

The rehabilitation protocol begins preoperatively. The protocol should be explained to the patient, including the importance of rehabilitation and the role the patient must play. The patient must understand that his cooperation and effort are necessary for success. Preoperative instructions, including exercises for the perioperative period, instructions for the neuromuscular stimulator, and instructions for the use of the rehabilitative brace, are given at this time. Counseling as to the mechanism of injury, pathomechanics of reinjury, and importance of activity modification is given. Preoperative tests are performed, including instrumental laxity testing, strength testing, and measuring range of motion and thigh girths. The therapist fits the patient for the rehabilitative brace for later use. With elective surgery, a strengthening program is started that consists of isotonic and isokinetic exercise. In the acute injury, straight leg raising exercises and isometrics are instituted to help preserve muscle tone.

Immobility phase

The surgeon's goal should be to eliminate the immobility phase through appropriate anterior cruciate ligament graft selection, placement, and fixation. However, on occasion this cannot be achieved, and it is necessary to immobilize the limb for a brief period of time. This is necessary in order to control forces and prevent disruption of a suture line or ligament attachment site. The most frequent reason to use immobility is when concomitant surgery is performed, especially multiple ligament repairs and meniscal repair. The reason for this is that the ability to reconstruct or repair multiple ligaments isometrically is difficult, and meniscal repairs are more easily disrupted by joint reaction forces produced with motion.

The immobility phase should never exceed 6 weeks and is generally no longer than 3 weeks. The immobilization angle will vary according to the surgery performed, but for anterior cruciate ligament reconstruction or repair we prefer to immobilize at 40 degrees of flexion, the angle at which the anterior cruciate ligament is most relaxed.[6] Equally important is the fact that in this flexed position the anterior cruciate ligament graft or repair is not stressed with quadriceps activity.[6,20,33] When immobilization is necessary, we prefer to use a rehabilitative knee brace that permits wound inspection, passive patellar mobilization, and progressive changes in the active range of motion.

Motion phase

The motion phase of rehabilitation begins as soon after surgery as possible. Strong repairs or grafts, isometrically placed and securely attached, can begin immediate *passive* range of motion. The judicious use of continuous passive motion devices will aid in preventing knee contracture and articular surface changes. The passive range of motion permitted is determined at the time of surgery when the repair or reconstruction can be observed or the tension measured as the knee is ranged. The graft is actually stronger at this point than it will ever be again. Nevertheless, fixation techniques and obligatory stress risers still prevent us from going to the extremes of knee flexion and extension early on; but in general, the more isometric the graft, the more passive motion is allowed.

Although the *passive* range of knee motion is generous and performed out of the brace, active range of motion exercises require protective bracing to control external forces that may lead to ligament deformation. *Active* knee extension is controlled and limited early because of anterior drawer forces present during the active leg extension exercise. Initially, the brace is set for 40 to 70 degrees of flexion. These parameters are gradually (and arbitrarily) increased as the strength of the healing ligament increases. By approximately the fourth postoperative week, advances in *active* motion at a rate of 5 degrees of extension and 10 degrees of flexion per 1 to 2 weeks are instituted until the desired range of motion is achieved. The settings for the brace reflect the desire for the active range of motion only. Passive range of motion exercises performed out of the brace will allow for more extension since the anterior drawer force produced by quadriceps activity is lacking. Resistive quadriceps exercises are not necessarily performed through the same range of motion allowed by the brace. We impose a terminal extension restriction on resistance quadriceps exercises, requiring a block on the leg extension machine or an adjustment made on the brace setting during exercise. (See the section on the isotonic phase that follows.)

Our goal is a *normal* range of knee motion. Knee motion less than −5 degrees of extension to +130 degrees of flexion is unacceptable. At least 90% of the normal range of motion should be achieved within the first 4 months following surgery. If a plateau in the passive range of motion occurs, then manipulation must be considered. Manipulation for complete range of motion can be employed at any time in the postoperative phase, given a strong repair has been placed isometrically. Loss of flexion can easily be corrected through manipulation; however, loss of extension is better corrected through the application of extension (drop-out) casts that gain extension gradually over a 1-week period of time.

If *patellar entrapment* occurs, as manifested by poor patellar mobility, quadriceps lag, and patellar pain, it is imperative that this be recognized early and that patellar mobilization techniques be reinforced. Early manipulation and/or arthroscopic debridement and release may be necessary.

Progressive weight bearing phase

Weight bearing is important since the integrity of the "chondral unit" is dependent not only on motion but also on weight bearing. However, the muscle movements necessary to control the knee during weight bearing are large and can definitely jeopardize the healing ligament if not appropriately controlled. Despite the development of elaborate bracing techniques, crutches are still our best ally in controlling these forces. Rehabilitative braces and functional braces help control flexion and extension movements, but their ability to control anterior and posterior translation is poor.[12,32] How much and how fast weight bearing can be allowed is determined by many factors, including the strength of the reconstruction or repair, the type of the ligament fixation, whether the graft is placed isometrically, active knee motion, quadriceps and hamstrings strength, and general knee alignment.

In general, the initiation of weight bearing begins at 6 to 8 weeks postoperatively. More weight bearing is allowed as the graft strength and fixation strength increase and as muscle strength and neuromuscular control improve. Given appropriate progression, weight bearing can be increased at approximately the rate of 25% of body weight per week until 75% weight bearing with one crutch is achieved. This level is maintained until (1) a near normal range of motion is achieved; (2) swelling is subsiding; (3) no quadriceps extension lag is present; and (4) quadriceps extension strength (demonstrated isotonically is at least 10% of body weight. Once these requirements are achieved, full weight bearing is allowed. At this point the patient changes from the rehabilitative brace to the functional brace. The functional brace should have an extension stop that prevents hyperextension during weight bearing. The patient continues to wear the functional brace for weight bearing activities until quadriceps strength is at least 60% and hamstring strength is at least 80% of the opposite limb (demonstrated by dynamometer); this usually occurs at around 20 to 24 weeks postoperatively.

Isometric phase

Isometric exercise, that is, muscle contraction without joint movement or change in the muscle fiber length, begins in the immediate postoperative period. The patient regularly performs quadriceps and hamstring isometrics as well as straight leg raising exercises. The power developed during an isometric contraction is limited in that only the muscle fibers active for that joint position are being maximally exercised. For this reason the isometric phase lessens but does not prevent muscle atrophy.

To be most effective, isometric exercise must be done constantly throughout the day and requires maximum patient cooperation. In that this is not always possible, neuromuscular stimulation is an important adjunct. It has been shown that neuromuscular stimulation will prevent the decrease in oxidative enzymes and will decrease the amount of muscle atrophy that occurs with immobility.[15] We recommend neuromuscular stimulation that generates peak muscle force rapidly and maintains that force for at least 10 seconds. The pads are placed so as to stimulate the vastus medialis obliquus, the rectus femoris, and the hamstring muscles. We recommend stimulation at 2-hour intervals, three to four times a day. Intermittent use prevents skin irritation and burns. We believe that the emphasis on *concomitant* quadriceps and hamstring stimulation, so as to prevent the anterior drawer force produced with quadriceps stimulation alone, has been overly emphasized and is not necessary if the knee is maintained at 40 degrees of knee flexion. Therefore quadriceps and hamstring stimulation may be done concomitantly or alternately.

Isometric exercise and neuromuscular stimulation is replaced with progressive resistance exercise once the patient can perform active voluntary muscle contractions and joint motion begins. However, spectrum isometrics, that is, isometric exercise at various degrees of knee flexion, may be required for a more extended period of time in those joints with patellofemoral joint disease, tibiofemoral athrosis, or patellar entrapment syndrome.

The effect of isometric exercise can be further enhanced through the use of "cross over effect." By vigorously exercising the well, contralateral leg a "cross over" strengthening effect can be obtained on the operated limb.[22,23,24] Animal studies have demonstrated as much as a 30% increase in strength as a result of cross over effects. Therefore, during the isometric phase, the opposite limb regularly performs strengthening exercises to take advantage of this effect. Stationary cycling with the well leg is also performed to maintain cardiovascular and neuromuscular endurance.

Isotonic phase

Isotonic exercise, that is, the movement of a load at constant resistance through an arc of motion, has been the foundation of limb rehabilitation since its introduction and popularization by DeLorme in 1945.[13] Although great gains in strength can be made with this form of exercise, there is one major disadvantage that must be addressed. A muscle cannot be loaded to maximum capacity during isotonic exercise because muscle strength varies with joint position, thus allowing the weaker position to limit the amount of weight that can be lifted. Maximum muscle tension cannot be developed for the stronger joint positions. Also, since muscle strength varies with joint position, the speed at which the exercise is performed varies, subject to either considerable acceleration or deceleration, making total muscle development unpredictable.

To compensate for these problems, variable resistance strength training modalities have been developed. These systems were developed to increase or decrease muscle tension throughout the range of motion in accordance with joint position. It is questionable how well these machines accomplish their goal in that muscle length-tension ratios vary from person to person. Nevertheless, these systems do emphasize flexibility and strength through a full range of motion, which is good, and they can generally be performed in the sitting or supine positions, which is safer than conventional free weights.

The isotonic phase of rehabilitation begins immediately upon the initiation of active joint motion. At this time a quadriceps progressive resistance exercise program to increase strength is performed. Up to 10% of body weight is allowed for quadriceps exercises through the complete range of active motion. This permits the patient to come off his crutches safely. However, progressive resistive quadriceps exercises beyond 10% of body weight are allowed only from 40 degrees to 110 degrees of knee flexion during the first 5 to 6 months postoperatively. This is the period during which the ligament repair or reconstruction is its weakest. After the quadriceps terminal extension limitation is ended, a full range of motion, progressive resistance, exercise program is instituted to develop strength and muscle bulk at low speeds. A minimum amount of strength must be developed isotonically through a complete range of motion so as to prevent joint contracture and cartilage degeneration and to allow for controlled weight bearing. Hip, calf, and hamstring isotonics are performed without weight limitations throughout the prescribed range of motion.

Isotonic exercises must be continued throughout a patient's lifetime to maintain muscle bulk and strength. It is necessary that muscle *bulk* be regained as well as peak strengths. It has been our observation that gains in strength without increases in bulk result in accelerated atrophy if progressive resistance exercises are stopped. We believe that muscle bulk is what enhances the ability of the muscle to maintain its strength during nonexercise periods.

Because of the specificity of strength training, both concentric and eccentric isotonic exercises should be performed. Concentric exercise, that is, shortening of the muscle during loading, is referred to as positive exercise. Eccentric or negative exercise is performed when the muscle lengthens while resisting a load. Strength gains in these two areas occur independently and at differing rates and therefore must be addressed separately.[7] The muscle develops selectively to either concentric or eccentric loading, and training with one mode fails to have a substantial effect on the other. For this reason, a specific program to include both concentric and eccentric exercise must be started early in the isotonic phase.

Isokinetic phase

If available, isokinetic strength training can be an integral component of the strength training program. This type of exercise is performed at a constant velocity of muscle contraction in which resistance varies.[34] The velocity of each contraction is identical, and the torque varies with each contraction as the muscle fatigues. Several disadvantages exist with this form of exercise as well. Because the resistance is variable and controlled by patient effort, load limitations about the knee become extremely difficult, if not altogether impossible, to control. The dynamometer can measure force, but it cannot control it; therefore the resultant vector forces placed on the healing ligament are unpredictable. This is particularly true when initiating leg extension exercises with a thrusting motion. If the resistance pad is placed lower near the ankle, the resultant lever arm and moment are greatly increased.

Besides the anterior drawer forces placed on the anterior cruciate ligament, the joint reaction forces in the patellofemoral joint are also of special concern. We believe isokinetic exercise should not be instituted until isotonic quadriceps exercises can be done pain free with smooth patellofemoral joint mechanics (i.e., dynamic patellar tracking, so as to prevent patellofemoral joint arthrosis). To initiate rapid motion or high-resistance quadriceps exercises before normal dynamic patellar tracking invites this problem. If at any time during the isokinetic phase patellofemoral symptoms develop and persist, these exercises must be reduced or stopped altogether.

Isokinetic exercises are initiated when the patient can perform isotonic exercises equal to 10% of body weight. Isokinetic exercises are initiated at high speeds only since the resistance will be less than at lower speeds, thus reducing patellofemoral joint reaction forces. Progression to lower-speed isokinetic exercises is done slowly as dynamic patella tracking improves. At the same time, isotonic exercises are continued that also augment slow-speed strength gains. The isokinetic leg extension exercise is performed through the prescribed range of motion using an extension block. Anti-shear pads must be used.

Isokinetic exercises are encouraged and maintained until the patient or athlete returns to full activity. However, the maintenance period does not contain isokinetic exercise because of the obligatory expense and limited access to the isokinetic machines. Maintenance is primarily through isotonic exercise since these machines are readily available.

Endurance phase

There are two types of endurance that must be developed during the rehabilitation process: cardiovascular endurance and muscular endurance. Cardiovascular conditioning decreases rapidly with a period of inactivity. These losses can be decreased by the early initiation of well leg stationary cycling. Once endurance exercises are initiated with the operated leg, the exercises to build muscular endurance will at the same time build cardiovascular endurance.

Exercises to build muscular endurance begin early in the rehabilitation process. It is the endurance capabilities of the muscle that are slowest in returning and that require the most time to regain. In general, repetitive high-speed exercises are designed to enhance muscle endurance not bulk. Gains in endurance occur concomitantly with initiation of isokinetic exercises being performed at high speeds. Augmenting isokinetic effects, and usually more convenient, is the use of a stationary bicycle. Cycling is initiated after 110 degrees of flexion is achieved and when at least 10% of body weight is being lifted isotonically. Like isokinetic exercise, bicycling should only be performed if pain free and without excessive knee crepitation. To enhance endurance capabilities, cycling activities should be performed at the initiation of the exercise period as well as at the end and should be performed to exhaustion. Cycling is begun with little or no resistance. If the terminal extension limitation is still in effect and if more resistance is added, the seat can be lowered to decrease knee extension. Swimming activities also enhance endurance capabilities and can be instituted simultaneously with the initiation of knee motion. Later in the rehabilitation program after adequate ligament and cartilage healing has occurred (4 to 6 months), a more vigorous outdoor cycling program may be performed as well as stationary track and rowing exercises. The endurance program can be alternated every other day with the strength training program.

Running phase

A progressive running program is initiated late in the rehabilitation process after adequate ligament healing and strength gains have been achieved (6 to 9 months). Hamstring/quadriceps muscle ratios must be near normal, and the strength of the involved quadriceps must be at least 75% of total body weight as demonstrated by peak muscle torques at both low and high speeds on the dynamometer. There should be little or no swelling in the knee. Running should be performed in a functional knee brace.

The initiation of the running phase is facilitated by the use of stretch cords. These devices help maintain body control while the patient runs in place.[37] The running program then progresses to a walk/jog protocol on level ground or on a track, running the straights and walking the curves. The workouts begin every other day and progress slowly to every day. Thirty yard sprints without sudden stops are initiated early and progress slowly over a 6 to 12 week period to 45 degrees angle cutting and figure-of-eight drills. Running inclines or stairs is not encouraged until late in the program, if at all.

If there has been a prior menisectomy or if joint arthrosis is present, the running program is specifically designed to return the patient to activities without encouraging running for endurance. In those knees with maintained joint surfaces and menisci and near normal stability, running for endurance is permitted.

Sports phase

The initiation of the sports phase should be determined by the absence of joint arthrosis and the presence of joint stability, not patient or physician desire.

High-velocity, high-risk sports that involve twisting, jumping, and pivoting, such as basketball and volleyball, are discouraged. Moderate risk activities such as raquetball, skiing, and softball can be resumed in most instances. Lifetime conditioning and maintenance sports such as biking, swimming, weight training, track skiing, and rowing are especially encouraged.

The sports phase is initiated at the completion of all of the other rehabilitation phases and usually begins between 9 to 15 months postoperatively. Neuromuscular coordination and enhancement occur slowly through the performance of skill drills specifically related to the sport that the patient is returning to. Functional knee braces are required for the first 24 months after surgery and then are used thereafter based on residual laxity and patient desires.

Patient and coach cooperation is mandatory on the patient's initial return to sports. If at any time the endurance of the limb is exceeded, play must stop since the neuromuscular system's ability to protect the knee is greatly compromised by fatigue. In our experience, the most common cause of reinjury is a failure to observe this simple rule. As endurance increases, so does playing time.

REFERENCES

1. Akeson, W.H., Amiel, D., and LaViolette, D.: The connective tissue response to immobility: a study of chondroitin-4 and -6 sulfate and dermation sulfate changes in periarticular connective tissue in control and immobilized knees of dogs, Clin. Orthop. 51:183-197, 1967.
2. Akeson, W.H., Amiel, D., LaViolette, D., et al.: The connective tissue response to immobility: an accelerated aging response? Exp. Gerontol. 3:289-301, 1968.
3. Akeson, W.H., Amiel, D., Mechanic, G.L., et al.: Collagen cross-linking alterations in joint contractions: changes in the reducible cross-links in periarticular connective tissue collagen after nine weeks of immobilization, Connect. Tissue Res. 5(1):15-20, 1977.
4. Akeson, W.H., Woo, S.L.-Y., Amiel, D., et al.: The connective tissue response to immobility: biochemical changes in periarticular connective tissue of the immobilized rabbit knee, Clin. Orthop. 93:356-362, 1973.
5. Alm, A., Ekstrom, H., Gillquist, J., et al.: The anterior cruciate ligament—a clinical and experimental study on tensile strength, morphology and replacement by patellar ligament, Acta Chir. Scand. (Suppl.) vol. 445, 1974.
6. Arms, S.W., Pope, M.H., Johnson, R.J., et al.: The biomechanics of anterior cruciate ligament rehabilitation and reconstruction, Am. J. Sports Med. 12:8-18, 1984.
7. Borde-Peterson, F., Knuttgen, H.G., and Nendrikisson, J.: Muscle metabolism during exercise with concentric and eccentric contractions, J. Appl. Physiol. 33:792-795, 1972.
8. Burks, R., Daniels, D., and Losse, G.: The effect of continuous passive motion on anterior cruciate ligament reconstruction stability, Am. J. Sports Med. 12(4):323-327, 1984.
9. Cabaud, H.E., Rodkey, W.G., and Feagin, J.A.: Experiment studies of acute anterior cruciate ligament injury and repair, Am. J. Sports Med. 7:18, 1979.
10. Clancey, W.G., Nanechania, R.G., Rosenberg, T.D., et al.: Anterior and posterior cruciate ligament reconstruction in Rhesus monkeys, J. Bone Joint Surg. (Am.) 63:12-70, 1981.
11. Daniels, D.: Evaluation of ligament fixation device, Eleventh annual meeting AOSSM, Nashville, Tenn. June 30-July 3, 1985.
12. Drez, D.: Evaluation of functional knee braces, Eleventh annual meeting AOSSM, Nashville, Tenn. June 30-July 3, 1985.
13. DeLorme, T.L.: Restoration of muscle power by heavy-resistance exercises, J. Bone Joint Surg. (Am.) 27:645-667, 1945.
14. Eriksson, E.: Sport injuries of the knee ligaments: their diagnosis, treatment, rehabilitation and prevention, Med. Sci. Sports Exerc. 8:133, 1976.
15. Eriksson, E., and Häggmark, T.: Comparison of isometric muscle training and electrical stimulation supplementing isometric muscle training in the recovery after major knee ligament surgery, Am. J. Sports Med. 7:169, 1979.
16. Evans, E.B., Eggers, G.W.N., Butler, M., et al.: Experimental immobilization and remobilization of rat knee joints, J. Bone Joint Surg. (Am.) 42:737-758, 1960.
17. Finsterbush, A., and Friedman, B.: Reversibility of joint changes produced by immobilization in rabbits, Clin. Orthop. 111:290-298, 1975.
18. Gelberman, R.H., Menon, J., Gonsalves, M., et al.: The effects of mobilization on the vascularization of healing flexor tendons in dogs, Clin. Orthop. 153:283-289, 1980.
19. Ginsberg, J.M., Eyring, E.J., and Curtiss, P.H.: Continuous compression of rabbit articular cartilage producing loss of hydroxyproline before loss of hemosamine, J. Bone Joint Surg. (Am.) 51:467-474, 1969.
20. Grood, E.S., Suntay, W.J., Noyes, F.R., et al.: Biomechanics of the knee-extension exercise, J. Bone Joint Surg. (Am.) 66:725-734, 1984.

21. Häggmark, T., and Ericksson, E.: Cylinder or mobile cast brace after knee ligament surgery: a clinical analysis and morphologic and enzymatic studies of changes in the quadriceps muscle, Am. J. Sports Med. 7:48, 1979.
22. Hellebrandt, F.A., and Waterland, J.C.: Indirect learning: the influence of unimanual exercise on related muscle groups of the same and the opposite side, Am. J. Phys. Med. 41:45-55, 1962.
23. Hellebrandt, F.A., Houtz, S.J., and Kirkorian, A.M.: Influence of bimanual exercise on unilateral work capacity, J. Appl. Physiol. 2:452-466, 1950.
24. Hellebrandt, F.A., Houtz, S.J., Parrish, A.M., et al.: Tonic neck reflexes in exercises of stress in man, Am. J. Phys. Med. 35:144-159, 1956.
25. Henning, C.E., Lynch, M.A., and Glick, K.R.: An in vivo strain gauge study of elongation of the anterior cruciate ligament, Am. J. Sports Med. 13(1):22-26, 1985.
26. Hirsch, E.F., and Morgan, R.H.: Causal significance to traumatic ossification in tendon insertions, Arch. Surg. 39:824-837, 1939.
27. Kennedy, J.C., Weinberg, H.W., and Wilson, A.S.: Anatomy and function of the anterior cruciate ligament, J. Bone Joint Surg. (Am.) 56:223, 1974.
28. Morrison, J.B.: The mechanics of the knee joint in relation to normal walking, J. Biomech. 3:51-61, 1970.
29. Morrison, J.B.: The forces transmitted by the human knee joint during activity, Doctoral Thesis, University of Strathclyde, Glasgow (1967).
30. Noyes, F.R., Torvik, P.J., Hyde, W.B., et al.: Biomechanics of ligament failure. II. An analysis of immobilization, exercise and reconditioning effects in primates, J. Bone Joint Surg. (Am.) 56:1406-1418, 1974.
31. Noyes, F.R., Butler, D.L., Grood, E.S., et al.: Biomechanics analysis of human ligament grafts used in knee-ligament repairs and reconstructions, J. Bone Joint Surg. (Am.) 66:344-352, 1984.
32. Paulos, L.: Clinical and functional assessment of functional knee bracing, ACL study group, Steamboat Springs, Colorado, 1983.
33. Paulos, L., Noyes, F.R., Grood, E., et al.: Knee rehabilitation after anterior cruciate ligament reconstruction and repair, Am. J. Sports Med. 9:140-149, 1981.
34. Perrine, J.J., and Edgerton, V.R.: Muscle force, velocity and power velocity relationships underisokinetic loading, Med. Sci. Sport Exerc. 10:159-166, 1978.
35. Salter, R.B., Simmond, D.F., Malcolm, D.W., et al.: The biological effect of continuous passive motion on the healing of full-thickness defects in articular cartilage, J. Bone Joint Surg. (Am.) 62:1232-1251, 1980.
36. Smidt, G.: Biomechanical analysis of knee flexion and extension, J. Biomech. 6:79-92, 1973.
37. Steadman, J.R.: Personal communication, February 1984.
38. Troyer, H.: The effect of short-term immobilization on the rabbit knee joint cartilage: a histochemical study, Clin. Orthop. 107:249, 1975.
39. Walker, P.S.: Human joints and their artificial replacements, Springfield, Illinois, 1977, Charles C Thomas, Publisher.
40. Winston, T.B., and Walmsley, R.: Some observations on the reaction of bone and tendon after tunneling of bone and insertion of tendon, J. Bone Joint Surg. (Br.) 42:377-386, 1960.
41. Woo, S.L.-Y., Matthews, J.V., Akeson, W.H., et al.: The connective tissue response to immobility: a correlative study of the biomechanical and biochemical measurements of the normal and immobilized rabbit knee, Arthritis Rheum. 18:257-264, 1975.

20

The future of anterior cruciate surgery

DOUGLAS W. JACKSON

Clinicians caring for the knee with a compromised anterior cruciate ligament have realized two principles: (1) the anterior cruciate ligament is an integral part of normal knee function and (2) a knee without a functioning anterior cruciate ligament can be improved with a successful replacement. Surgeons treating the anterior cruciate deficient knee realize the present shortcomings. There is the almost world-wide recognition and identification of present problems and this usually precedes major breakthroughs. Anterior cruciate deficient knee surgery is on the verge of exciting new improvements that will be seen to various degrees in the following categories:

1. Instrumentation in diagnosis and documentation
2. Arthroscopically assisted precision graft placement
3. Tensioning of the graft at surgery
4. Fixation of the graft
5. New grafts that more closely duplicate the ligament's properties
6. More selective use of bracing
7. Shortened time away from sports and work following an anterior cruciate ligament reconstruction

Multiple factors will continue to be involved in deciding how the anterior cruciate ligament disruption is best managed, including the patient, the associated injury complex, the surgeon treating the patient, and the future demands on the knee.

The basis for any treatment will remain accurate diagnosis of all the manifestations of the cruciate deficient knee, including assessment of the associated injuries to the articular cartilage, menisci, capsule, and other ligaments. Currently, the lack of standard instrumentation to document and quantitate the altered degrees of freedom following knee injury limits communication of clinical results. The available technology must be developed and applied so that instrumented knee testing will be easily reproduced by different testers, be available in the office and clinic settings and be time and cost efficient. Instrumented documentation will be necessary to aid in specific protocols that attempt to reproduce normal joint kinematics.

With the recent widespread application of arthroscopically assited positioning of the anterior cruciate replacement, more attention is being given to the precise placement of the graft. Future graft placement will further refine and address the different lengths of the individual fibers of the graft. During the range of motion, the configuration of the replacement anterior cruciate ligament will need to not only accommodate differing lengths as well as tensions within the bulk of the ligament. If the graft is not positioned properly, the forces generated during the range of motion will lengthen or rupture any biological or synthetic material. If the improperly placed replacement fibers do not rupture or stretch, they will alter the joint in a manner that it will probably be more deleterious than beneficial. Significant improvements have been made regarding placement of the graft to control the anterior displacement of the tibia. However, future requirements of the different components of the cruciate ligament will attempt to reestablish the factors affecting rotation as well as the anterior displacement throughout the range of motion.

Tensioning at surgery becomes an important consideration if there is accurate placement of the graft. The appropriate tension in the ligament is necessary when duplicating the restraints of a normal ligament on the knee. However, if the tensioning is too tight, in a short period of time with the cyclic loading of normal knee motion, the forces generated will alter the length of the graft. If the replaced knee ligament is too lax, it will fail to offer the restraint required in the normal ligament. Devices will be forthcoming to assist the surgeon in operative tensioning of the graft throughout the range of motion.

Fixation also becomes more important as new grafts that more closely duplicate the normal anterior cruciate ligament are developed, properly placed, and tensioned. If the graft is placed so that there is minimal change in the length of the individual fibers during knee motion, then holding the ligament in this position under desired tension until bony ingrowth and more permanent fixation occur becomes desirable. New fixation devices must be able to withstand repeated cyclic loading, resistance to weightbearing loads, and unexpected types of trauma, such as the patient slipping. This desired fixation during the postoperative phase is critical until its funtion is replaced by bony ingrowth. Future fixation devices may be biological, biodegradable, or continue to consist of hardware that may or may not need to be removed.

A significant portion of this text has been devoted to information regarding biological and prosthetic graft selection. It appears that in the future new ligaments must more closely duplicate the original anterior cruciate ligament. Since the time necessary for revascularization and replacement of a biological tissue is quite long, the associated activity restriction prevents the vast majority of patients with cruciate deficient knees from having surgery. The search for methods of augmentation of biological grafts and/or prosthetic ligaments to shorten recovery time will continue. New types of biological enhancement as well as mechanical enhancement of autografts and allografts may open new avenues in the use of biological tissue. Present grafts will become obsolete within 5 to 10 years as technologies develop from multiple disciplines. One problem in developing new grafts relates to the economics of new ligament research and development. FDA requirements placed on new materials require long, arduous, and expensive testing. These requirements will need to be clearly delineated so that a product can be more specifically tested to a set of guidelines once the adequate follow-up demonstrates that it is functional.

The time consuming rehabilitation following present day anterior cruciate ligament surgery will decrease as fixation, tensioning, and graft materials improve so that there is essentially immediate motion, reestablishment of normal muscle function, and weight-bearing. The exercises will be done by the patient with supervision by the physician and therapist.

Bracing has been primarily on an empirical basis. More information is needed on its efficacy. A good prophylatic knee brace in high-risk sports would be desirable. Future studies involving the use of braces will emphasize indications for use in different settings—postoperatively, during rehabilitation, and during sports participation.

How fast a person can return to work and sports remains a major consideration for the future. It calls for an optimal ligament and a procedure that can be performed on an outpatient basis with minimal time off work and with the capability of returning to vigorous labor and athletics in a shorter period of time than present procedures allow. If this procedure develops, there are large numbers of patients with anterior cruciate deficient knees that will undergo

surgery. It is apparent at this time from the research that is underway that the following will occur in the future.
1. More anterior cruciate ligament surgery will be performed.
2. Surgical techniques will have less morbidity.
3. Weightbearing, range of motion, and strengthening will be as immediate as pain and swelling allow.
4. Return to work and sports will be much earlier.
5. Rehabilitation will be greatly simplified.
6. New prosthetic and/or augmented biological material and technology will be developed.
7. The prevention of rupture of the anterior cruciate will occupy more of the research effort.

Index

A

Abrasion, definition of, 241, 262
Allograft(s)
  anterior cruciate ligament, 211-224, 216-218
    irradiation of, 219-220
    preservation of, 211-220
    procurement of, 218-219
    storage of, 220-221
    surgical considerations for, 222-224
  azothioprine and, 214
  bone-anterior cruciate ligament bone, 217-218
  fascia lata, 215-216
  freeze-drying, 214, 220-221
  freezing, 220-221
  immune responses to, 213-214
    reduction of, 214-215
  patellar tendon-bone complex, 215, 216
  revascularization of, 48-49
  soft-tissue, 215-218
  sterilization of, 219-220
  types of, for anterior cruciate ligament repair, 215-218
ALRI; see Anterolateral rotatory instability
AMRI; see Anteromedial rotatory instability
Anterior cruciate deficient knee, anteroposterior testing of, 97-100
Anterior cruciate ligament(s)
  anatomy of, 17-25
    functional, 58
    interstitial, 20-22
  biomechanics of, 53-71
  deficiency of, 97-100
  disruption of, 69-70
  embryology of, 18
  femoral origin of, 18-19
  function of, 173
  functional anatomy of, 58
  healing parameters of, 293-295
  injuries to, diagnosis of, 193-198
  insertion of
    initial point-selection for, 107
    isometric sites for, 103-111
    technique for, 103-105
  instability of; see Anterior cruciate ligament instability
  insufficient, 55
  interstitial anatomy of, 20-22
  isometric attachment points for, verification of, 107-110
  laxity of
    examination for, 72-88
    quantitative, 90-100
  microstructure of, 22-24
  normal, 102-103
  and pivot-shift phenomenon, 86
  primary repair of, suture technique for, 115
  reconstruction of; see Anterior cruciate ligament reconstruction
  replacements for, revascularization of, 41-51
  ruptured
    arthroscopic surgery for, 129-130
    management of, 127-140
    nonoperative management of, 127-128
    surgical treatment of, 130
  and soft-tissue fixation; see Soft-tissue fixation
  subsitution of; see also Anterior cruciate ligament prostheses; Anterior cruciate ligament substitutes
    by arthroscopy, 274-284
    extra-articular surgery following, 284
    by gracilis tendon, 160-162
    rehabilitation following, 296-298
  tensile strength of, in domestic animals, 267
  tibial insertion of, 19
  vascular response of, to injury and repair, 35-41
  vascularity of, 27-53
  working loads on, 230-231
Anterior cruciate ligament instability
  chronic, arthroscopic reconstruction of, 203-205
  diagnosis of, 273-274
  extra-articular procedures for, 168-189
  functional, chronic, 198
  intra-articular procedure for, biomechanical considerations of, 198-199
  surgical indications for, 171-172
Anterior cruciate ligament prostheses
  animal model for, 266-267
  creep rupture of, 259
  creep testing of, 257-259
  design considerations for, 254-270
  femoral insertion of, 264-265
  modified over-the-top placement of, 266
  resistance of
    to abrasion, 262-263
    to fatigue, 260-262

Anterior cruciate ligament prostheses—cont'd
　strength requirements for, 260
　and stresses at sharp edges, 262
　surgical routing of, 263-266
　tensile strength of
　　postoperative, 267-269
　　ultimate, 255-260
　tibial placement of, 263-264
Anterior cruciate ligament reconstruction, 24-25, 70, 130-140
　acute, 135-136
　arthroscopic, 203-205, 273-285
　autografts for, 144-163
　bone-block iliotibial band transfer for, 154-157
　chronic, 137-140
　combined intra-articular and extra-articular, 181-182
　complications with open arthrotomy techniques for, 164-165
　and concomitant surgery, rehabilitation following, 301-312
　extra-articular, 131-135
　Hey Groves technique for, 154
　intra-articular, 135-140
　　historical review of, 142-144
　　materials for, 130-131
　intra-articular iliotibial band for, 154-157
　intra-articular semitendinosus, 157-159
　mensci for, 162-163
　osseous tunnels for, 147, 165
　patellar tendons for, 144-153
Anterior cruciate ligament repair, acute, and patellar tendon graft augmentation, 202-203
Anterior cruciate ligament stabilization, intra-articular, biological substitutes for, 206
Anterior cruciate ligament substitute(s)
　arthroscopic placement and fixation of, 283-284
　biological, synthetic augmentation of, 226-238
　fixation of, and rehabilitation, 298-299
　healing time for, 294
　ideal, 211
　intra-articular
　　biomechanical placement of, 201-203
　　pitfalls of, 206-207
　isometric placement of, 102-112
　placement of, and rehabilitation, 299-301
　and rehabilitation, 296-298
　success of, 244-247
　tension of, 316
　tunnel placement of, 110
Anterior cruciate ligament surgery
　goal of, 198
　rehabilitation after, 291-292
Anterior cruciate ligament tear, acute third degree, 197-198
Anterior drawer test, 82

Anterolateral rotatory instability, 169, 172-173
　extra-articular procedures for, principles of, 174
Anteromedial rotatory instability, 169
　surgery for, 187
Arthroscopy
　for anterior cruciate ligament reconstruction, 203-205, 273-285
　and anterior cruciate ligament substitution, 274-284
　diagnostic, for anterior cruciate ligament instability, 273-274
　for ruptured anterior cruciate ligament, 129-130
Arthrotomy techniques, complications with, in anterior cruciate ligament reconstruction, 164-165
Artificial ligament(s), 208
　biomechanics of, and associated problems, 239-270
　fixation of, 124-125
　proper tensioning of, 245, 247
　types of, 247-252
Autografts
　for anterior cruciate ligament reconstruction, 144-163
　anterior cruciate ligaments, 193-208, 211-212
　revascularization of, 41
Axes of knee motion, 3
Axis of rotation, 3
Azathioprine and allografts, 214

B

Biological degradation, definition of, 242
Bone
　fixation of, to bone, 122-123
　healing of, role of soft tissue in, 52-53
Bone-block iliotibial band transfer, 154-157
Bone tunnels
　and anterior cruciate ligament substitutes, 244-245
　preparation of, 282
　size of, and graft size, 247
Brace(s), 317
　definition of, 286
　knee; see Knee braces
　for weight-bearing phase of rehabilitation, 306-307

C

Carbon fiber ligament, 251
Cartilage, articular, 55
Clinical laxity grade, definition of, 14-15
Compliance, definition of, 242
Compliance measurement, definition of, 15
Condyles, femoral, 56-57
Constant load creep, definition of, 241-242

Constrain, definition of, 4
Couple, definition of, 4-5
Creep, definition of, 11, 241-242, 255
Creep rupture of anterior cruciate ligament prostheses, 259
Creep testing of anterior cruciate ligament prostheses, 257-259
Cyclic creep, definition of, 242

D

Deformation, plastic, 11
Degree of freedom, definition of, 2
Dexon graft, 251
Dimethylsulfoxide, 220
Displacement force, definition of, 15
DMSO; see Dimethylsulfoxide
Double loop suture technique, 122-123
Double weave suture technique, 122-123
Drawer test, flexion-rotation, 78-80
Drugs, immunosuppressive, and allografts, 214-215

E

Elastic deformation, definition of, 239
Elastic-region, definition of, 11
Elongation, equation for, 258-259
Endurance, development of, following ACL repair, 311
Ethylene oxide for sterilization of allografts, 220
Exercise
  isokinetic, 310
  isometric, following anterior cruciate ligament repair, 307-308
  isotonic, following anterior cruciate ligament repair, 308-309
Extra-articular osseous tunnels, site selection of, 276-277

F

Fatigue
  definition of, 260
  resistance to, of anterior cruciate ligament prostheses, 260-262
Fatigue strength, definition of, 239, 241
Fixation of anterior cruciate ligament substitutes, 245
Fixation post technique, 117-118
Flexion, 3
Force, definition of, 9
Four-bar linkage and knee motion, 65
Freeze-drying allografts, 220-221
Freezing allografts, 220-221

G

Gamma radiation for sterilization of allografts, 220
Gortex, 247

Gracilis tendon for anterior cruciate ligament substitution, 160-162
Graft(s)
  augmentation of; see Graft augmentation
  anterior cruciate ligament
    augmented and unaugmented, 233-234
  biological, synthetic augmentation of, 226-238
  Dexon, 251
  fixation of, 316-317
  Gortex, 247
  Meadox, 249-250
  patellar tendon
    strength of, 199
    vascular studies of, 199-201
    vascularized, 47
  placement of, 316
  quadriceps-patellar tendon, 201
  synthetic, and rehabilitation, 298
Graft augmentation, 317
  synthetic; see also Synthetic augmentation devices
    biomechanics of, 227-230
    principles of, 226-227
Guide pins
  femoral, placement of, 227-281
  placement of, confirmation of, 281-282

H

Healing, ligament, parameters of, 293-295
Hey Groves technique for anterior cruciate ligament reconstruction, 154
Hysteresis, definition of, 11

I

Iliotibial band
  intra-articular, 154-157
  and pivot-shift phenomenon, 84
  tenodesis of, 182-186
    modifications of, 186
  in extra-articular procedures for anterolateral rotatory instability, 174
  in lateral pivot-shift phenomenon, 173
Immobility and anterior cruciate ligament repair, 292, 293, 304-305
Immunogenicity, sources of, 212
Implants, biological, for anterior cruciate ligament reconstruction, 70
Infrapatellar fat pad, vascularity of, 32
Injury, mechanism of, definition of, 14
Injury activity, definition of, 14
Injury event, definition of, 14
Instability
  definition of, 14, 73
  functional, definition of, 16
  rotatory, anterolateral; see Anterolateral rotatory instability
  rotatory, anteromedial; see Anteromedial rotatory instability

Instability—cont'd
  rotatory, posterolateral; see Posterolateral rotatory instability
Instruments for anterior cruciate ligament insertion, 103-105
Intercondylar femoral notchplasty, 245
Intercondylar notch
  debridement of, arthroscopic, 274
  preparation of, arthroscopic, 274-276
Interference fitscrew technique, 123
Intra-articular procedure for anterior cruciate ligament instability, 198-199
Isometric, definition of, 7-8
Isometric exercise following anterior cruciate ligament repair, 307-308
Isometric point, selection of, 277
Isometric tension device, 281-282

J

Joint with pure rolling motion, 60-62
Joint displacement measurements, definition of, 15
Joint laxity
  normal, definition of, 15
  pathological, definition of, 16

K

Knee(s)
  anterior cruciate deficient, laxity and stiffness of, 95
  anterior stiffness of, definition of, 92
  axes of, 3
  constraint of, 4-6
  coupled motion of, 4-7
  displacement of, vectors of, 73
  flexion of, 3
  functional anatomy of, 55-60
  instability of, classification of, 169-171
  instant center of, 3
  mechanics of, 81-86
  motion of; see Knee motion
  normal, laxity and stiffness of, 92-93
  vascular soft tissues of, and revascularization, 49
Knee braces
  functional, 288-289
  prophylactic, 286-287, 289
  rehabilitative, 287-288, 289
Knee motion
  characteristics of, 60-65
  coupled, 4-7
  external constraints and, 5-6
  terminology for, 1-16

L

Lachman test, 75, 82
  for anterior cruciate ligament injury, 193-194

LAD; see 3M/Kennedy Ligament Augmentation Device
Laxity
  anterolateral rotatory, tests for, 76-81
  definition of, 73
  of ligaments, 8-13
Laxity test(s)
  definition of, 15
  passive, definition of, 15
Laxity testing conditions, definition of, 15
Leeds-Keio ligament, 248-249
Ligament(s), 81
  anterior cruciate; see Anterior cruciate ligament(s)
  carbon fiber, 251
  cruciate, 55-56
    healing of, 35
    vascularity of, 27-32
  injury of, clinical terminology for, 14-16
  laxity of, 8-13
  Leeds-Keio, 248
  mechanical properties of, 239-244
  patellar, vascularity of, 35
  Proplast, 250
  Richards Polyflex, 250
Ligament augmentation device, 124-125, 208
Ligament injury grade, definition of, 14
Losee procedure, 175-177
Losee test, 77-78

M

MacIntosh procedure, modified, 179-181
Meadox graft, 249-250
Menisci, 58
  for anterior cruciate ligament reconstruction, 162-163
Moment, definition of, 9
Motion
  after anterior cruciate ligament repair, 305-306
  constrained, 4-6
  coupled, 4-7
  of knee; see Knee motion
  pure gliding, 60
  pure rolling, 60-62
Movement, translation, definition of, 74

N

90-degree anterior drawer test, 75
Notchplasty
  arthroscopic, 275
  intercondylar femoral, 245

O

Osseous tunnels
  for anterior cruciate ligament reconstruction, 147, 165
  extra-articular, site selection of, 276-277

Index

P

Patellar ligament, vascularity of, 35
Patellar tendon
 as anterior cruciate ligament graft, 122-123
  for anterior cruciate ligament reconstruction, advantages of, 144-145
  central one third of, for anterior cruciate ligament reconstruction, 144-147
  middle third of, for anterior cruciate ligament reconstruction, 147-151
Patellar tendon grafts, vascularized, 152-153
Pivot-shift phenomenon, 83-86, 172-174
Pivot-shift test, 76-77, 194
 true vs. reversed, 87-88
Plastic deformation, 11
 definition of, 239
PLRI; *see* Posterolateral rotatory instability
Polyvinylpyrrolidone, 220
Polyprophylene for ligament augmentation device, 231-234
Posterior cruciate ligament, functional anatomy of, 58, 60
Posterolateral rotatory instability, 169, 171
 surgery for, 187-188
Proplast ligament, 250
Prostheses
 anterior cruciate ligament; *see* Anterior cruciate ligament prostheses
 synthetic, revascularization of, 49
PVP; *see* Polyvinylpyrrolidone

R

Range of motion, passive after anterior cruciate ligament repair, 305
Relaxation, definition of, 11, 13
Restraints, 81
Rehabilitation
 after anterior cruciate ligament reconstruction, 205-206
 after anterior cruciate ligament surgery, 291-312
 after anterior cruciate ligament substitution, 296-298
 and anterior cruciate ligament substitute fixation, 298-299
 and anterior cruciate ligament substitute placement, 299-301
 endurance phase of, 311
 immobility phase of, 304-305
 isokinetic phase of, 310
 isometric phase of, 307-308
 isotonic phase of, 308-309
 motion phase of, 305-306
 phases of, 302-312
 preoperative phase of, 304
 running phase of, 311-312
 sports phase of, 312

Rehabilitation—cont'd
 weight-bearing phase of, 306-307
Rehabilitation prescription, 302-312
Richards Polyflex Ligament, 250
Right hand rule, definition of, 2
Rotation
 automatic, of tibia, 68
 definition of, 1, 74
 instant center of, 60
Running following anterior cruciate ligament repair, 311-312

S

Screw(s)
 cog-type, fixation with, 153
 for soft tissue fixation to bone, 117, 118-119, 120, 122
"Screwing-home mechanism" of tibia, 68
Semitendinosus, intra-articular, for anterior cruciate ligament reconstruction, 157-159
Six degrees of freedom, definition of, 2
Slocum test, 80-81
Soft tissue(s)
 fixation of, 114-125
  to bone, 117-122
 role of, in healing of bone, 52-53
 suturing of, to bone, 117, 120
 suturing of, to soft tissue, 114-116
 suturing techniques for, 116
Soft-tissue fixation, 114-115
Sports after anterior cruciate ligament repair, 311-312
Stability, definition of, 14, 73
Staples for soft tissue fixation to bone, 117-118, 119-120
Sterilization, secondary, of allografts, 219-220
Strain, definition of, 9
Stress, definition of, 9
Surgery
 extra-articular, for anterolateral rotatory instability, 174-186
 for ruptured anterior cruciate ligament, 130
Suture(s), excursion of, measurement of, 104-105
Suture techniques
 for bone to bone fixation, 122-123
 for primary repair of anterior cruciate ligaments, 115
 for soft tissue fixation to bone, 117, 120
Synthetic augmentation devices
 advantages and disadvantages of, 236-237
 alternative, 234-236
 biomechanics of, 227-230
 material requirements for, 230-234
 polyprophylene, 231-234
 principles of, 226-227

T

Tendon(s)
  gracilis, for anterior cruciate ligament substitution, 160-162
  patellar
    advantages of, 211
    as anterior cruciate ligament graft, 122-123
    for anterior cruciate ligament reconstruction, 144-153; *see also* Patellar tendon for anterior cruciate ligament reconstruction
  semitendinous, for intra-articular anterior cruciate ligament stabilization, 206
Tenodesis
  iliotibial band, 132-134, 182-186
    modifications of, 186
  lateral, 177-179
Tensile strength
  of natural anterior cruciate ligament of domestic animals, 267
  postoperative, of anterior cruciate ligament prostheses, 267-269
  ultimate; *see* Ultimate tensile strength
Tensile testing of anterior cruciate ligament prostheses, 268-269
Test(s)
  for anterior cruciate ligament insufficiency, 193-198
  anterior drawer, 82
  for anterolateral rotatory laxity, 76-81
  creep, of anterior cruciate ligament prostheses, 257-259
  drawer, flexion-rotation, 78-80
  Lachman, 75, 82, 193-194
  laxity, definition of, 15
  Losee, 77-78
  90-degree anterior drawer, 75
  pivot-shift, 76-77, 194
    true vs. reversed, 87-88
  for pivot-shift phenomenon, 173-174

Test(s)—cont'd
  Slocum, 80-81
  tensile, of anterior cruciate ligament prostheses, 268-269
  for translation, 75
3M/Kennedy Ligament Augmentation Device, 251-252
Tibial tunnels in intra-articular anterior cruciate ligament stabilization, 206-207
Tibial plateau, 57-58
Tissue(s), soft; *see* Soft tissues
Translation
  definition of, 74, 75
  tests for, 75
Translocation, definition of, 74
Tunnel divergence angle and rehabilitation, 301

U

UCLA portable instrumental clinical knee testing apparatus, 90-92
Ultimate tensile strength
  of anterior cruciate ligament prostheses, 255-260
  definition of, 239

V

Vascular leash and patellar ligament, 35
Viscoelastic body, 13
Viscoelasticity, 255

W

Weightbearing following anterior cruciate ligament repair, 306-307

X

Xenotech, 250-251

Y

Yield point, definition of, 239